Equine Dentistry and Oral Surgery

Editors

EDWARD T. EARLEY
ROBERT M. BARATT
STEPHEN S. GALLOWAY

VETERINARY CLINICS OF NORTH AMERICA: EQUINE PRACTICE

www.vetequine.theclinics.com

Consulting Editor
THOMAS J. DIVERS

December 2020 • Volume 36 • Number 3

ELSEVIER

1600 John F. Kennedy Boulevard • Suite 1800 • Philadelphia, Pennsylvania, 19103-2899

http://www.vetequine.theclinics.com

VETERINARY CLINICS OF NORTH AMERICA: EQUINE PRACTICE Volume 36, Number 3
December 2020 ISSN 0749-0739, ISBN-13: 978-0-323-72222-3

Editor: Katerina Heidhausen
Developmental Editor: Donald Mumford

Veterinary Clinics of North America: Equine Practice (ISSN 0749-0739) is published in April, August, and December by Elsevier Inc., 360 Park Avenue South, New York, NY 10010-1710. Business and Editorial Offices: 1600 John F. Kennedy Blvd., Suite 1800, Philadelphia, PA 19103-2899. Subscription prices are $290.00 per year (domestic individuals), $585.00 per year (domestic institutions), $100.00 per year (domestic students/residents), $334.00 per year (Canadian individuals), $737.00 per year (Canadian institutions), $365.00 per year (international individuals), $737.00 per year (international institutions), $100.00 per year (Canadian students/residents), and $180.00 per year (international students/residents). To receive student/resident rate, orders must be accompanied by name of affiliated institution, date of term, and the signature of program/residency coordinator on institution letterhead. Orders will be billed at individual rate until proof of status is received. Foreign air speed delivery is included in all *Clinics* subscription prices. All prices are subject to change without notice. **POSTMASTER:** Send address changes to *Veterinary Clinics of North America: Equine Practice*, 3251 Riverport Lane, Maryland Heights, MO 63043. Customer Service (orders, claims, online, change of address): Elsevier Health Sciences Division, Subscription **Customer Service, 3251 Riverport Lane, Maryland Heights, MO 63043. Tel: 1-800-654-2452 (U.S. and Canada); 314-447-8871 (outside U.S. and Canada). Fax: 314-447-8029. E-mail: journalscustomerservice-usa@elsevier.com (for print support);** E-mail: **journalsonlinesupport-usa@elsevier.com (for online support).**

Reprints. For copies of 100 or more of articles in this publication, please contact the Commercial Reprints Department, Elsevier Inc., 360 Park Avenue South, New York, NY 10010-1710. Tel.: 212-633-3874; Fax: 212-633-3820; E-mail: reprints@elsevier.com.

Veterinary Clinics of North America: Equine Practice is covered in *MEDLINE/PubMed (Index Medicus), Excerpta Medica, Current Contents/Agriculture, Biology and Environmental Sciences,* and *ISI*.

Contributors

CONSULTING EDITOR

THOMAS J. DIVERS, DVM
Diplomate, American College of Veterinary Internal Medicine; Diplomate, American College of Veterinary Emergency and Critical Care; Steffen Professor of Veterinary Medicine, Department of Clinical Sciences, Section of Large Animal Medicine, College of Veterinary Medicine, Cornell University, Ithaca, New York, USA

EDITORS

EDWARD T. EARLEY, DVM
Diplomate, American Veterinary Dental College, Equine; Large Animal Dentistry, Equine Farm Animal Hospital, Cornell University, Ithaca, New York, USA

ROBERT M. BARATT, DVM, MS
Diplomate, American Veterinary Dental College, Small Animal/Nonspecies; Diplomate, American Veterinary Dental College, Equine; Salem Valley Veterinary Clinic, Salem, Connecticut, USA

STEPHEN S. GALLOWAY, DVM
Diplomate, American Veterinary Dental College, Small Animal/Nonspecies; Diplomate, American Veterinary Dental College, Equine; Animal Dental Care Specialist, Somerville, Tennessee, USA

AUTHORS

ROBERT M. BARATT, DVM, MS
Diplomate, American Veterinary Dental College, Small Animal/Nonspecies; Diplomate, American Veterinary Dental College, Equine; Salem Valley Veterinary Clinic, Salem, Connecticut, USA

IAN BISHOP, DVM
Kirkfield, Ontario, Canada

LUIS CAMPOY, LV, CertVA, MRCVS
Diplomate of the European College of Veterinary Anaesthesia and Analgesia; Clinical Professor in Anesthesiology and Pain Medicine, Department of Clinical Sciences, College of Veterinary Medicine, Cornell University, Ithaca, New York, USA

ELAINE F. CLAFFEY, DVM
Diplomate, American College of Veterinary Surgeons, Large Animal; Cornell Ruffian Equine Specialists, Elmont, New York, USA

ALLISON R. DOTZEL, DVM
Laurel Highland Veterinary Clinic, Williamsport, Pennsylvania, USA

NORM G. DUCHARME, DVM, MS
Diplomate, American College of Veterinary Surgeons; Cornell Ruffian Equine Specialists, Elmont, New York, USA; Department of Clinical Sciences, Cornell University, College of Veterinary Medicine, Ithaca, New York, USA

EDWARD T. EARLEY, DVM
Diplomate, American Veterinary Dental College, Equine; Large Animal Dentistry, Equine Farm Animal Hospital, Cornell University, Ithaca, New York, USA

JACK EASLEY, DVM, MS
DABVP (Eq Practice), Diplomate, American Veterinary Dental College, Equine; Shelbyville, Kentucky, USA

ERIN EPPERLY, DVM
Diplomate, American College of Veterinary Radiology; Instructor, Cornell University College of Veterinary Medicine, Ithaca, New York, USA

STEPHEN S. GALLOWAY, DVM
Diplomate, American Veterinary Dental College, Small Animal/Nonspecies; Diplomate, American Veterinary Dental College, Equine; Animal Dental Care Specialist, Somerville, Tennessee, USA

JON M. GIECHE, DVM
Diplomate, American Veterinary Dental College, Equine; Owner/President, Kettle Moraine Equine Hospital & Regional Equine Dental Center, Whitewater, Wisconsin, USA

TRAVIS HENRY, DVM
Diplomate, American Veterinary Dental College, Small Animal/Nonspecies; Diplomate, American Veterinary Dental College, Equine; Midwest Veterinary Dental Services, Assistant Adjunct Professor, University of Wisconsin, Madison, Wisconsin, USA

LEAH E. LIMONE, DVM
Diplomate, American Veterinary Dental College, Equine; Owner, Northeast Equine Veterinary Dental Services, LLC, Topsfield, Massachusetts, USA

JOHN PIGOTT, DVM, MS
Diplomate, American College of Veterinary Surgeons, Large Animal; Cornell Ruffian Equine Specialists, Elmont, New York, USA

JEFFREY D. REISWIG, DVM, MS, PhD
Diplomate, American Veterinary Dental College, Equine; Veterinary, Equine Veterinary Dental Services, LLC, Granville, Ohio, USA

SAMANTHA R. SEDGWICK, DVM
Resident in Anesthesiology, Department of Clinical Sciences, College of Veterinary Medicine, Cornell University, Ithaca, New York, USA

CLAUDIA K. TRUE, DVM
Woodside Equine Clinic, Ashland, Virginia, USA

JUSTIN A. WHITTY, DVM
Department of Clinical Sciences, Cornell University College of Veterinary Medicine, Ithaca, New York, USA

Contents

Equine dentistry has been practiced for almost 3000 years, making it one of the oldest areas of equine health care. Progress has been slow and mirrored changes seen in human medical care. Many horsemen practiced equine dentistry during the late nineteenth and early twentieth centuries. Most of what was known then concentrated on sharp enamel points and abnormal dental occlusal wear. This changed slowly in the late twentieth century as research in equine dentistry increased. Today, veterinarians performing equine dentistry focus on detailed oral examination and base treatment for proper diagnosis of orthodontic, endodontic, periodontal, or other forms of dental disease.

 Video content accompanies this article at http://www.vetequine. theclinics.com.

Oral endoscopy is a valuable addition to the equine dental examination process. It enables veterinarians to visualize subtle oral disorders and is a useful client education tool. There are several commercially available oral endoscopic systems on the market. Practitioners can also assemble their own systems. An oral endoscope is used to perform a thorough and systematic oral examination and to visualize normal oral structures as well as oral disorders. It is also used to guide instrument placement during oral surgeries and other dental procedures.

Radiography is an important imaging modality and is available to most equine veterinarians providing primary care. Diagnostic radiographic imaging of the equine skull and dentition requires careful positioning and technique. This article is aimed at providing the veterinarian with instructions and guidelines for obtaining diagnostic skull and dental radiographs and a discussion of the radiographic signs of dental disease with case-based examples. The limitations of radiography are discussed with regard to determining the need for adjunct diagnostic techniques and more advanced imaging techniques, such as computed tomography.

Procedural sedation has become popular for describing a semiconscious state that allows patients to be comfortable during certain surgical or diagnostic procedures. Sedation may be enhanced by locoregional anesthetic techniques to produce sufficient analgesia and muscle relaxation for surgery to occur. Sedation and local anesthesia for standing diagnostic and surgical procedures on the horse's head circumvents the potential complications of general anesthesia (particularly, complications related to recovery). However, the implementation of a locoregional anesthetic technique requires a thorough understanding of the anatomy to maximize success and minimize possible complications.

Odontoplasty (floating and occlusal equilibration) is the most commonly performed procedure in equine dentistry. From an anatomic perspective, an irregular occlusal surface, prominent cingula, transverse ridges, and enamel points all contribute to the function, form, and longevity of the equine cheek tooth. With limited reserve crown available and an average functional life range between 18 and 25 years, removal of tooth structure should be conservative. The authors consider a quality oral examination to be the most important dental procedure performed in the horse. Individual tooth evaluation should lead to a specific diagnosis and treatment plan. Tooth odontoplasty should be site-specific.

Computed tomography (CT) has revolutionized the veterinarian's ability to image the equine skull and led to improved diagnostic accuracy and clarity for surgical planning. The increased cost for this evaluation is offset by more accurate diagnosis and targeted therapy. As novel technology is developed that allows for increased availability of equine head, the price will continue to decrease and more examinations will be performed. New skills are needed for the veterinarian to accurately interpret this modality. This article reviews the normal CT appearance of the equine skull and presents examples and key features of several common diseases.

 Video content accompanies this article at http://www.vetequine. theclinics.com.

This article serves as a template for equine veterinarians to become proficient in basic intraoral premolar and molar extraction techniques of Equidae. Indications, equipment, and methodology are described. Numerous photos and videos are included to achieve a more immersive learning experience than can be accomplished with the written word alone.

Clinicians performing these techniques will continue to improve their skill-sets to achieve positive outcomes as case specifics become more challenging.

Adjunct extraction techniques are used when the shape or integrity of the tooth, the shape or size of the patient's oral cavity, the location of the tooth, or the location of the proximal teeth prevents or complicates standard oral extraction. Techniques described and discussed include partial coronectomy, tooth sectioning, minimally invasive buccotomy, transbuccal screw extraction, and commissurotomy.

Dental repulsion techniques reported in the past decades have a high incidence of complications. Although the practice of surgical extractions in horses is limited because of the training, instrumentation, and experience required to perform these techniques, veterinarians should be aware these procedures are available, general anesthesia is not required, and when performed by skilled veterinary dentists, have low complication rates. Surgical techniques are often used after failure of other extraction techniques to remove retained tooth root and fragments or to debride chronically contaminated orofacial lesions. However, surgical extractions should be considered during initial treatment planning of all complicated cases.

The anatomy of the equine paranasal sinuses is critical to understand to assess the extent of the disease process, the optimal surgical approach, and the ability to drain through the normal nasomaxillary pathway. By following established anatomic landmarks, direct sinus access can be used to further explore the sinus compartments, remove compromised cheek teeth, remove any purulent debris or feed contamination, and establish drainage. Many complications can be avoided or minimized by thoroughly evaluating all sinus compartments and critically assessing the ability of the sinus to drain.

Oral extraction has become the most popular extraction technique owing to its high rate of success with minimal major complication. Repulsion continues to produce unacceptably high iatrogenic complication rates. As an alternative to tooth repulsion, veterinary dentists have introduced procedures to facilitate difficult intraoral extractions and surgical extraction techniques. Minimizing complications is best achieved preoperatively. A comprehensive preoperative evaluation and treatment plan allows the dentist to predict intraoperative complication and prepare for procedures to produce the best outcome. With proper case selection and adherence to extraction principles, the primary veterinarian and the veterinary dentist can perform equine tooth extractions with minimal complications.

Elaine F. Claffey and Norm G. Ducharme

 Video content accompanies this article at http://www.vetequine. theclinics.com.

The nasal conchal bullae (dorsal and ventral) are separate, air-filled structures within their respective dorsal and ventral nasal conchae. Computed tomography scans have assisted with the increasing diagnosis of empyema of the nasal conchae. This condition is usually associated with dental or sinus disease. Drainage of affected bullae is considered critical for resolution of clinical signs. The ventral conchal bullae can be easily viewed with a standard 10 mm diameter flexible endoscopy via the middle nasal meatus. This approach can also be used for fenestration of the bullae, using a diode laser, equine laryngeal forceps, or bipolar vessel sealing device.

Leah E. Limone

 Video content accompanies this article at http://www.vetequine. theclinics.com.

Equine odontoclastic tooth resorption and hypercementosis (EOTRH) is a progressive, painful disease, affecting incisors, canines, and cheek teeth. Examination findings include gingival inflammation, gingival recession and/or hyperplasia, subgingival swelling, bulbous enlargement of teeth, associated periodontal disease, pathologic tooth fracture, and/or tooth mobility and loss. Current hypotheses include biomechanical stresses and secondary bacterial involvement. Early recognition allows case management, but it is a progressive disease. Owner education is crucial; horses with complete or multiple extractions have a favorable prognosis. Human oral and dental health may be affected by bisphosophonate use; long-term effects of these drugs are currently unknown in horses.

VETERINARY CLINICS OF NORTH AMERICA: EQUINE PRACTICE

RELATED SERIES

Veterinary Clinics of North America: Food Animal Practice

Preface

Snapshot of Equine Dentistry: Past, Present, and Future

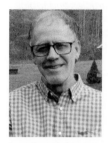
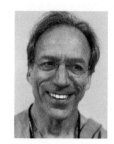
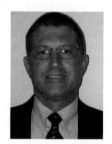

Edward T. Earley, DVM, AVDC/Eq

Robert M. Baratt, DVM, MS, AVDC, AVDC/Eq

Stephen S. Galloway, DVM, AVDC, AVDC/Eq

Editors

A lecture on Equine Dentistry given by Dr Mike Lowder almost 20 years ago was titled "Who's Floating Who?" At the time, the *experts* were mostly charismatic lay *"Equine Dentists,"* and the dental procedures being taught had not significantly changed, other than improved instrumentation, during the previous century. Furthermore, almost all of the procedures being performed at that time had no scientific basis. Some commonly practiced procedures did not correct the indicating problems, and some procedures were actually harmful to our patients.

During the first decade of this century, it is fair to credit Drs Paddy Dixon and Jack Easley with leading a concerted effort to transform Equine Dentistry from a livestock management service into a scientific health care discipline. As well, during this decade, Dr David Klugh promoted changing the focus of Equine Dentistry from a finite set of predetermined dental procedures performed on all horses into the application of dental treatment principles prescribed to benefit the unique *individual horse*. These efforts planted the seeds for specialty training in and professional recognition of Equine Veterinary Dentistry in North America.

Currently, many dental procedures that have been performed on the horse for decades are being scrutinized. Procedures, such as canine reduction, wolf tooth extraction, cheek tooth equilibration, incisor leveling, tooth repulsion, bit seats of premolars, and even enamel point reduction, have been questioned as to their validity and merit as dental procedures. There is presently a paradigm shift toward conservative procedures that would preserve and prolong dental health for the life of the horse. The intent of this *Veterinary Clinics of North America: Equine Practice* 2020 issue is to highlight topics with recent progression in Equine Dentistry. Authors were selected based on their advanced understanding of the selected topics, creating a unique combination

Vet Clin Equine 36 (2020) xi–xiii
https://doi.org/10.1016/j.cveq.2020.10.001
0749-0739/20/© 2020 Published by Elsevier Inc.

and perspective of Equine Dentistry within 1 article. The editors and authors look forward to the continued innovation and understanding of this discipline.

The examination process is the foundation for the practice of veterinary medicine and specifically equine dentistry. With advancements of imagery, such as endoscopy (oral, sinus, and nasal), radiography, and computed tomography, our comprehension of dental disease has dramatically improved over the last several years. The most appropriate treatment is based upon diagnostic accuracy and the current understanding of a disease process and pathology. The articles and topics covered in this 2020 Veterinary Clinics of North America: Equine Practice issue collectively demonstrate the most current perspectives in Equine Dentistry. A special thank you of appreciation is given to the contributing authors and coeditors for making this issue possible.

—Edward T. Earley, Editor

While equine dentistry has over the years been neglected by veterinarians in general practice, and given sparse treatment in the veterinary school curriculums, during the last decade, we have seen significant developments. The widespread use of digital radiography in general practice, the availability of oral endoscopy, the increasing availability of computed tomography, and new instrumentation and techniques for facilitating oral extraction of cheek teeth have greatly improved the quality of dental care in the horse in the last decade. This updated Veterinary Clinics of North America: Equine Practice/Equine issue should provide equine practitioners with a "state-of-the-art" reference for equine dentistry.

—Robert M. Baratt, Coeditor

Equine Dentistry can be characterized during the second decade of this century as a period of constantly increasing research, procedural improvements, and advances in training opportunities. However, while our scientific basis for treatments has exponentially improved, we are only beginning the process of critical review; therefore, we still fall short of the goal of practicing evidence-based dentistry. Best practices largely remain a matter of opinion; therefore, individual treatments should be based upon the operators personal training, competency, and experience. With the continued study of Equine Dentistry, I am grateful for the colleagues who have and continue to teach me, and I hope other veterinarians find this study as fulfilling and rewarding.

—Stephen S. Galloway, Coeditor

Edward T. Earley, DVM, AVDC/Eq
Large Animal Dentistry
Equine Farm Animal Hospital
Box 24, C3 Hallway CPC
Ithaca, NY 14853, USA

Robert M. Baratt, DVM, MS, AVDC, AVDC/Eq
Salem Valley Veterinary Clinic
12 Centre Street
Salem, CT 06420, USA

Stephen S. Galloway, DVM, AVDC, AVDC/Eq
Animal Dental Care Specialist
8565 Highway 64
Somerville, TN 38068, USA

E-mail addresses:
ete9@cornell.edu (E.T. Earley)
robert.baratt.dvm@gmail.com (R.M. Baratt)
achvet@yahoo.com (S.S. Galloway)

A Brief History of Equine Dental Practice

Jack Easley, DVM, MS

KEYWORDS

• Dentistry • Horse • Equine • History • Change • Antiquity • Veterinary

KEY POINTS

- Equine dentistry has a long and interesting history, being one of the earliest areas of equine health care.
- Equine dentistry was a neglected area of veterinary and animal husbandry research during the twentieth century.
- Great progress has been made by veterinarians and equine medical researchers over the past 30 years in improving understanding of equine dental disease.
- New and innovative equine dental diagnostic and therapeutic techniques have been developed in the twenty-first century, based on evidence from clinical and bench research.

INTRODUCTION

Historically, equitarians always have been aware of the benefits of good dental care to improve performance of the equine athlete and extend the useful life span of the horse. Recent archeozoological data from equine skeletal remains show that horse dentistry took root in the tribes of nomadic pastoralists living on the steppes of Mongolia and northeast Asia during the Bronze age (ca.750 BCE). The inception of dentistry within the tribes occurred following the introduction of using a metal bit to control horses.[1] For the next 2000 years, medical and dental practice was focused on physical techniques, such as farriery and barber surgery, and the Hippocratic-based theory of disease. This theory taught that disease was caused by an imbalance of the 4 humors: black bile, yellow bile, phlegm, and blood. These humors were associated with the 4 seasons of the year and the 4 known elements (air, earth, fire, and water). For centuries, this theory of disease was combined with the belief in good and evil spirits to derive medical advice and base treatments. New discoveries around the seventeenth

The author (J. Easley) has no commercial or financial conflicts of interest or any funding sources outside of a private equine dental veterinary practice.
PO Box 1075, Shelbyville, KY 40066, USA
E-mail address: easleydvm@aol.com

century began the Age of Enlightenment, which slowly changed the thinking about health and disease.

Equine dentistry was a pillar of veterinary practice at the turn of the twentieth century. By 1905, 4 complete textbooks (**Box 1**) dedicated to equine dentistry were in print. Merillat[2] stated, "the principal objective of dentistry is to promote the general health (of the horse) by improving mastication and by relieving pain." Equine clinicians today agree that the goal of dentistry remains the same. Merillat's text described how to float enamel points, manage deciduous teeth, and extract terminally diseased teeth.[2] With the exception of the outstanding clinical work of Erwin Becker (1898–1978),[3] some 50 years later, the standard of equine dental care saw minimal change through most of the twentieth century. Many of the procedures described by Merillat, such as wolf tooth extraction, canine teeth reductions, and bit seat application, now are commonly practiced—100 years later, with the continued practice of potentially harmful procedures that have no scientific validation.

Today, equine dentistry is one of the most common tasks performed by large animal veterinary practitioners. New discoveries in medical and dental science and species-specific dental research have opened eyes and minds to a better understanding of equine dentition in health and disease. These advances in understanding of equine dentistry have led to the abandonment of old procedures and techniques. Other techniques have been reinforced and/or improved on because of enhanced understanding of equine dental anatomy, physiology, and dental disease. Better methods of restraint and improved diagnostic equipment and techniques have allowed for a more accurate diagnosis to be made, which enables treatments to be more precisely planned and carried out.

EQUINE RESTRAINT

Prior to 1950, most horses requiring dental care were restrained by physical means (halter and lead, twitch, stocks with ropes, double side lines, or casting ropes). For dental procedures, cocaine-based local/regional anesthesia was used in combination with and to augment physical restraint. Tranquilizers, such as phenothiazine derivatives (Thorazine, Sparine, Tranvet, and acepromazine), rauwolfia derivative (reserpine), and propanediol derivatives (Equanil), were in common use. By the end of the twentieth century, most of these drugs no longer were on the medical drug market because their use in horses was not entirely satisfactory.[4] Xylazine was discovered as an antihypertensive agent in 1962 by Farbenfabriken Bayer in Leverkusen, Germany. Before the discovery that xylazine was effective as an equine sedative, there were no sedatives approved for use in horses.[5]

Box 1
Four books on equine dentistry published before 1900

The Horse's Mouth. Edward Mayhew, MRCVS. Published by Messrs. Fores, 41, Piccadilly, London, 1850

Veterinary Surgery, Vol I, Animal Dentistry and Diseases of the Mouth. Merillat LA. Published by Haussmann and Dunn Co., Chicago, IL, 1905.

Horses Teeth. Clark HD. Published by WK Jenkins, New York, 1886

Veterinary Dental Surgery. Prof. Hinebauch TD, Published by Purdue University Press, La Fayette, IN, 1889

By the early twentieth century, general anesthesia was used in equine veterinary surgery but muscle-relaxing drugs (choral hydrate/magnesium sulfate and succinylcholine), hypnotic drugs (thiopental and thiamylal), and gases (chloroform) were associated with high morbidity rates. By 1980, xylazine was in popular use and short-term anesthesia with intravenous combinations of xylazine/diazepam/guaifenesin/ketamine and better inhalant agents were used safely in equine practice. This changed equine dental practice more than any other single factor. Safe equine restraint and the ability to perform an oral examination with minimal complications were the beneficial results. A detailed dental examination could be performed safely in the field with use of a full-mouth speculum, dental mirror or endoscope, and dental picks and probes.

The next 25 years brought the introduction of other α_2 adrenergic receptor agonists (detomidine and romifidine) and opioid-based analgesics (butorphanol) as well as more refined and safer methods of local and regional anesthesia Such combinations have revolutionized working in the standing horse's mouth and opened the door to better diagnostic techniques and advanced imaging in the standing horse. Treatment options, such as novel oral extraction techniques, infundibular restorations, and endodontic treatments, also have evolved.

DENTAL EQUIPMENT AND INSTRUMENTATION

In 1648, the Dutch painter Paulus Potter produced "A Farrier's Shop" showing a farrier working in a horse's mouth with what appears to be a rasp or float (**Fig. 1**). In 1664, Jacques de Sollysel complained of people "bishoping" lower incisor teeth, which changed the shape of the dental spot to appear like a cup in order to make a horse appear younger. Several types of jewelers' drills were used throughout Europe to alter incisors. Many veterinary texts published over the next 200 years carefully documented the process of aging horses by dentition and the importance of not being fooled by "low dealers," who would perform this unethical practice. Professor Havemann from the Hannover Veterinary School introduced the technique and instrumentation for repelling teeth in 1805. In England, the Arnold and Sons Steel Works began manufacturing dental horse floats and other equipment. And, by 1844, Sharp & Smith in Chicago were in the equine dental tool manufacturing business. Friedrich and Karl Guenther were veterinary surgical pioneers in Germany. By 1859, they had developed

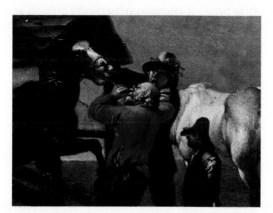

Fig. 1. A Farrier's Shop," 1648, by the Danish painter Paulus Potter. This oil shows a horse having a dental procedure performed while brutally restrained with a stocks and lip twitch.

a full mouth speculum and had constructed more than 36 different dental instruments including 19 different extraction forceps.[6]

In North America, after the civil war (1865) until the 1920s, there was no regulation of veterinary practice. Many imposters claiming to be veterinarians, or "hos docs," were working on horses and other animals. This period has been referred to as the "Time of Quackery." During this time period, C.D. House was a retired US Army Cavalryman who promoted himself and his equine dental techniques. He claimed to perform dental procedures without a speculum and routinely reduced the incisors claiming to bring the horse "into balance." In 1895, Hermann Haussmann, Chicago, IL patented the first speculum with removable incisor plates followed by J. Gordon McPherson's model, which still is in use today.[6–8]

During the early years of the twentieth century and after the introduction of affordable bicycles, automobiles, and tractors, horse numbers and economic interest declined. In North America, between 1880 and 1925, more than 100 veterinary and equine dental schools had opened and closed their doors. By this time human and veterinary medicine were rapidly changing for the better with the revolutionary discoveries of scientists, veterinarians, and physicians, such as Louis Pasteur, Fleming, Lister, and McFadyean.

The world still depended heavily on horse-drawn power for transportation, manufacturing, and military dominance until World War II. During the 1930s, the German engineer and veterinarian Becker (1898–1978) made significant contributions to modern equine dentistry that are still felt today. Becker was the nephew of Helmar Dun, a renowned private equine veterinary practitioner and promoter of veterinary dentistry. Portable stocks and head supports, use of the full-mouth speculum and head light, electric-powered and water-cooled dental grinders, dental records that allowed compilation of types and incidences of disease, and documentation of dental conditions with impressions and plaster models are just a few of Becker's contributions. Professor Becker had a long academic career in Berlin and after the war became a leader in the institute of roentgenology, veterinary dentistry, and veterinary surgery at the Berlin Free University. His scientific work includes 59 publications as well as approximately 400 educational and operating films produced in his film department.[9,10]

In the 1990s, Americans began to improve equine dental equipment. Donnie Matlock and Rich Capps manufactured carbide float blades replacing the steel interchangeable blades that had been used for 100 years. Frank Alberts, Dale Jeffery, and Herb Harlton's tools began to improve on the quality of floats and other equipment that had previously been utilized. Estrada, an Argentinean veterinarian, developed and marketed an electric portable flexible shaft float (**Fig. 2**). Dr Clay Stubbs perfected the

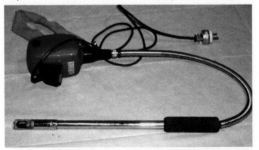

Fig. 2. The portable electric powered flexible cable tooth grinder developed by Estrada; an Argentinian veterinarian. This and many other improved dental instruments were introduced to the North American Veterinary market between 1970 and 2000.

motorized oscillating float and the use of air-powered tools in equine dentistry and Dennis Rach a Canada veterinarian developed a rotary float system (PowerFloat, PowerFloat Inc. Calgary, Alberta, Canada). Veterinarians could now safely sedate and examine the horse's mouth and with proper instruments almost effortlessly carry out occlusal corrective procedures. The next step in the scientific method was to test the procedures that had been performed on teeth since 1600 AD and to determine which ones were of value to the horse and/or rider. In 1993 an editorial by Professor P. M. Dixon[11] at Edinburgh University challenged the veterinary profession to research this neglected area of practice. This began the present age of scientific progress in the field of equine dentistry and oral health.

DENTAL DISEASE AND ITS CORRELATION TO DENTAL CORRECTIVE PROCEDURES

Dental corrective procedures have been performed on the horse's mouth for centuries without any real understanding of the disease or condition being treated. As early as 1350, a book by Abu Bekr Ibn Bedr contains drawings of horses having teeth extracted and the breaking or cutting of elongated teeth. In 1550, Rabelais wrote, "He always looked a given horse in the mouth." It was evident that good horsemen of that day understood a little about the appearance of incisor teeth and their relationship to age. Until the late nineteenth century, however, age-related changes on the incisor surface was thought to be due to excretion of material up through the tooth to change its shape and consistency, not occlusal wear. Much of the knowledge of the day was based on superstition and no place was this more evident than in training and bitting horses. Wolf teeth removal was thought to be necessary to prevent moon blindness or to prevent the cavalry horse from seeing the "wolf in battle." Before the first formal veterinary school was established in Lyons, France, in 1761, there were no standards or accountability for the veterinary profession. The first real anatomy course for veterinarians was conducted at the second school in Alfort, France, but dentistry was not at the forefront. Through the nineteenth century "bleeding" and "burning the lampas" (**Box 2**)were common professional practices.[10] In 1879, W. H. Clark[12] in his book *Horse Teeth* makes a reference to the difference between "skill vs brutality." This text was one of the first to properly describe horse dentition and disease processes. Professor T. D. Hinebauch[13] at Purdue University wrote *Veterinary Dental Surgery* in 1889 and covered most of the dental disease conditions seen in veterinary practice today. Much of the literature published for the next 50 years contained little new or researched information. Colyer, Hofmeyer, and Honma published original works on dental disease and pathology in the middle 1900s.[14–16] Becker's German work on more than 50,000 horses was published in the 1940s but because of World War II, laid almost unnoticed in the English-speaking world for approximately 50 years. In the 1970s, Gordon Baker[17] presented his PhD thesis on equine dental disease and continued to publish on this area of equine practice until his retirement in 2009.

Box 2
Definition of lampas

Lampas is an antiquated term for mucosal thickening or inflammation of the hard palate just behind the upper incisors. This is a normal feature in young horses that are erupting permanent dentition. Thickening of the palate mucosa also can be seen in horses that have been on soft grass forage that are suddenly brought into confinement and fed very course forage or chaff. This condition is self-limiting but for centuries was treated with caustic agents, lancing with differ blade devices ∖, or soft tissue charring with thermocautery. All of these so-called methods of therapy were brutal and inhumane

The equine tooth is complex and unique in that the occlusal surface and exposed crown is ever changing due to occlusal wear as the horse ages and the root constantly is remodeling. This makes radiographic based imaging necessary for evaluating the subgingival portion of the tooth and surrounding periodontium. Radiographic imaging has changed dramatically over the past century since the discovery of x-rays by Wilhelm Röntgen a German physics professor in 1895. This soon was followed by the introduction of contrast agents in 1916. Film-based systems have been replaced by computerized and digital systems using phosphor sensing detectors and digital sensors. Nuclear medicine became possible in the 1950s and was in common use in veterinary medicine by the 1980s. Ultrasonography was developed in the 1960s based on the principles of sonar developed during World War II. The use of 3-dimensional imaging (computed tomography and magnetic resonance imaging) was developed in the 1970s and has revolutionized understanding of dental anatomy and pathology. These advanced imaging techniques have allowed for a more accurate diagnosis of dental disease and specific treatments.

Oral extraction of diseased teeth was practiced by a few brave practitioners for centuries but was limited mainly to loose teeth. There were high mortality and complication rates associated with this procedure.[18,19] The extraction forceps introduced by Gunther and Hauptner in the late 1800s stimulated the development of better forceps by Robertson, Gowing, Sharp & Smith, and Frick by 1912.[20] Even with better equipment oral extraction proved to be unsuccessful in many cases. With the addition of safer general anesthesia and radiographic support, retrograde repulsion techniques for removal of diseased cheek teeth gained popularity in the veterinary surgical community in the twentieth century. Even with these improvements, the tooth repulsion technique often was found to be unsuccessful and carried a high rate of surgical complications.[21] Veterinary training and literature had shifted by 1950 putting less emphasis on equine and more on canine and feline care.[22] As equine dental care improved in the late twentieth century and, as veterinarians gained a better understanding of dental pathophysiology, new and improved techniques for tooth removal and preservation have been developed.

The expanded array of techniques to treat diseased teeth introduced in the twenty-first century include orthograde and retrograde endodontic procedures and infundibular restorations to preserve diseased teeth. Extraction techniques have expanded to include surgical extractions through buccal and lateral alveolar approaches for incisors, canines and cheek teeth. Minimally invasive buccal approaches have been introduced to better access cheek teeth to aid in extractions or restorations. Equine dental instruments and equipment have been developed to allow right angled burs and elevators to be used to section and remove cheek teeth intraorally.

All aspects of dental care have improved over the past century but also progress has been made in the diagnosis and treatment of secondary or associated conditions that often accompany dental disease. Sinusitis secondary to dental disease has always been a recognized comorbidity and often led to the demise of the horse. The knowledge to trephine and drain the sinus compartments was described and referred to in the early veterinary literature as "nasal Gleet."[8] At that time, it was observed that in chronic sinus infections "the pus hardens and concretes, until by degree the cavities are filled with a foul and solid matter."[23] Treatment of secondary sinus disease has become a less invasive and more controlled procedure with the advent of flexible fiberoptic endoscopes introduced to veterinary practice in the 1960s. More recently, these therapeutic and diagnostic sinus surgeries are performed commonly as standing outpatient procedures. This allows samples for bacteriologic culture and histopathology to be taken more easily, which leads to more accurate diagnosis and treatment.

To master these new and innovative equine dental techniques efforts have been made in the veterinary medical community to better train students and equine practitioners to treat dental cases. Efforts began in the late twentieth century by the American Association of Equine Practitioners (AAEP) and the British Equine Veterinary Association with sponsorship from the equine dental manufacturing community to offer continuing education of lecture seminars and wet laboratories for veterinarians and veterinary students. Hundreds of these programs have provided training to equine veterinarians over the past 30 years. Veterinary school curriculums have been ungraded to provide better dental training to students with the help of the veterinary dental specialty colleges (American Veterinary Dental College and European Veterinary Dental College).

In 2017, Professor Dixon was invited to present the Frank J. Milne State-of-the-Art Lecture at the AAEP annual meeting.[24] He presented a lecture entitled "The Evolution of Horses and the Evolution of Equine Dentistry" to a crowd of more than 2000 equine veterinarians. He addressed the progress made in this area of veterinary practice and was able to reference more than 100 papers that had been published since his editorial addressing the lack of attention to equine dentistry in 1993.[11] He described several new disease processes that had been described only in the twenty-first century (equine odontoclastic tooth resorption and hypercementosis, infundibular cement hypoplasia, peripheral cemental caries, and peripheral caries of cheek teeth). He also brought attention to the new molecular bacteriologic techniques that have been used to map the normal and abnormal microbiome of the horse's mouth.

SUMMARY

It should be clear to anyone who has kept up with the current veterinary literature that equine dental disease is more prevalent and more wide ranging than once thought. The complete and detailed oral examination is critical to diagnosing and planning treatment of any dental pathologic condition. Dentistry no longer can be approached from the standpoint of being concerned only with abnormalities of occlusal wear and sharp enamel points.

In the late 1980s, a new revival in equine dentistry became evident. The conflict between lay dental care providers (LDCPs) and veterinarians began in earnest at this time. Most LDCPs had worked for veterinarians who had trained them to float teeth during the slow times at the racetrack. Seeing the opportunity for more money as independent operators outside the supervision of a veterinarian, new equine dental groups began to emerge. This trend set back the scientific and medically sound practice of equine dentistry. Dental care is an integral part of overall equine health care. It is a professional veterinary practice, not simply an animal husbandry task.

In the past 2 decades, equine veterinarians have expanded the scientific knowledge about equine dental anatomy, aging by dentition, dental and masticatory physiology, and pathophysiology of dental disease and have improved diagnostic and treatment techniques more than at any time in the past 4 centuries. This information is the foundation for this equine dentistry edition of *The Veterinary Clinics* and many other recent equine veterinary dental texts and publications. Let us continue this progress and not be the generation that relinquishes equine dentistry to untrained, uneducated, nonscientific-thinking yeomen. Such would not be in the best interest of the horse or the veterinary profession.

REFERENCES

1. Taylor WTT, Bayarsaikhan J, Tuvshinjargal T, et al. Origins of equine dentistry. Proc Natl Acad Sci U S A 2019;115(29):E6707–15.
2. Merillat LA. Veterinary surgery, Vol I, animal dentistry and diseases of the mouth. Chicago: Haussmann and Dunn Co; 1905. p. 13.
3. Becker E. Handbuch der Speziellen Pathologischenm, Anatomie der Haustiere, VolV. 3rd edition. Berlin: Paul Porey; 1962.
4. Muir WW, Hubbell JAE. History of equine anesthesia. In: Muir WW, Hubbell JAE, editors. Equine anesthesia: monitoring and emergency therapy. 2nd edition. St Louis (MO): Saunders/Elsevier; 2009. p. 1–9.
5. Greene SA, Thurmon JC. Xylazine–a review of its pharmacology and use in veterinary medicine. J Vet Pharmacol Ther 1988;11(4):295–313.
6. Easley J, Hatzel J. The history of equine dentistry. In: Easley J, Dixon PM, Schumacher J, editors. Equine dentistry. 3rd edition. Edinburgh (Scotland): Saunders/Elsevier; 2011. p. 11–25.
7. Easley K. Veterinary Dentistry: It's Origin and Recent History. J Hist Dent 1999; 47(2):83–5.
8. Harvey CE. The history of veterinary dentistry, part one: from the earliest record to the end of the 18th century. J Vet Dent 1994;11(4):135–9.
9. Schaffer HJ, Frerking H. Prof. Dr. Med. Vet. Erwin Becker (1898-1978) Leben und Werk, Inaugural-Dissertation (Dr. med. Vet.). Germany: Hanover University; 2001.
10. Fahrenkrug P. The history and future of equine dental care. In: Proceedings from the North Am Vet Conf January 15, 2005; Orlando, 151-154.
11. Dixon PM. Equine Dental Disease: a neglected field of study. Equine Vet Educ 1993;6:285–6.
12. Clark WH. Horses teeth. 3rd edition rev. New York: WK Jenkins; 1886.
13. Hinebauch TD. Veterinary Dental Surgery. IN: La Fayette, IN; 1889.
14. Miles AEW, Grigson C. Colyer's Variations and diseases of the teeth of animals. Cambridge: Cambridge University Press; 1960.
15. Hofmeyer CFB. Comparative dental pathology. J S Afr Vet Med Assoc 1960;29: 471–80.
16. Honma K, Yamalawa M, Yamauchi S, et al. Statistical study on the occurrence of dental caries in domestic animals. The Horse. Jpn J Vet Res 1962;10:31–6.
17. Baker GJ. A study of dental disease in the horse. PhD thesis. Glasgow (Scotland): University of Glasgow; 1979.
18. Blundeville T. The Fowler Chiefyst Offices Belonging to Horsemanshippe. London; 1566
19. Cadiot PJ. Clinical veterinary medicine and surgery Translated and edited by JAW Dollar. New York: Wm R Jenkins Co.; 1908. p. 8–14.
20. Dollar JAW. Regional veterinary surgery and operative techniques (Incorporating H Muller's veterinary surgery). New York: Wm R Jenkins; 1912. p. 271–357.
21. Prichard MA, Hackett RP, Erb HN. Long term outcome of tooth repulsion in horses: a retrospective study of 61 cases. Vet Surg 1992;21:145–9.
22. O'Conner JJ. Dollar's veterinary surgery. 4th ediiton. Chicago: Alexander Eger; 1950. p. 590–601.
23. Mayhew E. The Illustrated horse Doctor. Philadelphia: JB Lippincott; 1888. p. 91–4.
24. Dixon PM. The Evolution of Horses and the Evolution of Equine Dentistry. In: Proceedings of the 63rd Annual American Association of Equine Practitioners Convention, December 17-21, 2007; San Antonio, TX.

Equine Oral Endoscopy

Claudia K. True, DVM[a], Allison R. Dotzel, DVM[b],*

KEYWORDS

- Oral endoscopy • Oral endoscope • Oral examination • Equine dentistry

KEY POINTS

- An oral endoscopic system can be created that provides a high-resolution image at an economical price.
- Oral endoscopic examination in the horse includes a detailed evaluation of the clinical crown (cementum, dentin, enamel, pulp horns, and infundibula) and the surrounding soft tissue structures (eg, gingiva, mucosa, tongue, hard/soft palate, salivary ducts).
- Oral endoscopy is useful for detailed evaluation and treatment of dental/oral disorders such as dental fractures/defects, periodontal disease, oral fistula, and tumors.
- Precise placement and use of dental instrumentation are accomplished when aided with oral endoscopy.
- Oral endoscopy can easily be adapted for use in both a large animal mobile practice as well as a clinical hospital environment.

Video content accompanies this article at http://www.vetequine.theclinics.com.

INTRODUCTION

In this era, most equine practitioners understand the importance of the thorough oral examination, not only when checking for potential oral abnormalities or disease but also before any routine dental procedure. To perform such an examination, the following is essential: (1) an adequately sedated patient, (2) a full-mouth speculum, (3) a good light source, and (4) a mirror to visualize the entire oral cavity. The addition of an oral endoscopic examination not only helps the practitioner in discovering subtle disorders that may have been missed but can also add value for the client, who can now visualize what the practitioner is seeing. Use of an endoscope often allows superior visualization compared with a mirror because of both magnification and resolution of the image. In addition, many horses seem to object less to the endoscope in the caudal portions of the oral cavity. Oral endoscopy is extremely helpful when

[a] Woodside Equine Clinic, PO Box 989, Ashland, VA 23005, USA; [b] Laurel Highland Veterinary Clinic, 2586 Northway Road Ext, Williamsport, PA 17701, USA
* Corresponding author.
E-mail address: ardotzel@laurelhighland.com

Vet Clin Equine 36 (2020) 433–443
https://doi.org/10.1016/j.cveq.2020.07.001
0749-0739/20/© 2020 Elsevier Inc. All rights reserved.

vetequine.theclinics.com

performing instrumented periodontal and endodontic procedures, extractions, and surgical techniques.

ORAL ENDOSCOPIC EXAMINATION

An oral endoscopic examination should consist of a thorough and systematic assessment of the dental soft and hard tissues. The soft tissues examined include the oral mucosa, gingiva, tongue, lips, and salivary ducts.[1] The occlusal surface of the equine cheek tooth consists of an in-folding pattern of enamel, dentin, and cementum (**Figs. 1–3**). The areas of dentin and cementum are softer and wear at a faster rate than the enamel, causing the formation of enamel ridges. The maxillary cheek teeth have mesial and distal infundibulae that are filled with cementum in mature horses. Centrally within the infundibulum is a variably sized channel (or channels) that are a remnant of the former site of blood vessels supplying the developing (unerupted) tooth. The ridges on the buccal aspect of the maxillary cheek teeth are normal anatomic structures called cingula. Enamel points may develop on the occlusally located portions of the cingula of the maxillary cheek teeth as well as on the lingual aspect of the mandibular cheek teeth.[2]

As the occlusal surface wears, secondary dentin is laid down to protect the pulp from exposure.[3] The secondary dentin overlying the pulp horns tends to stain darker because of the dentinal tubules absorbing pigments from the diet (eg, forage, hay). Indications of pulp exposure or insult include white mineralization of the pulp horn, pitting or dull surface of dentin, and food impaction. The pulp horns of each cheek tooth are numbered using a system described by DuToit.[3,4] The pulp horns of the maxillary cheek teeth are identified starting on the buccal aspect of the tooth. The mesiobuccal pulp horn is numbered 1 and the distobuccal pulp horn is numbered 2. Numbering then moves to the next row of 2 pulp horns with the mesial pulp horn numbered 3 and the distal pulp horn numbered 4. The most palatal pulp horn is numbered 5 (**Fig. 4**A). The pulp horns of the mandibular cheek teeth are numbered starting on the buccal aspect of the tooth. The mesiobuccal pulp horn is numbered

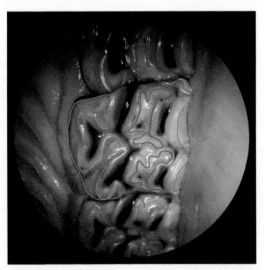

Fig. 1. Cementum component of an equine maxillary cheek tooth. Peripheral cementum outlined in orange; central (infundibular) cementum outlined in red.

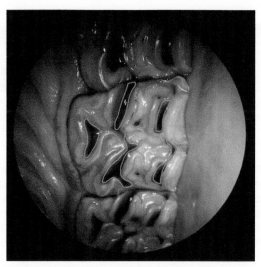

Fig. 2. Dentin component of an equine maxillary cheek tooth (*green*).

1 and the distobuccal pulp horn is numbered 2. The row of lingual pulp horns of the mandibular cheek teeth are numbered from mesial to distal (3, 4, and 5) (**Fig. 4**B). The second premolar and third molar teeth (Triadan number 06 and 11) have additional pulp horns numbered 6, 7, and 8 (see **Fig. 4**).[4]

Equine teeth are identified using the Triadan system of dental nomenclature. The system consists of a 3-digit number unique to each tooth. The first digit refers to the quadrant, where 1 indicates the right maxillary arcade, 2 the left maxillary arcade, 3 the left mandibular arcade, and 4 the right mandibular arcade.[2] Numbering begins at the central incisor and progresses distally along the arcade. The cheek teeth include

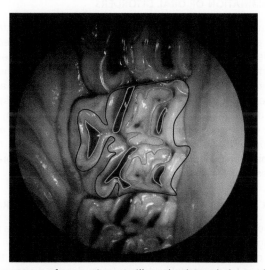

Fig. 3. Enamel component of an equine maxillary cheek tooth (enamel outlined in *blue*; dentin outlined in *green*, and infundibular cementum outlined in *orange*).

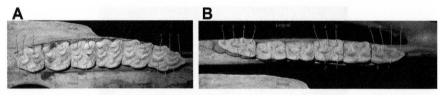

Fig. 4. (*A*) DuToit numbering system for pulp horns of equine maxillary premolars and molars. (*B*) DuToit numbering system for pulp horns of equine mandibular premolars and molars.

tooth 06 through 11 in each of the 4 arcades. Triadan number 05 refers to the first premolar, or wolf tooth, which may or may not be present in normal adult horses.

The equine endoscopic examination should include careful assessment of the occlusal, mesial, distal, lingual/palatal, and buccal aspects of each tooth as well as all the soft tissue structures. The endoscope is positioned between the right maxillary and mandibular arcades so that the occlusal surface of 106 is in the field of view. For the best imaging quality of the occlusal surface, place the optical lens of the scope approximately 2 cm below (maxillary cheek teeth) or above (mandibular cheek teeth) the occlusal surface. The endoscope is then advanced caudally to evaluate the occlusal surface of each tooth in the arcade. When the distal aspect of 111 is reached, the endoscope is repositioned to visualize the palatal aspect of 111 and then withdrawn in a rostral direction in order to examine the palatal mucosa and interdental spaces. When the mesial aspect of tooth 106 is reached, the endoscope is rotated to visualize the buccal aspect of the tooth and then advanced to the distal aspect of 111 in order to examine the buccal interdental spaces and buccal mucosa. The endoscope is then repositioned below the 200 arcade and the same systematic examination process is repeated. On completing the examination of the 200 arcade, the endoscope is rotated 180° and the 300 and 400 arcades are examined in a similar way (Video 1).

ENDOSCOPIC EXAMINATION OF ORAL DISORDERS

The enhanced image obtained when using an oral endoscope is extremely beneficial to the practice of equine dentistry because it can help clinicians identify and monitor subtle oral disorders.[5–10] The endoscope can be used to evaluate endodontic disorders such as cemental and enamel fissures, crown fractures, and pulp exposure (**Figs. 5–7**). Endoscopic examination also aids in the identification and classification of periodontal disease (**Fig. 8**). The endoscope can be used in combination with a periodontal probe to determine the extent of attachment loss caused by periodontal disease. Infundibular caries and peripheral cemental abnormalities can also be evaluated with oral endoscopy (**Fig. 9**). Other types of disorder that may be noted on an oral endoscopic examination include oral tumors, lingual and buccal abrasions or lacerations, and pustules of the mucous membranes (**Fig. 10**).[5]

USE OF THE ORAL ENDOSCOPE IN DENTAL AND ORAL SURGICAL PROCEDURES

An oral endoscope can be used to improve visualization and to guide the placement of instruments during dental procedures.[5,7,11,12] For instance, it can be used to obtain a better view when cleaning out periodontal pockets and help ensure that the pocket is thoroughly cleared of feed material and completely debrided after subgingival curettage (**Fig. 11**). The endoscope can also be used to ensure the proper placement of

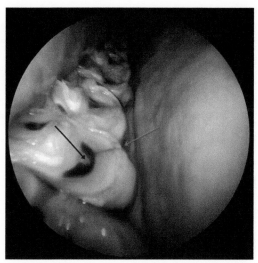

Fig. 5. Occlusal fissure of tooth 309 extending from the dentin (pulp horn 1) through the cementum and enamel (*red arrow*). Also note the calcification in pulp horn 1 (*blue arrow*).

the blades of a dental spreader during tooth extraction, preventing accidental damage to the tooth being extracted, the adjacent tooth, or the surrounding soft tissues (**Fig. 12**). It can help evaluate the quality of contact of dental extraction forceps, confirming a good fit and lessening the risk of damage to the tooth caused by instrument movement (**Fig. 13**). Progress of the extraction can be assessed by inserting the endoscope while the tooth is being manipulated in order to gauge the amount of movement as periodontal attachments are broken down. In procedures with dental fragments or retained root tips or in minimally invasive buccotomy procedures, the endoscope can

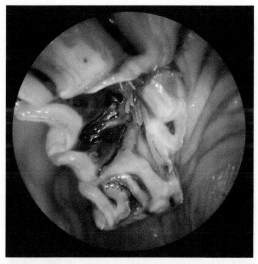

Fig. 6. Complicated crown fracture of tooth 109. Infundibular decay is present but the tooth is fractured through pulp horns 3 and 4.

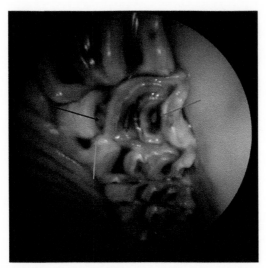

Fig. 7. Pulp exposure tooth 207 (pulp horn 1; *red arrow*). Also note the calcification of pulp horn 3 (*blue arrow*) and the occlusal fissure extending from pulp horn 3 to pulp horn 5 (*green arrow*).

aid in the proper positioning of elevators and small forceps.[5,12] Endoscopic guidance is also extremely helpful with high-speed burs when sectioning teeth and performing diastema procedures. It is useful for placement of instruments during restorative procedures (**Fig. 14**), debridement of oronasal or oroantral fistulae, and evaluation during sinus surgeries (**Fig. 15**).[5]

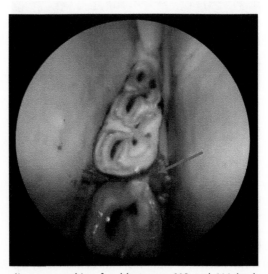

Fig. 8. Closed valve diastema packing food between 410 and 411 (*red arrow*).

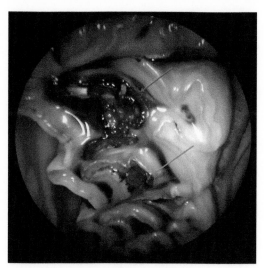

Fig. 9. Infundibular caries lesion of the mesial (*red arrow*) and distal (*green arrow*) infundibulae of tooth 109.

BUILDING AN ORAL ENDOSCOPE

An oral endoscope system can be built at a cost of around US$2000 to 2500. The components include a rigid endoscope (this is typically a human laparoscope) that is 10 mm in diameter and is ideally 40 to 60 cm in length. Although the angle of the lens at 70° is ideal for both general examination and in guidance and placement of instruments in dental procedures, the more widely available 45° endoscope works well for most purposes. These laparoscopes can be purchased new from the manufacturers or found on multiple Internet sites that sell used or refurbished medical instruments.

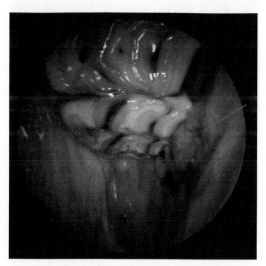

Fig. 10. Buccal abrasion at the level of the 211 tooth (*red arrow*).

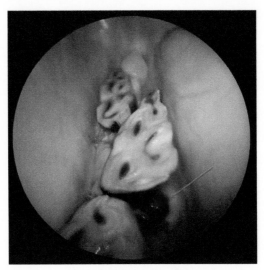

Fig. 11. Periodontal pocket on the lingual aspect of tooth 409 and 410 following debridement (*red arrow*).

A high-resolution, Wi-Fi–compatible digital camera needs to be modified by removing the lens and replacing it with a C-mount lens adaptor plate. Specifically, this needs to be a C-mount lens to micro4/3 M4/3 adapter. A video coupler connects the endoscope to the camera. A handheld, bright light source, either halogen or light-emitting diode, is essential for excellent image quality.

Any tablet with Wi-Fi capabilities greatly enhances the use of this system. Not only does it give the operator of the endoscope better visualization but it also allows clients to both easily view and better understand normal and abnormal findings. Another

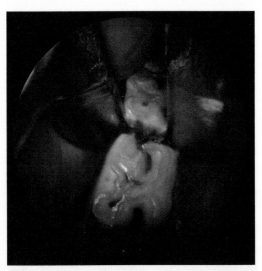

Fig. 12. Checking the placement of the blades of a dental spreader in the interdental space during extraction of tooth 309.

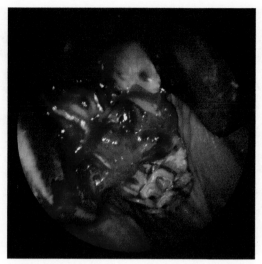

Fig. 13. Checking the fit of dental extraction forceps during extraction of tooth 109.

helpful feature of the tablet is that can be used to remotely take both photos and videos by downloading a camera-specific application. This feature makes recording the examination by an assistant holding the tablet more convenient than the endoscope operator using the camera buttons. If the oral endoscope is used in an ambulatory setting, it is recommended that a sturdy, water-resistant case be purchased to protect the tablet endoscopic system.

The settings on a single-lens reflex camera need to be adjusted so that it is set to shoot without a lens. Also, the record format is set for MP4 so that videos are saved as MP4 files. Photos and videos are taken with the intelligent auto mode on. This mode ensures proper light adjustment for inside the oral cavity.

Once the system is built, the focus of the endoscope is adjusted to approximately 2.0 to 2.5 cm from the object to be viewed, which is best done by holding the

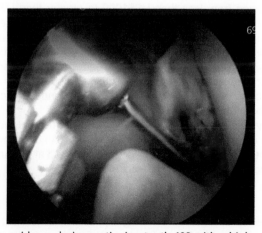

Fig. 14. Endoscopic guidance during sectioning tooth 409 with a high-speed bur.

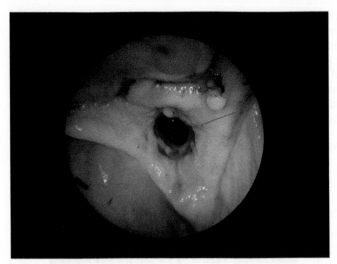

Fig. 15. Oroantral fistula following extraction of tooth 111 (*red arrow*).

endoscope lens over any small text before the endoscope is used in the oral cavity. The focus ring on the video coupler is rotated in either direction until the text comes into focus. Next, the Wi-Fi must be switched on in order to transmit the image to the tablet. Any pictures or videos taken are saved on the camera's SD (secure digital) card, which can then be added to the patient's records.

In a clinic setting, a monitor may be used for greater magnification and visualization. A compatible monitor may be linked through an application to the camera's Wi-Fi. If the goal is to view the real-time image simultaneously on both the tablet and a monitor, a high-definition multimedia interface (HDMI) cable is used that is specific to the tablet's HDMI adaptor.

COMMERCIAL ORAL ENDOSCOPES

Endoscopes that are marketed for equine oral examinations and procedures have become more common over the last several years. Picture quality, ability to capture images (both still and video), ease of use, durability, and portability vary widely among the units. Costs range from less than US$1000 to greater than US$10,000. Practitioners should consider these features and decide which instrument best fits their needs. For example, consider portability and ease of use if the endoscope will be used in a strictly ambulatory setting. One such endoscope is advertised for its portability. For a clinic setting where multiple types of endoscopes are used, a system that integrates a camera, insufflation pump, light source, video recorder, and image capture in 1 unit may be more beneficial. In addition, an oral endoscopic irrigation sheath is available that could be helpful during dental procedures.

If good-quality videos and pictures are necessary for medical records or publications, be sure the unit can take high-resolution images. An overview of the some of the oral endoscopes on the market was recently presented at the American Association of Equine Practitioners annual conference.[13]

SUMMARY

In the past few decades, research involving equine dentistry has greatly expanded, creating a need to better identify and treat oral disorders. At the same time, more equine dental continuing education is being offered, which helps disseminate this research to practitioners. As veterinarians realize the additional disorders that can be found through a thorough oral examination, the need to have the appropriate equipment becomes paramount. Although the dental mirror is inexpensive, it has limitations and is difficult to use for imaging. An oral endoscope is easier to use, has superior visual enhancement, and images are recordable.[8] As the paradigm in equine veterinary dentistry shifts from dental filing to oral examination, oral endoscopes will give practitioners an improved capacity to diagnose and treat equine oral disorders.

DISCLOSURE

The authors do not have any commercial or financial conflicts of interest or any funding sources to disclose.

SUPPLEMENTARY DATA

Supplementary data related to this article can be found online at https://doi.org/10.1016/j.cveq.2020.07.001.

REFERENCES

1. Menzies RA. Oral examination and charting setting the basis for evidence based medicine in the oral examination of equines. Vet Clin North Am 2013;29:325–43.
2. Easley KJ. Dental and oral examination. In: Easley KJ, Dixon P, Schumaker J, editors. Equine dentistry. 3rd edition. New York: Elsevier; 2011. p. 185–98.
3. Dixon PM, DuToit M, Staszyk C. A fresh look at the anatomy and physiology of equine mastication. Vet Clin North Am 2013;29:257–72.
4. DuToit N, Kempson SA, Dixon PM. Donkey dental anatomy. Part 1: gross and computed axial tomography examinations. Vet J 2008;176:338–44.
5. Dotzel AR. How to use an oral mirror and endoscope. Proceedings Am Assoc Equine Pract 2018;64:25–9.
6. Easley KJ. How to properly perform and interpret an endoscopic examination of the equine oral cavity. Proceedings Am Assoc Equine Pract 2008;54:383–5.
7. Griffin C. How to incorporate oral endoscopy into an equine dental examination. Proceedings Am Assoc Equine Pract 2014;60:464–9.
8. Goff C. A study to determine the diagnostic advantages of oral endoscopy for the detection of dental pathology in the standing horse. Am Assoc Equine Pract Focus 2006;266–8, 264–6.
9. Razman PHL. Oral endoscopy as an aid to diagnosis of equine cheek tooth infections in the absence of gross oral pathological changes: 17 cases. Equine Vet J 2009;41(2):101–6.
10. Simhofer H, Griss R, Zetner K. The use of oral endoscopy for the detection of cheek teeth abnormalities in 300 horses. Vet J 2008;178(3):396–404.
11. Galloway SS, Easley J. Incorporating oral photography and endoscopy into the equine dental examination. Vet Clin Equine 2013;29:345–66.
12. Razman PHL, Dallas RS, Palmer L. Extraction of fractured cheek teeth under oral endoscopic guidance in standing horses. Vet Surg 2011;40(5):586–9.
13. Henry TJ. How to make dental endoscopy part of routine oral examination. Proceedings Am Assoc Equine Pract 2017;63:39–45.

Dental Radiography and Radiographic Signs of Equine Dental Disease

Robert M. Baratt, DVM, MS

KEYWORDS

- Dentistry • Equine • Radiography • Extraoral • Intraoral • Positioning
- Radiographic signs • Dental disease

KEY POINTS

- Diagnostic-quality equine dental radiographic examination requires multiple radiographic views.
- A diagnostic equine dental radiographic study includes at least 6 standard views. Additional views, or further diagnostics, frequently are required for accurate diagnosis and therapeutic planning.
- Radiographic signs of dental disease include, but are not limited to, periapical alveolar bone lysis and/or sclerosis, widening of the periodontal ligament space, blunting of tooth roots, reserve crown-root resorption and/or hypercementosis, tooth or root fragmentation, and tooth malformation or malpositioning.
- The 3-dimensional anatomy of the teeth is difficult to assess with standard radiography. There are cases in which computed tomography is required to fully assess the nature of dental disease and the frequently associated sinus disease.

INTRODUCTION

Today's equine veterinarians in general practice have access to high-quality portable digital radiography systems, and most have acquired the necessary skills to produce diagnostic radiographs of the horse's limbs. With a modest investment in additional equipment, the same digital radiographic systems can be used for imaging of the head. This article focuses on

- Proper positioning for each of the standard radiographic projections of the head, with an emphasis on the teeth and paradental sinuses
- A review of the radiographic anatomy of the head
- The radiographic signs of dental disease and sinusitis of dental etiology

The author has no funding sources nor conflict of interest to declare.
Salem Valley Veterinary Clinic, 12 Centre Street, Salem, CT 06420, USA
E-mail address: robert.baratt.dvm@gmail.com

Vet Clin Equine 36 (2020) 445–476
https://doi.org/10.1016/j.cveq.2020.08.001
0749-0739/20/© 2020 Elsevier Inc. All rights reserved.

vetequine.theclinics.com

- The limitations of standard radiography and the indications for advance imaging procedures

INDICATIONS FOR DENTAL RADIOGRAPHY

Equine veterinarians have for decades stressed the importance of regular dental care in horses, and owners now expect that their horse's teeth require annual (or biannual) "floating." Many times, however, this largely unnecessary and often overzealous removal of enamel points is performed with a cursory oral examination or without any oral examination at all. Unfortunately, this service often is performed by

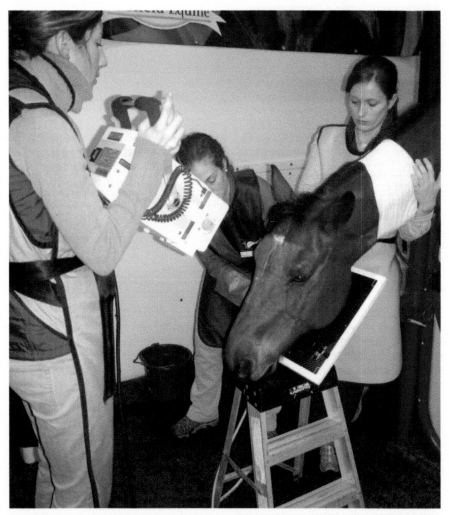

Fig. 1. The level of sedation allows the horse to quietly rest its head on a low support. Motion artifact largely is eliminated by resting the DR sensor on the same object and having an assistant steady the head/neck. With the head in a low position, the clinician can comfortably hold the x-ray generator and look directly over it for proper positioning.

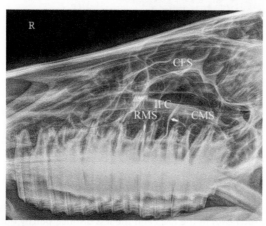

Fig. 2. The latero-lateral view is used primarily for evaluation of the paradental sinuses. This is the right lateral view obtained by placing the sensor on the right side of the horse's head with the center of the plate and central beam on the rostral aspect of the facial crest, which is about in the center of the maxillary arcade. In this view, the right and left infraorbital canals (IFC) are superimposed. The right and left conchofrontal sinuses (CFS), caudal maxillary sinuses (CMS), and rostral maxillary sinuses (RMS) are superimposed. Arrow indicates the maxillary septum separating the RMS from the CMS. The RMS also is superimposed on the VCS.

nonveterinarian dental providers (lay floaters). A thorough oral examination with a good light source, dental mirror (or preferably an oral endoscope), an explorer, and periodontal probe, with findings documented with photographs and a dental chart, is the current standard of care. This type of examination detects more oral pathology that is an indication for dental radiography:

- Clinical crown fractures, most of which involve the pulp horns and/or infundibula
- Malpositioned teeth, often with associated periodontal disease
- Missing teeth and supernumerary teeth

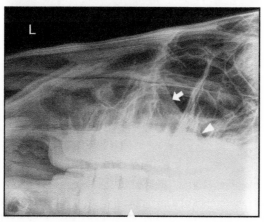

Fig. 3. A distinct fluid line present in the RMS (*arrow*), and a smaller volume of fluid in the CMS (*arrowhead*). A 15-year-old warmblood gelding.

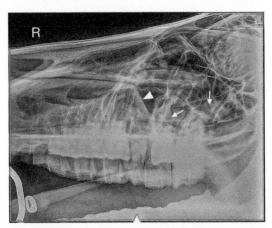

Fig. 4. An 18-year-old Hanoverian mare with malodorous right nasal discharge. Note the distinct fluid line (*arrowhead*) in the RMS and the less distinct, patchy fluid densities within the CMS (*arrows*).

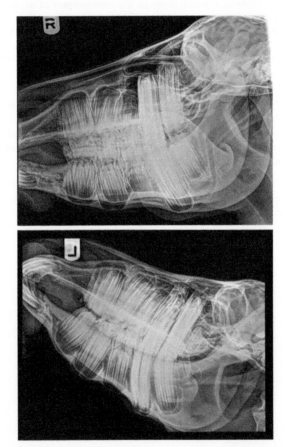

Fig. 5. Latero-lateral radiographs of a miniature horse colt at 2 years, 2 months (*top*), and at 4 years, 5 months (*bottom*). The patient had developed right mucopurulent nasal discharge at the age of 4. Note the degree to which the reserve crowns of the molars occupy the sinuses.

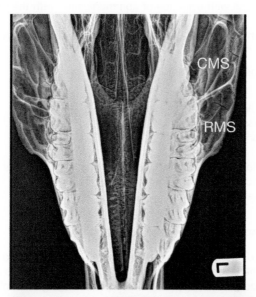

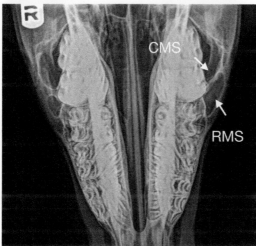

Fig. 6. DV view of an adult dry skull (*top*) and a 2-year-old miniature horse (*bottom*). The maxillary septum is a well-defined bony septum between the RMS and the CMS.

- Defects in occlusal secondary dentin overlying the pulp horns of the cheek teeth
- Deep caries lesions of the infundibula
- Gingival recession on the vestibular or lingual aspect of the cheek teeth
- Diastemata that predispose to feed impaction and periodontal disease
- Oral masses (non-neoplastic and oral tumors)
- Periodontal lesions with evidence of communication with the nasal passage or sinuses
- Abnormalities in the occlusal surface anatomy and premature attrition of the cheek tooth

Obvious indications for dental radiography include

- Facial swelling
- Cutaneous fistulas, oral fistulas
- Malodorous nasal discharge
- Quidding, dysphagia
- Bitting issues
- Abnormalities found on the examination of the diastema (bars) rostral to the mandibular second premolars, for example, blind wolf teeth
- Suspected facial fractures

SEDATION, RESTRAINT, AND EQUIPMENT CONSIDERATIONS

The sedation required for dental radiography generally is equivalent to that required for oral examination. Whenever possible, the author prefers to place the patient in examination/treatment stocks. This keeps the horse from swaying or leaning forward with heavy sedation.

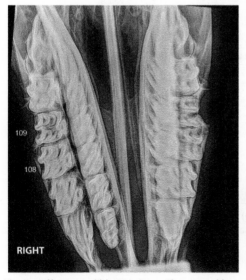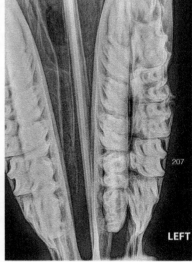

Fig. 7. Offset mandible DV views. The central beam is perpendicular to the palate. Note that the beam is parallel to the long axis of the 108, 109 (*left*), and the 207 (*right*), with some obliquity evident in the other maxillary cheek teeth. Because the mandibles are at a slight angle to the sagittal plane, these teeth also exhibit obliquity.

The author prefers a level of sedation that results in the horse resting his chin on a low support (**Fig. 1**). A large halter with multiple sites of adjustment is preferable. If the patient is in stocks, the halter often can be removed so that it does not have metal components in the area of interest. Some radiographic images require opening the mouth fully or lateral distraction of the mandibles. Standard full-mouth speculums may have too much metal that interferes with imaging. Aluminum speculums are radiolucent enough to permit diagnostic imaging of the head in most instances. The mouth also can be held wide open with a 4-in × 4-in block of wood, polyvinyl chloride pipe, or a large Kong chew toy[a].

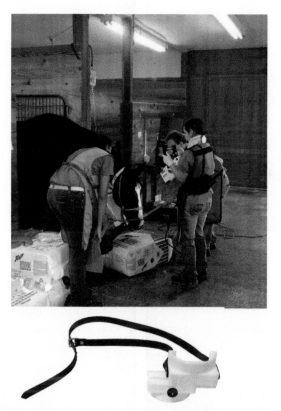

Fig. 8. To better isolate the cheek teeth in the DV views, the mandibles can be offset right and left. Note that the clinician is holding the generator directly below her head so that the central beam is perpendicular to the sensor. The assistants are pulling the mandible and maxilla gently in opposite directions (*top*). Alternatively, a commercially available adjustable gag (Juliuster, MXR Podoblock, USA) can be used (*bottom*). (Bottom image courtesy of Podoblock USA LLC, Hobe Sound, FL; with permission.)

---

[a] Kong (hyperlink).

STANDARD RADIOGRAPHIC PROJECTIONS FOR DENTAL ASSESSMENT

The basic radiographic study of the skull and cheek teeth can be performed with a minimum of 6 views:

- Latero-lateral
- Dorsoventral (DV)
- Right and left lateral dorsal 30° ventral oblique (RtD30°-LeVO, LeD30°-RtVO), with the mouth wide open
- Right and left lateral ventral 50° dorsal oblique (RtV50°-LeDO, LeV50°-RtDO), with the mouth wide open.

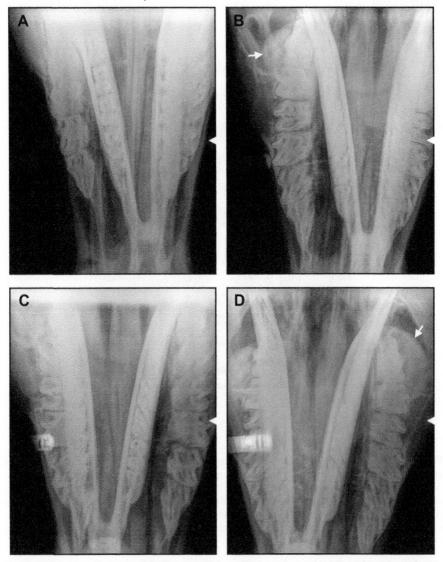

Fig. 9. Dorsoventral views with the mandibles offset to the right (A) and to the left (B). Offset mandible DV views with varying rostrocaudal angulation of the central beam. This 13-year-old warmblood gelding had bilateral maxillary sinusitis. Note the soft tissue opacities present int he right and left caudal maxillary sinuses (*arrows* [*B, D*]).

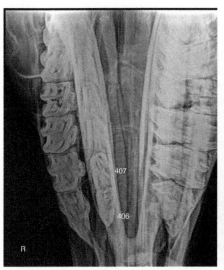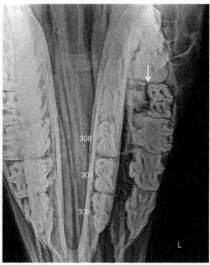

Fig. 10. Dorsoventral views with the mandibles offset to the left (left panel) and to the left (right panel) in a10-year-old warmblood gelding There was a sagittal fracture of the left maxillary second molar (arrow). Note that only the rostral mandibular cheek teeth (306, 307, 406, and 407) are oriented parallel to the central beam. Imaging of the caudal mandibular cheek teeth would require shifting the generator to shoot in a more rostral-caudal angle.

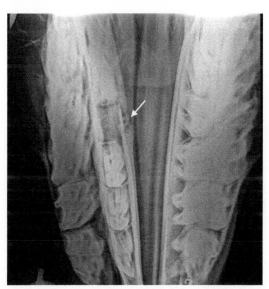

Fig. 11. Offset DV radiograph of a 7-year-old Westfalia gelding with prior repulsion of a fractured and apically abscessed right mandibular first molar (409). The rostra-caudal angulation of the central beam has resulted in significant obliquity of the maxillary molars and the mandibular second and third premolars (406, 407). Note the fracture of the medial cortex of the mandible (*arrow*).

The American College of Veterinary Radiology uses the convention that the presentation of radiographs of the skull is with the animal always facing the viewer's left. The right-left marker is determined by the side of the horse's head that is closest to the sensor. The American Veterinary Dental College (AVDC) uses the convention where the horse faces the viewer's right for those views in which the sensor is on the right side of the head. To avoid confusion, right-left markers should be used routinely. In survey radiographs of the skull, the central beam is directed at the level of the rostral end of the facial crest, which usually is approximately midpoint in the maxillary cheek teeth arcade (**Fig. 2**). Due to superimposition of the cheek teeth, the lateral view is used primarily for evaluation of the sinuses. The right and left sinus structures, however, also are superimposed, and pathology noted in the lateral view cannot readily be localized without the orthogonal (DV) view. The rostral sinus compartment is composed of the ventral conchal sinus (VCS) and the rostral maxillary sinus (RMS), which share a common space dorsal to the infraorbital canal, also referred to as the conchomaxillary opening. Dorsally, this compartment is bounded by the thin, dome-shaped bulla of the maxillary septum. Ventral to the infraorbital canal, the VCS is separated from the RMS by a bony septum. The maxillary septum separates the rostral sinus compartment from the caudal sinus compartment. The rostral and caudal compartments have separate sinonasal channels that join in a common sinonasal channel, which empties into the middle nasal meatus via the nasomaxillary aperture, commonly referred to as the drainage angle.[1] The dorsal location of the common sinonasal channel predisposes to the accumulation of fluid when there is sinus infection, which is manifested as distinct fluid lines in the lateral radiographic projection (**Fig. 3**). When inspissated pus is the predominant component of sinus empyema, there is patchy soft tissue density within the normally air-filled sinus compartment (**Fig. 4**). In a horse less than 6 years of age, the developing permanent fourth premolar and molars occupy a large space, which gradually becomes the air-filled RMS and CMS because these teeth erupt and the reserve crowns shorten. The reserve crowns of the molars in the miniature horse are particularly large in proportion to the size of the head (**Fig. 5**) and predispose to

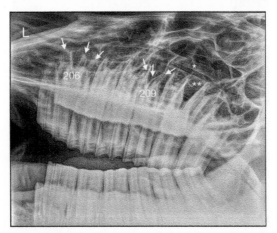

Fig. 12. RtD30-LeVO, open-mouth. The apices of the left maxillary cheek teeth and the crowns of the left mandibular cheek teeth are isolated in this view. The left infraorbital canal (*asterisk*) is projected dorsal to the right infraorbital canal (*double asterisk*). With the mouth wide open, this view isolates the crowns of the left mandibular cheek teeth. The roots of 206 and 209 are identified (*arrows*).

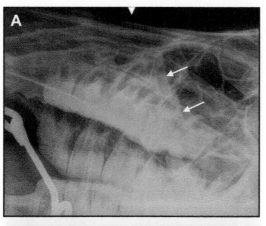

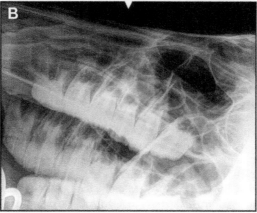

Fig. 13. A 15-year-old warmblood gelding with left maxillary sinusitis secondary to a sagittal fracture of the left maxillary first molar (209). (*A*) While the fluid lines in the maxillary sinus systems are quite evident in the initial RtD30-LeVO view (*arrows*), by altering the beam angle slightly in a caudo-rostral angle, (*B*) the obliquity of the left maxillary cheek teeth was eliminated.

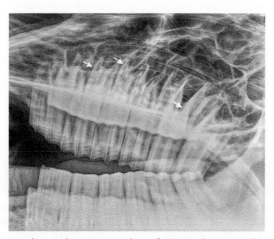

Fig. 14. The PDL space (*arrows*) represents the soft tissues between the reserve crown and roots and the alveolar bone. This includes the PDL made up of Sharpey's fibers and the lymphatics, blood vessels, and nerves. The radiodense alveolar bone adjacent to the PDL is termed, cribriform plate or lamina dura.

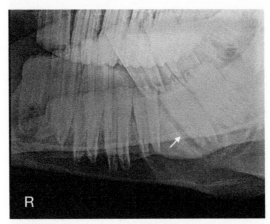

Fig. 15. Widening of the PDL space is associated with periodontal disease of the right mandibular second molar (410) in this 6-year-old Oldenburg gelding (*arrow*).

malpositioning/impaction of these teeth, periodontal disease, sinusitis, and nasal obstruction. Because the right and left maxillary sinus systems are superimposed in the lateral-lateral projection, the orthogonal DV projection is required to localize radiographic abnormalities noted in the lateral view. With adequate sedation, the horse rests its head on a low support and the assistant can place the sensor against the ventral aspect of the head, resting on the same support, thus reducing the chance for motion artifact. The technique for this projection is significantly stronger than that for the lateral projection. For a typical 454 kg horse, using a portable generator, the lateral x-ray technique is approximately 80 kVp, 2.5 mAs, whereas the DV view might be obtained with settings of 90 kVp to 100 kVp, at 3.6 mAs to 4.0 mAs. The operator should look directly over the generator when positioning for the DV view (see **Fig. 1**). If the horse has a normal occlusion, this results in the nasal septum situated midway between the mandibles and right-left symmetry of the skull (**Fig. 6**).

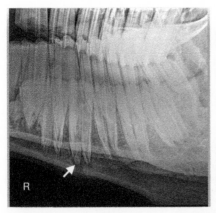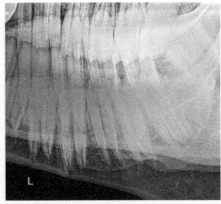

Fig. 16. RtV60°-LeDO (*left panel*) and LeV60-RtDO (*right panel*) of the mandibles of a 9-year-old Dutch warmblood mare with painful swelling of the right mandible and a crown fracture of the right mandibular fourth premolar (408). There is periapical alveolar bone lysis (left panel,arrow) and subtle periosteal reaction on the ventral mandible. Compare with the unaffected left mandible (right panel).

The offset mandible DV views are recommended for better isolation of the cheek teeth (**Fig. 7**). The positioning for this view is same as for the DV view, except that the mandibles are distracted to the right then left. The mandibles can be distracted either by 2 assistants using gauze bandage looped around the mandible and maxilla or with a commercially available device[b] (**Fig. 8**). Due to the angulation of the maxillary and mandibular cheek teeth, the DV view with the central beam directed along the long axis of the central cheek teeth (4th premolar, 1st molar) usually exhibits obliquity of the other 4 cheek teeth. In order to align the central beam down the long axis of the maxillary 2nd and 3rd premolars, there needs to be some rostral to caudal angulation of the central beam. Alternatively, for the maxillary 2nd and 3rd molars, the beam angle is shifted caudal to rostral. The opposite adjustments in beam angulation are necessary for the DV view of the mandibular cheek teeth (**Fig. 9**).

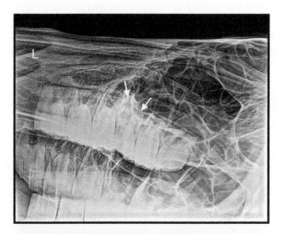

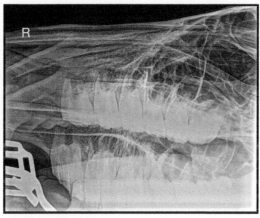

Fig. 17. This 18-year-old warmblood gelding was referred for evaluation of a fractured left maxillary first molar (209). The RtD30-LeVO view (*top*) reveals fragmentation of the reserve crown, and periapical alveolar bone sclerosis (*arrows*), without radiographic evidence of sinus infection. Compare to the LeD30-RtVO (*below*).

---

[b] Juliuster, MXR Podoblock USA (hyperlink).

The mandibles are angled slightly away from each other, with the width between the dorsal mandibles slightly greater than that at the ventral aspect. Thus, the offset mandible DV view with the central beam perpendicular to the palate results in obliquity of the mandibular cheek teeth. To align the central beam parallel to the long axis of the mandibular cheek teeth, the angle is changed from 90° to the plane of the palate to approximately 85° (**Fig. 10**). The rostral and caudal mandibular cheek teeth also frequently are angled and require a shifting of the central beam to a caudo-rostral direction to align parallel to the long axis of the rostral premolars or a rostra-caudal direction to better image the caudal molars (**Fig. 11**).

OBLIQUE LATERAL VIEWS

The DV and VD lateral oblique views are performed best with the mouth wide open. This eliminates much of the overlap of the arcades and allows for isolation of the maxillary apices in the VD projection. The length of the reserve crown in the young horse (<7 years old) may make isolation of the maxillary apices in the VD lateral open-mouth view impossible, even with a steep angle of the central beam. The average

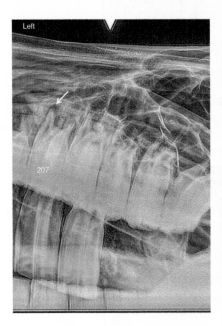
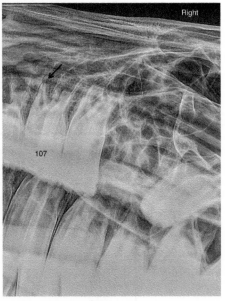

Fig. 18. Acute onset of left facial swelling rostral to the facial crest in a 12-year-old warm-blood mare. There is periapical sclerosis and alveolar bone lysis (halo) at the mesiobuccal root of 207 (*[left] white arrow*). This is appreciated more readily by comparison with the contralateral view of 107 (*[right] black arrow*).

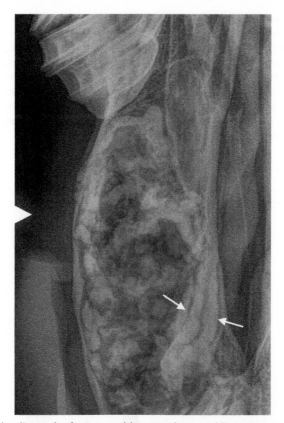

Fig. 19. Intraoral radiograph of a 7-year-old quarter horse gelding presented for swelling of the right maxilla rostral to the second premolar (106). Incisional biopsy was reported as odontogenic cyst (presumed dentigerous cyst) with chronic-active inflammation and sclerotic bony capsule. The unerupted right maxillary canine tooth (104) is indicated by the arrows.

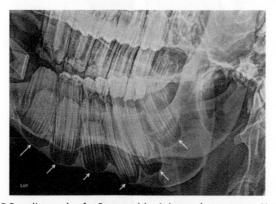

Fig. 20. RtV60-LeDO radiograph of a 3-year-old miniature horse mare. Note the prominent apical alveolar bone lucency of all of the left mandibular cheek teeth (*arrows*). This so-called eruption cyst is a normal radiographic feature of the immature permanent premolar and molar associated with the presence of the dental sac (dental follicle).

ventral-dorsal angle for isolation of the apices of the maxillary cheek teeth is approx-imately 50°; however, the required angle is dependent on the age of the horse.

The DV lateral oblique positioning should be obtained by first directing the central beam perpendicular to the long axis of the head (as for the straight lateral view) and then raising the generator dorsally approximately 30°. Depending on the age of the horse, the D30°-V lateral oblique view frequently isolates the individual roots of the maxillary cheek teeth (**Fig. 12**). Slight repositioning in a caudo-rostral or rostro-caudal direction may be required to eliminate obliquity and overlapping adjacent maxillary cheek teeth (**Fig. 13**).

RADIOGRAPHIC SIGNS OF DENTAL DISEASE

The normal alveolar radiographic anatomy includes the periodontal ligament (PDL) space, which is occupied by the PDL as well as nerves, blood vessels, and lymphatics

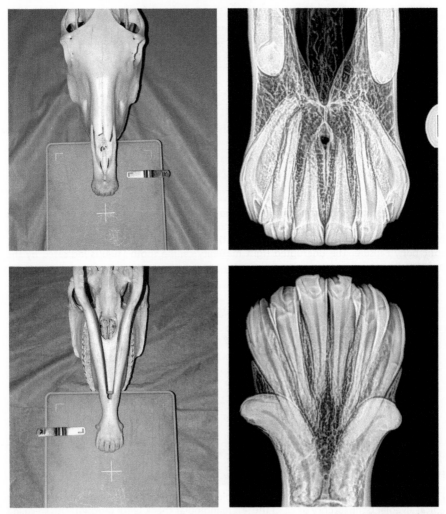

Fig. 21. Intraoral imaging of the maxillary (top left and right) and mandibular (bottom left and right) incisors using a standard DR sensor. The sensor usually can be inserted only to the mesial aspect of the second premolars, which limits complete imaging of the maxillary canine teeth.

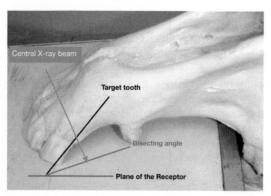

Fig. 22. Demonstration of the bisecting angle technique. The central beam is directed perpendicular to the plane that bisects the angle between to the tooth and the receptor. This results in an image of the tooth that is neither foreshortened or elongated.

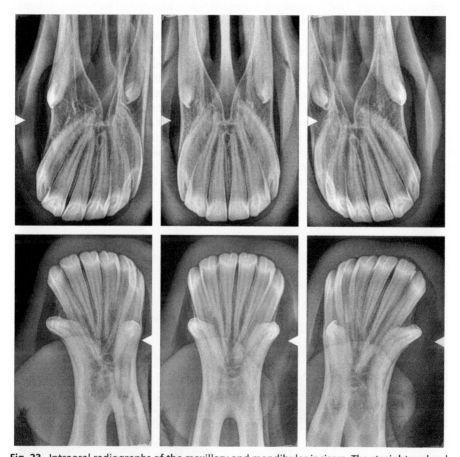

Fig. 23. Intraoral radiographs of the maxillary and mandibular incisors. The straight occlusal view of the maxillary (upper middle) and mandibular (lower middle) incisors has some overlap of the lateral (3rd) incisors and the 2nd incisors. Isolation of the right and left 3rd incisor roots is achieved with an oblique angle of about 15 degrees to the horse's right (upper and lower left panels) and to the horse's left (upper and lower right panels). The horse's right is on the viewer's left for all images.

(**Fig. 14**). The PDL space is obscured when the imaging of cheek teeth results in overlapping. The PDL is widened with periodontal disease (**Fig. 15**). The thin, compact radiodense alveolar bone adjacent to the reserve crown root is called the lamina dura. Although periodontal disease frequently results in lysis of this bone and inability to identify this structure on radiographs, its absence may be due to positional effects rather than pathology. The apical alveolar bone frequently undergoes changes in its radiographic appearance with endodontic and/or periodontal diseases. Pulpitis resulting in the formation of an apical granuloma or abscess may result in periapical alveolar bone lysis, or halo (**Fig. 16**). Alveolar bone sclerosis (also termed, condensing osteitis) is another radiographic sign of periapical inflammatory disease (**Fig. 17**). It is important to remember that these radiographic signs may not be detected readily early in the disease process. Some cases of acute facial swelling may have subtle radiographic signs, requiring careful comparison to the contralateral side (**Fig. 18**).

The nomenclature of cystic structures associated with teeth in the horse is confusing. In older literature, the term, dentigerous cyst, refers to what is now termed, temporal teratoma. This presents as a draining fistula associated with ectopic dental material at the base of the ear in young horses. This also has been termed, heterotrophic polyodontia, in some publications and commonly is referred to as an ear tooth.[2] In the human literature, and likewise for brachydont species, the term, dentigerous cyst, refers to a developmental cyst that surrounds and envelops the crown of an unerupted tooth.[3] The dentigerous cyst is lined by odontogenic epithelium and is noninflammatory. Using this definition, there are scant reports of dentigerous cysts in the horse[4] (**Fig. 19**). Eruption cysts are a nonpathologic, noninflammatory enlargement of the dental sac (follicle) of the immature permanent cheek tooth in the horse (**Fig. 20**). Eruption cysts present as nonpainful enlargements of the maxilla or mandible without evidence of fistulation, and there generally is resolution by the time the horse is 5 years to 6 years of age. Radicular cysts have been defined in the human and small animal veterinary literature as inflammatory cysts associated with the apex of the root (apical

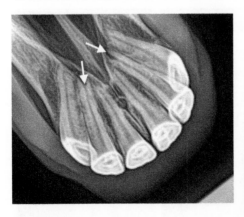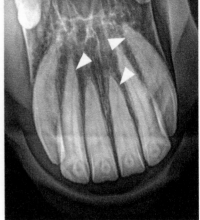

Fig. 24. Comparison of the incisor anatomy of an adult (approximately 12-year-old quarter horse mare [*left*]) and a geriatric horse (20-year-old warmblood gelding [*right*]). Note the centrally located apices and wider root canals of the mature incisors (*arrows*) versus the lateralized narrow apical foramen of the geriatric incisors (*arrowheads*).

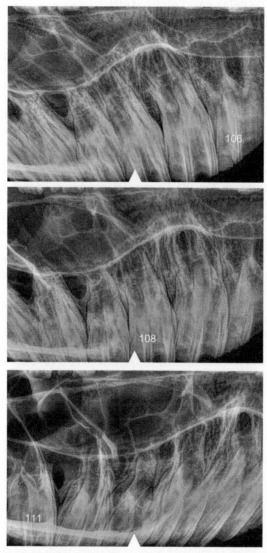

Fig. 25. Intraoral views of the right maxillary cheek teeth. In this horse, it was not possible to image all 6 cheek teeth in a single projection. In the top image the central beam is slightly rostra-caudal and in the bottom image it is slightly caudo-rostral. The middle image is with the central beam perpendicular to the long axis of the head.

periodontal cysts), whereas lateral periodontal cysts occur in a more coronal relationship with the root.[5] This type of cyst rarely has been reported in the horse.[6]

IMAGING OF THE INCISORS AND CANINE TEETH

Imaging of the incisors is performed best using the intraoral placement of the sensor. DR sensors used for imaging the extremities typically are 8-in to 12-in width and can be used to image the incisors (**Fig. 21**). A radiolucent tunnel or a speculum with radiolucent bite plates[c] should be used to protect the DR sensor. The bisecting angle technique is used to eliminate artifactual foreshortening or elongation of the incisors. Because the incisors are at an oblique angle to the intraorally placed sensor, a slight rostral-caudal angulation of the central beam (from the position starting perpendicular to the sensor) directs it perpendicular to the plane that bisects the angle between the incisor and the receptor (**Fig. 22**). The convergence of the roots of the incisors can result in overlap of the apical radiographic anatomy of adjacent teeth. Therefore, it may be necessary to obtain slightly oblique intraoral occlusal views to isolate the apices of the third incisors (**Fig. 23**). Incisor radiographic anatomy is less complicated than that of the premolars and molars. The incisors also are radicular hypsodont teeth with enamel extending the entire length of the reserve crown of the tooth. The cemento-enamel junction marks the transition between reserve crown and root. As normal attrition occurs with age and the reserve crown length shortens, the root elongates, with no further addition of enamel. The apical foramen is very large in the immature permanent incisor, and with age it becomes smaller and located laterally on the root (**Fig. 24**).

Digital intraoral dental radiography initially was available only in computed radiography (CT) systems that utilized phosphor plates for image capture. Some DR systems have complementary metal–oxide–semiconductor sensors designed for intraoral use [d,e]. For the intraoral radiographs of the cheek teeth, the sedation must be adequate to prevent chewing and tongue movement. The bisecting angle technique also is used

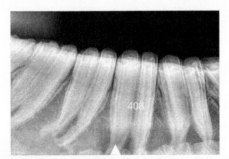

Fig. 26. Intraoral imaging of the right mandibular cheek teeth using the bisecting angle technique. Even in the geriatric horse with short reserve crowns, it is difficult to image the entire tooth, necessitating extraoral imaging techniques.

[c] XtandR. Podoblock USA

[d] Cuattro (Heska). https://www.heska.com/product/cuattro-hub/dentipod/.

[e] myvet imaging. https://myvetimaging.com/news/exhibit/myvet-imaging-highlights-large-format-equine-intraoral-sensor-at-aaep-2018/.

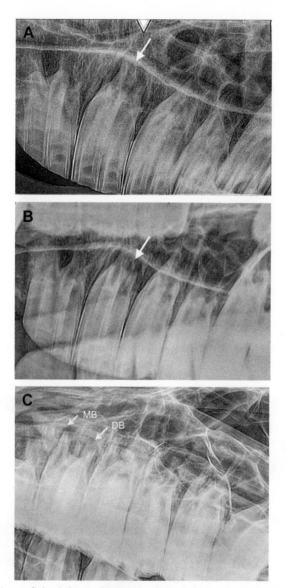

Fig. 27. Comparison of the (*A*) intraoral view of the left maxillary premolars with the (*B*) RtV60-LeDO extraoral view. A 12-year-old warmblood mare with apically infected 207; these views isolate the palatal root (*arrows*), whereas the (*C*) Rt3D30-LeVO view isolates the buccal roots. DB, distobuccal root; MB, mesiobuccal root.

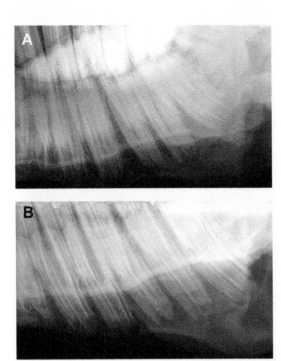

Fig. 28. A 3-year-old Thoroughbred gelding. (*A*) RtV50-LeDO view of the left mandibular cheek teeth; the sensor is placed against the left side of the head. (*B*) In the LeD45-RtVO view, the sensor is place flat against the ventral aspect of the mandibles, and the central beam is directed at the left mandible (generator on the left side of the horse). These are equivalent images of the mandibular cheek teeth apical reserve crowns.

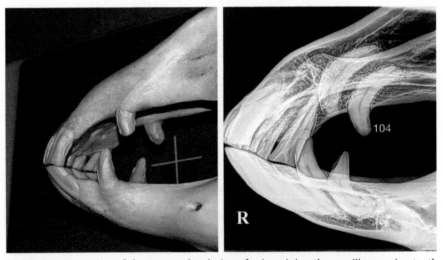

Fig. 29. Demonstration of the extraoral technique for imagining the maxillary canine teeth. This is an LeV10°Cd10°-RtDRO projection, which adequately separates the maxillary canine teeth from overlapping and allows the clinician to identify which is right and left. Dry skull (left panel) and radiographic projection (right panel) in which the right maxillary canine tooth (104) is projected below and behind the left maxillary canine tooth.

for the intraoral views of the maxillary cheek teeth. Using a full mouth speculum, the intraoral sensor is positioned between the tongue and the palate. For imaging the right maxillary cheek teeth, the positioning is right dorsal 50 degree to left ventral oblique (RtD50°-LeVO) (**Fig. 25**). The presentation of intraoral radiographs follows the AVDC labial mounting convention. The intraoral views of the right maxillary and mandibular cheek teeth are presented with the anterior cheek teeth on the viewer's right. The maxillary incisors are presented with the crowns down, and the mandibular incisors with the crowns up; the horse's left is on the viewer's right is both cases (see **Fig. 23**). Intraoral views of the mandibular cheek teeth are obtained with the sensor in the mouth, with the sensor facing ventrally, resting on the crowns of the mandibular cheek teeth. The bisecting angle is used again, but, due to the narrower space between the mandibles, imaging of the entire reserve crown and roots often is not possible (**Fig. 26**).

In the absence of an intraoral DR sensor, similar imaging can be obtained with the extraoral open-mouth lateral oblique views. The direction of the central beam essentially is opposite of that used for the intraoral imaging of the maxillary cheek teeth, so the images are similar, with isolation of the palatal root (**Fig. 27**). To image the crowns of the mandibular cheek teeth, the open-mouth, DV lateral oblique positioning is used (see **Fig. 12**), whereas the ventro-dorsal view is used to isolate the reserve crown roots (**Fig. 28**A). Alternatively, the mandibular cheek teeth reserve crown roots can be imaged with the sensor placed under the head (as for the DV view) and the central beam directed in a DV direction using the bisecting angle technique (**Fig. 28**B).

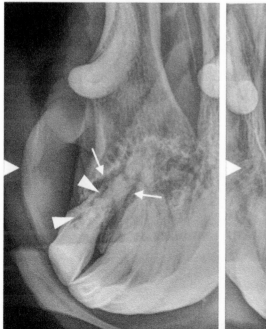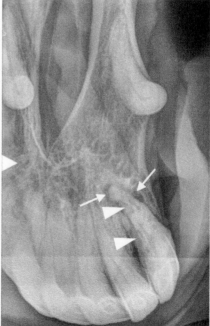

Fig. 30. A 22-year-old Dutch warmblood gelding. The use of an intraoral DR sensor improves the ability to capture the entire maxillary canine tooth. These images are slightly obliqued to better isolate the maxillary third incisors and canine teeth. There is marked external tooth resorption (*arrowheads*) with inflammatory alveolar bone lysis (*arrows*) of the maxillary third incisors 103 (left panel), and 203 (right panel).

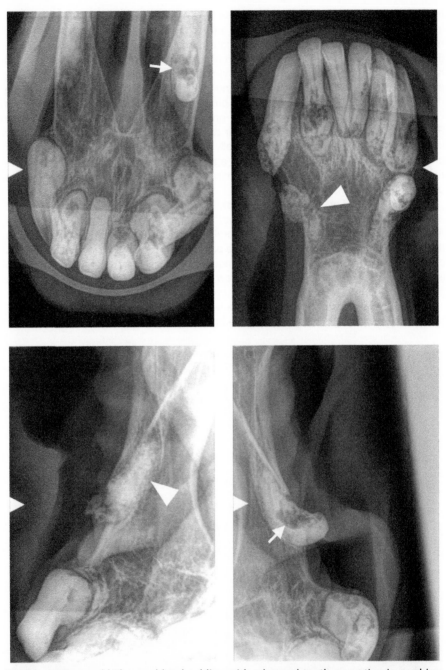

Fig. 31. A 29-year-old Thoroughbred gelding with advanced tooth resorption in combination with hypercementosis involving all incisors and canine teeth. In many cases of hypercementosis is predominant, the tooth is extruded and there is minimal alveolar osteomyelitis. Note that cervical inflammatory tooth resorption of the canine teeth (arrows, upper left and lower right panels) can occur with replacement resorption of the apical portion of the tooth (arrowheads, upper right and lower left panels).

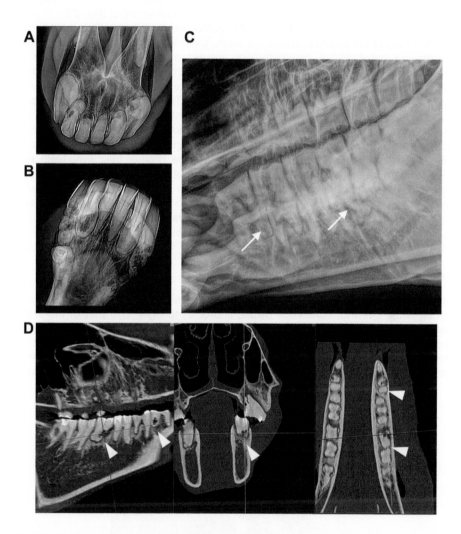

Fig. 32. (*A*, *B*) Intraoral occlusal radiographs of a geriatric warmblood gelding with incisor and canine tooth resorption and hypercementosis. (C) In the RtV45°-LeDO view, there is blunting of tooth roots with areas of decrease radiopacity (arrows).(D) Multiplanar reconstruction of the CT scan which is much more sensitive for identification of tooth resorption (arrows) in cheek teeth. In this horse, there was evidence in the CT scan of tooth resorption in nearly all of the cheek teeth.

Intraoral radiographic imaging of the maxillary canine teeth with standard DR sensors not always is possible due to the restriction of the commissures of the lips. If intraoral sensors are not available, then extraoral techniques can be used. The sensor is placed with the middle portion against the side of the head centered on the first cheek tooth. The generator initially is lined up for a straight lateral view (perpendicular to the sagittal plane), then lowered slightly and directed a bit from caudal to rostral (**Fig. 29**).

Equine odontoclastic tooth resorption and hypercementosis is one of the most common diseases of the incisors and canine teeth. Multiple studies have described the radiographic abnormalities, histopathology, incidence of this syndrome, and to a limited extent the etiopathogenesis.[7–12] Physical examination often reveals bulging of the incisive bone with gingival recession and incisor extrusion and multifocal mucogingival pustules and draining tracts over tooth roots. The clinical diagnosis of incisor tooth resorption is confirmed with intraoral radiographs, which often reveal a mix of external tooth resorption, inflammatory tooth resorption with lysis of alveolar bone, and hypercementosis (**Fig. 30**). This terminology is adapted from human and small animal dentistry and appears to be applicable to the horse.[13] When the canine teeth are affected, there frequently is inflammatory tooth resorption in the cervical third of the tooth and replacement resorption of the apical third (**Fig. 31**). Although there are few reports of tooth resorption in equine cheek teeth,[14] this probably reflects the relative insensitivity of standard radiography to detect these changes. CT is significantly more sensitive than digital radiography in the detection of and characterization of cheek tooth resorption (**Fig. 32**).

IMAGING OF THE TMJ

The temporomandibular joint (TMJ) is an occasional site of pathology that can present as facial swelling, cutaneous fistula, and/or dysphagia. This part of the skull anatomy is difficult to evaluate, however, with standard radiography, and CT should be considered if there is a high index of suspicion of pathology in this region. In the straight lateral-lateral view, there is superimposition of the right and left TMJ, so this is not a productive view (**Fig. 33**). Isolation of the TMJ can be improved by directing

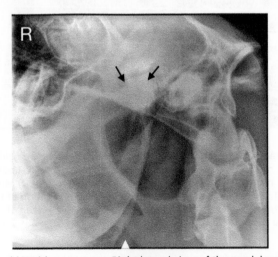

Fig. 33. A 9-year-old Welsh pony mare. Right lateral view of the caudal mandible. The TMJs are superimposed, with the left mandibular condyle (*arrows*) having the larger size due to magnification.

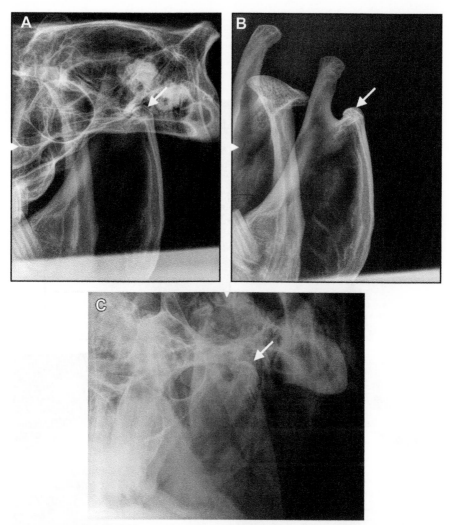

Fig. 34. LeV15Cd15-RtDRO. (*A*) Dry skull, with (*B*) removal of the upper jaw and (*C*) in a cadaver specimen. The arrow points to the right mandibular condyle in each image.

the central beam from a slightly ventro-dorsal and caudo-rostral angle (**Fig. 34**). Tangential views also can be used to isolate the lateral aspect of the TMJ (**Fig. 35**).[15,16] CT is very much the imaging modality of choice, however, for the TMJ in the horse, as in other species.

Malformed and malpositioned teeth can be identified easily on routine radiographic studies of the skull. CT imagining with multiplanar reconstructions, however, often is of value in surgical planning (**Fig. 36**). Cemental hyperplasia often distorts the normal anatomy of the tooth, sometimes with marked enlargement of the reserve crown root (**Fig. 37**). Even with modest hypercementosis of the reserve crown root of a diseased tooth, problems with standard intraoral extraction can be anticipated (**Fig. 38**).

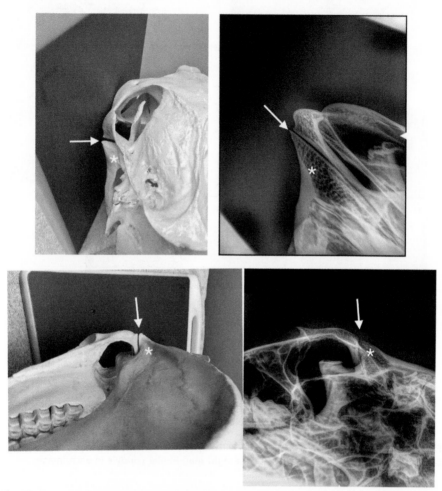

Fig. 35. Tangential views of the left TMJ compared. The left DV, caudo-rostral oblique view is obtained with the sensor on the left side of the horse's head (*top photo* and *top radiograph*), whereas the left ventro-dorsal, rostro-caudal view is obtained with the sensor positioned on the poll (*bottom photo* and *bottom radiograph*). Arrows indicate the TMJ, and the asterisk indicates the mandibular condyle.

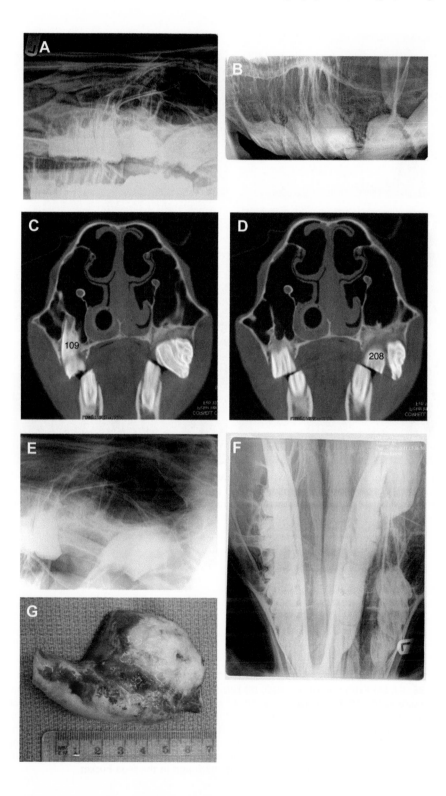

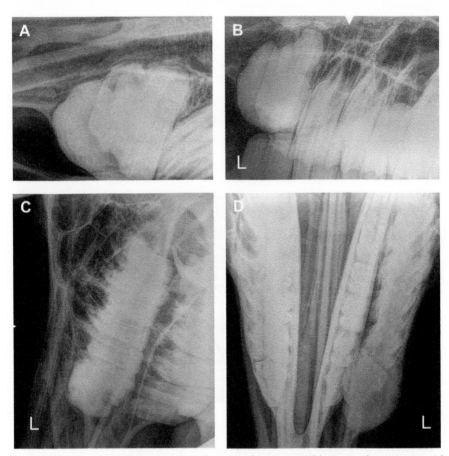

Fig. 37. (*A*) Intraoral and (*B–D*) extraoral views of a 15-year-old quarter horse mare with facial swelling over the left maxillary second premolar (206). There was oral exposure of the ventral aspect of the cementoma. No abnormal probing depths were noted and there was no evidence of periodontal disease at this examination.

Fig. 36. CT. (*A*) Extraoral RtD30-LeVO, (*B*) LeD-50-RtVO, intraoral, and (*C*) CT images transverse slice at 109; (*D*) transverse slice at 208 of a 14-year-old warmblood gelding with a malformed and malpositioned left maxillary first molar (209). There was extensive sclerosis of the surrounding maxillary bone and the left maxillary sinuses remained involved. The abnormal 209 also was displaced in the buccal direction with a projection overlapping the fourth premolar (208). Over time, the malformed 209 loosened and fell out. (*E*) RtD30-LeVO, (*F*) DV view, and (*G*) malformed 209 found in the feed bucket.

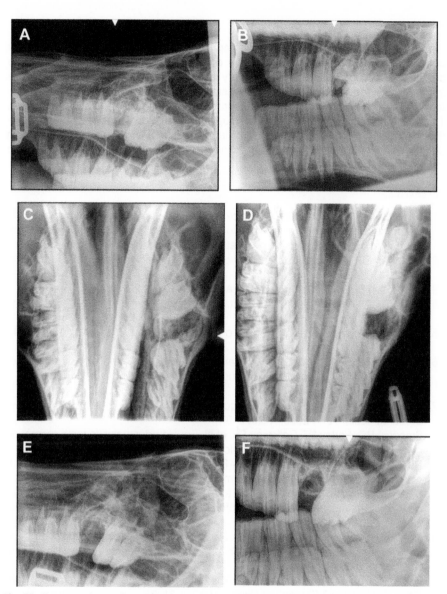

Fig. 38. Preoperative and postoperative radiographs of a fractured left maxillary first molar (209) with secondary left maxillary sinusitis. Preoperative radiographs: (A) RtD30-LeVO, (B) RtV50-LeDO, and (C), DV, mandibles offset to the right; although the remaining 209 reserve-crown was somewhat fragmented, the mesial drift of the second molar (210) had narrowed the coronal aspect of the 209 alveolus, necessitating sectioning of the large palatal fragment for oral extraction. Postoperative radiographs: (D) offset mandible DV, (E) RtD30-LeVO, and (F). RtV50-LeDOL. The left maxillary sinuses were subsequently débrided and lavaged via trephination of the left conchofrontal sinus.

SUMMARY

Proper positioning for the various radiographic projections of the teeth is critical for obtaining diagnostic-quality images. The equine veterinarian or technician should practice obtaining these views on a dry skull or cadaver head. Multiple views frequently are required for accurate assessment and treatment planning. It is important to radiograph the unaffected (contralateral) arcades for comparative purposes. This aids in the diagnosis of subtle pathology and in the identification of bilateral pathology. Due to the complicated and overlapping sinus anatomy and the difficulty in obtaining radiographs of the TMJ, CT scans may be required for treatment planning in challenging cases.

REFERENCES

1. Brinkschulte M, Bienert-Zeit A, Lüpke M, et al. The sinonasal communication in the horse: examinations using computerized three-dimensional reformatted renderings of computed-tomography datasets. BMC Vet Res 2014;10(1):1–20.
2. Gaughan EM. Dentigerous cysts: congenital anomaly of many names. Equine Vet Educ 2010;22:279–80.
3. Thompson LDR. Dentigerous cyst. Ear Nose Throat J 2018;97:57.
4. Delaunois-Vanderperren H. Congenital odontogenic keratocyst in a filly. Equine Vet Educ 2013;25:179–83.
5. Beckman BW. Radicular cyst of the premaxilla in a dog. J Vet Dent 2003;20(4): 213–7.
6. Poore LA, Scase TJ, Kidd JA. Surgical enucleation of unilateral mandibular radicular cysts in an 11-year-old Thoroughbred mare. Equine Vet Educ 2019;31: 286–91.
7. Staszyk C, Bienert A, Kreutzer R. Equine odontoclastic tooth resorption and hypercementosis. Vet J 2008;178:372–9.
8. Smedley RC, Earley ET, Galloway SS, et al. Equine odontoclastic tooth resorption and hypercementosis: histopathologic features. Vet Pathol 2015;52(5):903–9.
9. Rehrl S, Schröder W, Müller C, et al. Radiological prevalence of equine odontoclastic tooth resorption and hypercementosis. Equine Vet J 2018;50:481–7.
10. Earley ET, Rawlinson JR, Baratt RM, et al. Hematologic, biochemical, and endocrine parameters in horses with tooth resorption and hypercementosis. J Vet Dentistry 2017;34(3):155–60.
11. Henry TJ, Puchalski SM, Arzi B, et al. Radiographic evaluation in clinical practice of the types and stage of incisor tooth resorption and hypercementosis in horses. Equine Vet J 2017;49:486–92.
12. Baratt R. Equine odontoclastic tooth resorption and hypercementosis (EOTRH): What do we know? Equine Vet Educ 2016;28:131–3.
13. Peralta S, Verstraete FJ, Kass PH. Radiographic evaluation of the types of tooth resorption in dogs. Am J Vet Res 2010;71:784–93.
14. Moore NT, Schroeder W, Staszyk C. Equine odontoclastic tooth resorption and hypercementosis affecting all cheek teeth in two horses: Clinical and histopathological findings. Equine Vet Educ 2016;28:123–30.
15. Townsend NB, Cotton JC, Barakzai SZ. A Tangential Radiographic Projection for Investigation of the Equine Temporomandibular Joint. Vet Surg 2009;38:601–6.
16. True CK, Bolam CJ, et al. Diagnostic imaging in veterinary dental practice. J Am Vet Med Assoc 2018;252(7):275–8.

Standing Sedation and locoregional Analgesia in Equine Dental Surgery

Luis Campoy, LV, CertVA, Dip ECVAA, MRCVS,
Samantha R. Sedgwick, DVM*

KEYWORDS

- Procedural sedation • Regional anesthesia • Maxillary nerve block
- Inferior alveolar nerve block • Mental foramen nerve block • Equine

KEY POINTS

- Because of the greater simplicity of standing procedural sedation combined with locoregional anesthesia, many orofacial maxillary surgical procedures are performed as same-day procedures.
- Typically, infusions of sedative drugs are administered to produce procedural sedation. Opioids may also be administered.
- Protocols including alpha2-adrenergic agonists are increasingly popular.
- Ordinarily, the coinfusions are enhanced by locoregional anesthetic techniques.
- The implementation of a locoregional anesthetic technique requires a thorough understanding of the anatomy to maximize success and minimize possible complications.

INTRODUCTION

Because of the greater simplicity of standing procedural sedation combined with locoregional anesthesia compared with a full general anesthetic, many surgical procedures, such as orofacial maxillary surgery, can be performed as same-day procedures. Procedural sedation has become popular for describing a semiconscious state that allows patients to be comfortable during certain surgical or diagnostic procedures. Procedural sedation has been defined as a technique of administering sedatives or dissociative agents with or without analgesics to induce a state that allows the patient to tolerate unpleasant procedures while maintaining the cardiorespiratory function and is intended to result in a depressed level of consciousness that allows the patient to maintain oxygenation and airway control independently. People under procedural sedation are usually able to respond to physical stimulation and basic verbal commands while maintaining an uninstrumented airway and breathing spontaneously.

Department of Clinical Sciences, College of Veterinary Medicine, Cornell University, Mailbox 32, Ithaca, NY 14853, USA
* Corresponding author.
E-mail address: luis.campoy@cornell.edu

Vet Clin Equine 36 (2020) 477–499
https://doi.org/10.1016/j.cveq.2020.08.009
vetequine.theclinics.com
0749-0739/20/© 2020 Elsevier Inc. All rights reserved.

Typically, coinfusions of sedatives and/or opioids are administered. Ordinarily, the coinfusions are enhanced by appropriate locoregional anesthetic to produce sufficient analgesia and muscle relaxation for surgery.

Equine veterinarians are presented with a specific challenge when recovering horses from general anesthesia. Recovery from anesthesia is still a particularly hazardous time for horses and can be associated with catastrophic injuries.[1] Seddighi and Doherty[2] (2012) compared the outcome of procedures under general anesthesia in geriatric horses and concluded that standing surgery avoids some of the problems associated with general anesthesia and recovery and, in this population of horses, should be considered when possible to help decrease the rate of adverse events. Dugdale and colleagues[3] (2016) retrospectively studied anesthesia-related equine deaths. These investigators found that fractures during recovery were responsible for 26% to 64% of all anesthesia-related fatalities. This figure increased to 71%, in which dislocations were included.[3–6] Presumably, using local anesthetic and sedation techniques would allow surgeons to perform many standing procedures, thus decreasing the morbidity/mortality by circumventing the need for recovering the horse from anesthesia.

The implementation of a locoregional anesthetic technique requires a thorough understanding of the anatomy to maximize success and minimize possible complications; therefore, a review of the relevant anatomy of each individual block is featured here for each technique.

PROCEDURAL SEDATION

Protocols including alpha2-adrenergic agonists are becoming increasingly popular. The quality of procedural sedation using constant infusions of detomidine or medetomidine has been studied in horses.[7–14] Goodrich and Ludders[15] (2004) recommended a dose regime for detomidine consisting of an initial loading intravenous (IV) dose of 8.4 µg/kg followed by an infusion at a rate of 0.5 µg/kg/min for the first 15 minutes, then the rate was recommended to be reduced to 0.3 µg/kg/min for the following 15 minutes. Subsequently, the constant-rate infusion (CRI) can typically be reduced to 0.15 µg/kg/min for the remainder of the procedure. However, these rates are to be taken as guidelines and should be adjusted to the individual patient. Profound sedation could lead to severe ataxia and possible collapse.

However, alpha-2 agonists possess some well-known side effects, such as reduced gastrointestinal motility,[16,17] hypertension, bradyarrhythmias, hyperglycemia, and polyuria.

Clinical examination, particularly of the cardiovascular system, is recommended before sedation. Caution is recommended in patients with a reduced systolic function, particularly on the left side, or in patients with high vagal tone. Oromaxillary and facial surgical procedures may be of long duration, thus, as a precaution, it is recommended that patients for all elective procedures be starved from all food, both roughage and concentrates, for a minimum of 12 hours. Administration of IV fluids at a rate of 5 mL/kg/h is also recommended. Urinary catheterization helps minimize patient discomfort from having to urinate frequently and should be considered as an alternative to free urination.

Ringer and colleagues[18] (2012) reported the use of xylazine for standing procedures. Romifidine was compared with xylazine and detomidine as a single bolus dose by Englad and colleagues[16] (1992) and Hamm and colleagues[19] (1995). These investigators claimed romifidine caused less ataxia and therefore may have a better profile for standing procedural sedation. The addition of butorphanol to romifidine as a single bolus was found to enhance the sedation quality.[20–23] Ringer and colleagues[18] (2012) published an infusion rate for romifidine with or without butorphanol. This same rate was successfully used by Marly and colleagues[24] (2014) in clinical standing dentistry and ophthalmologic procedures.

Incidentally, butorphanol has been published to cause side effects such as forward movement, increased locomotor activity, head shaking, and muzzle twitching.[20,25,26] Clark and colleagues[20] (1991) compared the addition of butorphanol to a detomidine infusion for dentistry procedures. More head shaking/twitching was noticed in the butorphanol group. However, the addition of butorphanol decreased the undesired tongue movement during intraoral manipulation. The head shaking was not considered severe enough to disturb the procedure and did not require intervention.

Müller and colleagues[27] (2017) compared the infusion of romifidine with the addition of butorphanol, midazolam, or ketamine during standing cheek tooth extraction. These investigators found that the use of romifidine alone resulted in increased cortisol levels compared with the addition of butorphanol. The regimen recommended by the investigators was a loading dose of romifidine and butorphanol of 80 µg/kg IV and 18 µg/kg IV, respectively, followed by an infusion rate of 29 µg/kg/h (20–60 µg/kg/h) and 25 µg/kg/h for romifidine and butorphanol, respectively.

These same investigators also evaluated the infusion of several drug combinations containing romifidine, including romifidine alone at a loading dose of 0.03 mg/kg, followed by a CRI of 0.05 mg/kg/h. Romifidine (same dose) with midazolam (0.02 mg/kg; CRI 0.06 mg/kg/h), or romifidine (same dose) with butorphanol (0.02 mg/kg; 0.04 mg/kg/h), and romifidine (same dose) with ketamine (0.5 mg/kg; CRI 1.2 mg/kg/h) were evaluated. The combination of romifidine and midazolam showed less chewing and tongue activity but showed significantly higher grades of ataxia. The romifidine and ketamine CRI combination had the lowest incidence of intervention because of patient cooperation. Although ketamine is an excellent drug for chronic pain and adds sedation to the alpha2-adrenergic agonist, more studies are needed to determine an appropriate infusion rate in standing horses sedated with detomidine, xylazine, or medetomidine because previously published doses in several clinical cases have led to profound ataxia and occasional collapse of patients within the stocks.

Appropriate patient monitoring should include (but not be limited to) respiratory rate and effort, electrocardiography, and blood pressure.

RELEVANT ANATOMY OF THE TRIGEMINAL NERVE

The major sensory innervation relevant to orofacial maxillary surgery is provided by cranial nerve V (trigeminal nerve) (**Fig. 1**). The trigeminal nerve divides into the ophthalmic, maxillary, and mandibular branches. Briefly, the ophthalmic portion of the trigeminal nerve branches dorsally to the maxillary branch and enters the superior orbital fissure. The ophthalmic nerve at this point becomes the frontal nerve and branches into the supraorbital nerve and the infratrochlear nerve. The supraorbital nerve exits through the supraorbital foramen and provides sensory innervation to the medial two-thirds of the upper eyelid. The infratrochlear nerve is smaller and provides sensory innervation to the medial canthus of the eye.

The maxillary branch is primarily sensory but does receive parasympathetic fibers via the pterygopalatine ganglion from the facial nerve. The maxillary nerve becomes the infraorbital nerve once it enters the maxillary foramen and continues into the infraorbital canal. Branches originating directly from the maxillary nerve from within the pterygopalatine fossa supply the most caudal molars, whereas the rest of the arcade is supplied by branches originating from within the infraorbital canal.

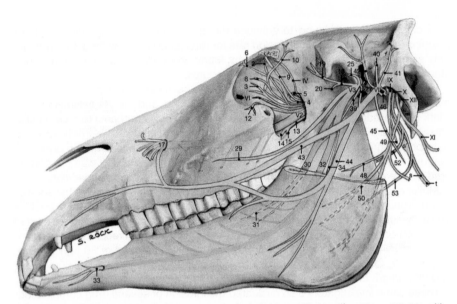

Fig. 1. Anatomy of the trigeminal nerve. V1: Opthalmic Nerve V2- Maxillary Nerve V3- Mandibular Nerve VII- Facial nerve IX: Glossopharyngeal nerve X: Vagus nerve XI: Accessory nerve XII: Hypoglossal nerve s: sympathetic trunk s': Cranial cervical ganglion t: Vagosympathetic trunk; 2. Dorsal branch (of the oculomotor nerve) 3. Ventral branch (of the oculomotor nerve) 4. Nasociliary nerve 5. Ethmoidal nerve 6. Infratrochlear Nerve; 8. Lacrimal nerve 9. Frontal nerve 10. Zygomaticotemporal branch of the opthalmic nerve; 13. Pterygopalatine nerve 14. Greater Palatine Nerve 15. Lesser Palatine Nerve 17. Infraorbital nerve 18. Masticatory nerve 19. Deep Temporal Nerve 20. Masseteric nerve; 25. Auriculotemporal nerve; 27. Communicating branch (of mandibular nerve); 29. Buccal nerve 30. Lingual nerve 31. Sublingual nerve 32. Inferior alveolar nerve 33. Mental Nerve 34. Mylohyoid nerve; 39. Chorda tympani (gustatory, psy) 40. Internal auricular br. 41. Caudal auricular nerve 42. Auriculopalpebral nerve 43. Dorsal Buccal branch (of Facial nerve) 44. Ventral buccal branch (of Facial nerve) 45. Cervical branch (of Facial nerve) 46. Digastric branch (of Facial nerve); 48. Pharyngeal branch (of glossopharyngeal) 49. Carotid sinus branch (of glossopharyngeal) 50. Lingual branch (of glossopharyngeal); 52. Pharyngeal branch (of the vagus) 53. Cranial laryngeal nerve.

The mandibular branch of the trigeminal nerve innervates the lower arcade, skin, and oral mucosa. The mandibular branch is not only sensory but contains some motor fibers that give rise to the masticatory nerve.

Any of the locoregional techniques described in this article can be performed with any local anesthetic, such as lidocaine, mepivacaine, bupivacaine, or ropivacaine. Lidocaine has a rapid onset (2–3 minutes) with a duration of effect of about 1 hour; mepivacaine lasts around 2 hours, bupivacaine has a slightly longer onset (6–10 minutes) of action but lasts 3 to 8 hours, and ropivacaine lasts around 6 hours. However, it is worth noting that volume and overall dose are directly related to duration. The block will be effective as long there is a critical mass of local anesthetic in direct contact with the nerve.

TECHNIQUES
Pterygopalatine Fossa Block (Maxillary Nerve Block)

Indications

- Dental extractions of the upper arcade

- Hard and soft palate surgery
- Maxillary or frontal sinus surgery
- Alar cartilage surgery
- Incisive maxillary fracture repair
- Rostral maxillary fracture repair
- Lacerations of the upper lip or face

Landmarks

- Facial crest
- Ventral border of the zygomatic process
- Pterygopalatine (also known as sphenopalatine) fossa
- Lateral canthus of the eye

Equipment

- Tuohy needle: 9 cm (3.5 inch), 18 to 20 gauge
- Loss of resistance syringe (optional)
- Extension set (T port)

Local anesthetic

- Between 20 and 30 mL of local anesthetic

Goal: diffusion of the local anesthetic within the pterygopalatine fossa, in direct contact with the maxillary nerve.

Complexity level: moderate to advanced.

WHAT IS ALREADY KNOWN?

Anesthesia of the equine maxillary nerve performed at the maxillary foramen was first described by Bemis in 1917. Several variations of Bemis's initial approach have been described since then. These variations can all be reviewed in articles such as Frank[28] (1947), Newton and colleagues[29] (2000), Fletcher[30] (2004), Stephenson[31] (2004), Schumacher[32] (2006), Tremaine[33] (2007), and Rice[34] (2017).

Tremaine[33] (2007) compared multiple of these different approaches. He concluded that the lateral approach was less precise, less repeatable, and therefore more likely to result in undesirable effects. Bardell and colleagues[35] (2010) compared 2 common approaches using methylene blue dye with dissection after injection to confirm perineural injection.

Staszyk and colleagues[36] (2008) reexamined the pterygopalatine fossa anatomy and compared 2 different needle depth insertions. A technique that avoided contact with the palatine bone was preferred because it seemed to carry less risk of vascular laceration.

Current research is focused on the equine maxillary nerve block to further decrease the complication rate. O'Neill and colleagues[37] (2013) described an ultrasonography-guided injection. Stauffer and colleagues[38] (2017) compared a surface landmark approach versus ultrasonography guidance for a maxillary nerve block in the horse performed by veterinary students on cadaver heads. The investigators concluded that ultrasonography guidance provided a significantly increased success rate (from 54% to 65.4%).

Nannarone and colleagues[39] (2016) performed computed tomography (CT)–guided retrograde maxillary nerve perineural injection of the infraorbital canal on equine cadavers. The study showed success of spread in cadaver heads but no further research has been published on efficacy in clinical patients.

INDICATIONS FOR THE BLOCK

This block is essential for performing dental extractions in the upper arcade, frontal or maxillary sinus surgery, alar cartilage surgery, and standing incisive or rostral maxillary fracture repair with wire fixation. In addition, lacerations involving the upper lips or face (rostral to the medial canthus of the eye and dorsal to the facial crest) as well as hard and soft palate surgery may also be performed.

CONTRAINDICATIONS

Skin infection at the puncture site
Bleeding diathesis
Peripheral neuropathy

CLINICAL ANATOMY

The maxillary nerve enters the pterygopalatine fossa at the rostral alar fissure and courses from caudal to rostral toward the maxillary foramen (**Figs. 2** and **3**). At the level of the caudal third of the pterygopalatine fossa, it gives out the pterygopalatine nerve. The greater and minor palatine nerves arise from the pterygopalatine nerve. The pterygopalatine ganglion is also located within the pterygopalatine fossa. The minor (lesser, also known as descending) palatine nerve exits the minor palatine foramen with the minor palatine artery supplying the sensory innervation to the soft palate and palatal gingiva. The major (also known as greater) palatine nerve continues its course rostrally and exits the major palatine foramen along with the major palatine artery, providing sensory innervation to the palatal soft tissues, whereas, still within the pterygopalatine fossa, the maxillary nerve continues as the infraorbital nerve. At this level, it gives rise to a branch that supplies the caudal superior molars (9–11) and their periodontium (the superior posterior alveolar branch). The infraorbital nerve exits the fossa via the maxillary foramen and continues into the infraorbital canal. Once the infraorbital nerve is inside the infraorbital canal, it gives off the middle superior alveolar branches, which enter the respective alveolar canals to supply the maxillary cheek teeth (5–8). Once it exits the canal, it gives rise to the rostral superior alveolar branches that supply the incisivomaxillary teeth (1–4).

The extraperiorbital fat pad is located immediately medial to the masseter muscle.

The periorbita is a dense connective tissue membrane that surrounds the orbit and is located in the dorsal aspect of the pterygopalatine fossa.

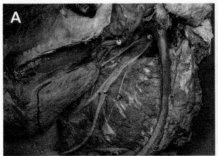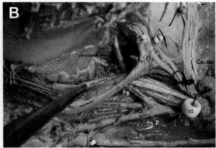

Fig. 2. (A, B) Anatomy of the pterygopalatine fossa.

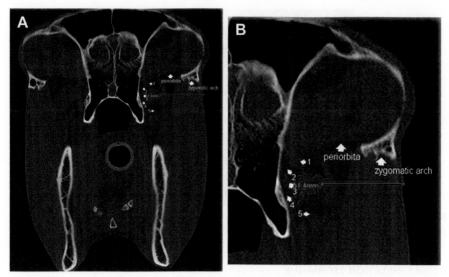

Fig. 3. (*A*) CT image of the pterygopalatine fossa. Note zoomed-in image (*B*). (1) Deep facial vein, (2) maxillary artery, (3) maxillary nerve, (4) major palatine artery, (5) buccal artery.

EXPECTED DISTRIBUTION OF ANESTHESIA

The infiltration of local anesthestic into the pterygopalatine fossa results in desensitization of the maxilla, premaxilla, and skin over the frontal sinus. It also desensitizes the mucosa of the lateral aspect of the nasal meatus (additional ethmoidal nerve block is necessary for complete ipsilateral desensitization of the nasal meatus, including the septum[40]). It desensitizes the superior incisors, canines, premolars, and molars as well as the associated alveoli and gingiva.

LOCAL ANESTHETIC: DOSE AND VOLUME

Bupivacaine or ropivacaine are typically used for the maxillary nerve block for an expected prolonged procedure time. Alternatively, mepivacaine can also be used. The recommended volume of local anesthetic is 20 to 30 mL.

Subzygomatic Approach

Patient preparation and positioning
With the sedated horse in the stocks, the puncture site should be surgically prepared. Local infiltration with 1% buffered lidocaine increases patient tolerance to the procedure.

Tip

This infiltration may block a branch of the facial nerve, causing transient ipsilateral facial paralysis.

SURFACE ANATOMY AND LANDMARKS

The puncture site is located approximately 1 cm ventral to the ventral rim of the zygomatic arch and approximately 2 to 3 cm caudal to the lateral canthus of the eye (**Fig. 4**).

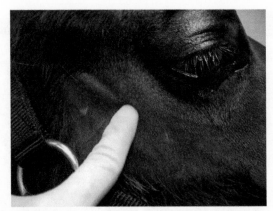

Fig. 4. The subzygomatic area of a horse. Note the index finger showing the ventral edge of the zygomatic arch. The puncture site should be located approximately 1 cm ventral to it and 2 to 3 cm caudal following the direction of the facial crest.

NEEDLE INSERTION TECHNIQUE

A Tuohy needle (8.9 cm [3.5 inch], 18–20 gauge) is inserted at the puncture site, lightly tapping the syringe plunger as the needle is advanced, feeling for the loss of resistance that indicates that the needle tip has entered the pterygopalatine fossa (**Fig. 5**). At a depth of approximately 4.5 to 5 cm in an adult horse, the tip of the needle goes through the medial fascia of the masseter muscle (a sudden increase in resistance should be noted). The penetration of this fascia is generally accompanied by

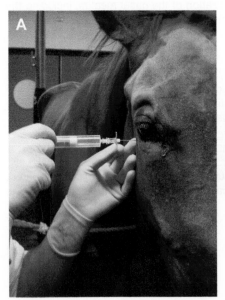
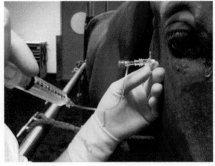

Fig. 5. (A) The Tuohy needle is advanced through the masseter muscle while gently tapping on the syringe plunger until a loss of resistance is felt, indicating penetration into the pterygopalatine fossa. (B) Injection of bupivacaine 0.5%. Before injection, negative blood aspiration must be documented.

a pop (fascial click) and a sudden loss of resistance. The needle should be further advanced an extra 0.5 cm. It is likely that the needle tip will end up located within the extraperiorbital fat pad.

Ultrasonography-Guided Technique

Patient preparation and positioning
With the sedated horse in the stocks, the puncture site should be surgically prepared. Local infiltration with 1% buffered lidocaine increases patient tolerance to the procedure.

Surface anatomy and landmarks to be used
The puncture site is located approximately 1 cm ventral to the zygomatic process of the temporal bone and approximately 2 to 3 cm caudal to the lateral canthus of the eye (**Fig. 6**).

Ultrasonography anatomy
The ultrasonography transducer should be placed immediately caudal to the extension of the facial crest, ventral to the zygomatic arch (temporal process), and ventral to an imaginary line connecting the medial and lateral canthi of the ipsilateral eye. The transducer should be tilted in a rostral and ventral direction, toward the contralateral last maxillary cheek tooth, until the maxillary bone plate is visualized. In an adult horse, the maxillary and pterygopalatine (sphenopalatine) fossa are approximately 6 cm deep.

The transducer can be tilted in a caudal direction to identify the basisphenoid, perpendicular plate of the palatine bone and the frontal bone plate. A cross section of the maxillary artery should be identified. The maxillary nerve is seen on ultrasonography as a hyperechoic structure (as is the extraperiorbital fat pad). Color flow can be used to identify the vasculature located within the fossa.

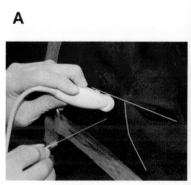
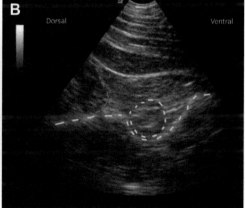

Fig. 6. (*A*) The transducer is positioned ventral to an imaginary line (*yellow*) connecting the medial and lateral canthi and extending caudal beyond the facial crest/zygomatic arch (*blue line*). (*B*) Ultrasonography imaging showing the deep facial vein (*yellow dashed line*), maxillary bone plate (*red*), and the cross section of the maxillary nerve (*blue circle*). (*From* O'Neill HD, et al. Ultrasound-Guided Injection of the Maxillary Nerve in the Horse. *Equine Veterinary Journal*, vol. 46, no. 2, 2013, pp. 180–184; with permission.)

Needle insertion technique

An 18-gauge, 8.9-cm (3.5-inch) Tuohy needle is introduced out of plane or in plane through the masseter muscle into the pterygopalatine fossa (a sudden increase in resistance and a pop (fascial click) should be noted as the needle goes through the medial fascia of the masseter muscle). The needle should be advanced toward the maxillary nerve approximately 4.5 to 5 cm.

Negative blood aspiration must be ensured and documented before injection. No resistance to injection should be encountered. Several negative blood aspirations should be verified during the injection process.

Block effects and patient management Proprioception to the arcade will be transiently lost. Therefore, caution must be observed and patients must be starved (prevented from chewing) until function is regained.

Potential complications

- Vascular laceration: if a hematoma rapidly forms, bulging of the supraorbital pouch may be observed. It is likely that the maxillary artery (or any of its branches), the infraorbital artery, the descending palatine artery, and the buccal artery may be involved. The needle should only be advanced approximately 0.5 cm once the pterygopalatine fossa is entered. Avoid deep needle insertions. The use of loss of resistance and of a Tuohy needle with depth markings or ultrasonography guidance helps reduce the possibility of vascular-needle contact. If the needle contacts bone at a depth of approximately 2 cm, it is likely that the needle is positioned too rostral and the maxillary bone has been contacted. If a hematoma forms or blood is detected on aspiration, it is likely that deep facial vein[41] has been punctured.
- Direct nerve contact (neuropraxia). The nerve can be visualized on ultrasonography and therefore avoided.
- Infection/abscess formation.
- Retrobulbar hematoma (if periorbita is entered inadvertently).
- Akinesia, blindness (if periorbita is entered inadvertently).
- Intravascular injection and possibly subsequent local anesthetic systemic toxicity with associated tachycardia, hypotension, arrhythmias, muscle twitches, tremors, seizures, collapse and possible death. To avoid this complication, the local anesthetic solution should be injected slowly. Ensure negative blood aspiration before the injection of local anesthetic. Frequent aspirations while injecting are strongly advised.

Infraorbital Nerve Block

Indications

- Maxillary arcade dental extractions (rostral to the site of the block)
- Surgical repair of skin of the upper lip
- Surgical incision or repair of the skin on the nose
- Alar fold resections
- Frontal sinusotomy
- Surgical incision or repair of the skin on the face to the level of the infraorbital foramen

Landmarks

- Nasomaxillary notch

- Rostral edge of the facial crest
- Levator labii superioris muscle

Equipment

- Needle: 13 mm (0.5 inch), 25 gauge
- Needle: 38 mm (1.5 inch), 20 to 22 gauge
- Extension set (T port)

Local anesthetic

- 5 mL of local anesthetic

Goal: the needle must engage the infraorbital canal. The local anesthetic should spread and migrate retrogradely while minimizing leakage onto the levator nasolabialis and labii superioris muscles.

Complexity level: moderate.

WHAT IS ALREADY KNOWN?

Wilkins[42] (1997) reported a high incidence of low tolerance (head tossing) to this procedure in the sedated horse as a result of needle-to-nerve contact (neuropraxia).

Berg and Budras[43] (2011) described the 3-fingers grip technique to locate the infraorbital canal. A thumb is placed in the nasomaxillary incisure and the middle finger on the rostral end of the facial crest. The index finger is then used to palpate the foramen, an area halfway between and 1.3 to 2.5 cm caudal to an imaginary line between these points.

In horses 5 years old or younger, there is a lateral concavity and a course near the dental alveoli. In horses greater than 5 years old, the concavity is within the maxillary sinus. With increasing horse age, proximal spread of the local anesthetic increases based on tomographic studies.[43] Nannarone and colleagues[39] (2016) reviewed the tomographic anatomy of the infraorbital canal. The foramen itself was found to have an elliptical cross section. The canal has a serpentine course and is approximately 12 to 13 cm in length. Nannarone and colleagues[39] (2016) and Liuti and colleagues[44] (2017) showed that the distance of the infraorbital canal in relation to the dental apices increases with age. They also showed the bony septum between cheek teeth alveoli and the canal increases in height with age. This finding may imply that the spread of the block could be altered with age, but further studies need to be performed to determine this.

Klugh[45] (2010), Coomer and colleagues[46] (2011), and Doherty[47] and Schumacher[48] (2011)[49] recommended an injected volume of 4 to 10 mL. Weber and colleagues[50] (2019) investigated the distribution of larger volumes of injectate (10 and 15 mL). In 90% of patients, 86.9% of the infraorbital canal was stained.

INDICATIONS FOR THE BLOCK

This block is essential for performing dental extractions of the superior incisors, canine tooth, and premolars on the ipsilateral side. This block may also be used for laceration repairs involving the superior lip, nostril, or skin up to the site of the performed block (where the nerve exits the alveoli).

CONTRAINDICATIONS

Skin infection at the puncture site

Bleeding diathesis
Peripheral neuropathy
Uncooperative horses

CLINICAL ANATOMY

The maxillary nerve gives rise to the infraorbital nerve still within the pterygopalatine fossa (**Fig. 7**). Within the infraorbital canal, the nerve sends off branches to the superior cheek teeth. Just before the infraorbital nerve exits the infraorbital canal at the infraorbital foramen, it divides into several fasciculi, namely, the external nasal branches, the internal nasal branches, the superior labial branches, and the rostral superior alveolar branches, which provide sensory function to the superior canine and incisor teeth and surrounding gingiva.

EXPECTED DISTRIBUTION OF ANESTHESIA

The infraorbital nerve block results in desensitization of the skin of the lip, nostril, and face up to the level of the foramen on the ipsilateral side, premaxillary incisors, canine tooth, premolars, plus or minus rostral molars (depending on how proximal the local anesthetic spreads), and associated alveoli and gingiva. Depending on how proximal the local anesthetic spreads, partial anesthesia of the ipsilateral nasal meatus may also be provided.

LOCAL ANESTHETIC: DOSE AND VOLUME

Bupivacaine or ropivacaine are typically used for the maxillary nerve block because they have a longer duration of action for an expected prolonged procedure time. Alternatively, mepivacaine can also be used. The recommended volume of local anesthetic is approximately 5 mL.

PATIENT PREPARATION AND POSITIONING

With the sedated horse in the stocks, the puncture site should be surgically prepared. Local infiltration with 1% buffered lidocaine increases patient tolerance to the procedure because needle-nerve contact with subsequent neuropraxia is likely.

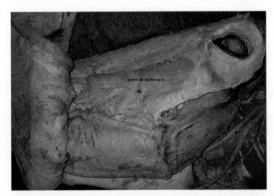

Fig. 7. Dissection of the infraorbital foramen area. Note the infraorbital nerve as it exits the infraorbital foramen (*arrowhead*) (partially covered by the levator labiis superioris muscle).

SURFACE ANATOMY AND LANDMARKS

The infraorbital foramen is relatively easy to palpate midway between the anterior edge of the facial crest and the nasomaxillary notch (formed by the nasal and the incisive bones) deep to the levator labii superioris and levator nasolabialis muscles when the anatomy is not disrupted (this may not be the case in the presence of local disorder). The levator labii superioris muscle should be retracted superiorly to allow for needle insertion.

NEEDLE INSERTION TECHNIQUE

The needle should be advanced into the foramen as flush to the maxillary bone as possible with a direction parallel to the facial crest to avoid contact the walls of the infraorbital canal.

Once the needle is in the canal, the local anesthetic can be injected. Always ensure a negative blood aspiration and absence of resistance to injection. The local anesthetic will redistribute proximally in the canal as it is injected. Following the injection, digital pressure onto the foramen should be applied to prevent backflow of the local anesthetic.

Block Effects and Patient Management

Leakage of local anesthetic can occur; the levator nasolabialis muscle may be directly infiltrated as a result and therefore temporarily paralyzed, resulting in the inability of the ipsilateral nostril to flare. Caution is needed in bilateral blocks. Nasal tubes may be needed if a bilateral nostril collapse is observed.

Potential Complications

- Neuropraxia: tissue infiltration with 1% buffered lidocaine increases patient tolerance.
- Because of the proximity of vasculature, there is great potential for inadvertent intravascular injection/vascular laceration and subsequent hematoma formation. Ensure negative blood aspiration before injection.
- A large volume may cause neural compression. Injection should be performed slowly to minimize pressure buildup inside the infraorbital canal.
- Nasolabialis levator muscle paralysis. Digital pressure after injection may minimize leakage. Avoid injection of large volumes.
- Patient compliance has been noted to prevent this block from being performed. Even when sedate, horses often toss their heads violently in response to blocking attempts.

Inferior Alveolar Nerve Block

Indications

- Dental extractions of the mandibular arcade
- Mandibular fracture repair
- Lacerations of the lower lip (chin)

Landmarks

- Medial aspect of the mandibular ramus
- Basihyoid bone
- Lateral canthus of the eye
- Facial crest

- Palpable buccal edge of the maxillary dental arcade

Equipment

- Insulated needle 150 mm, 21 gauge
- Peripheral nerve locator

Local anesthetic

- 20 mL of local anesthetic

Goal

- Lateral movement of the mandible pterygoid muscle in response to electrolocation

Complexity level: moderate/advanced.

WHAT IS ALREADY KNOWN?

Bemis (1917) is cited as the first to describe the topographic landmarks for the equine inferior alveolar nerve block.[48] In 1930, Boltz modified Bemis's approach in which the foramen was approached from the ventral border of ramus, rostral to the angle of the mandible.[48] An additional approach was described by Fletcher[30] (2004). Boltz's approach was further modified by Doherty and Schumacher[48] (2010).

Although there have been many modifications to the original approach, Henry and colleagues[51] (2013) described an intraoral approach to the inferior alveolar nerve similar to human dentistry. This approach requires special instruments but may minimize the risk of lacerating the mandibular artery.

There have been multiple publications comparing and contrasting new and different approaches. Harding and colleagues[52] (2012) compared the vertical and angled approaches. The investigators found no statistical difference in the accuracy and efficacy of the two approaches.

INDICATIONS FOR THE BLOCK

Indications are dental extractions of mandibular incisors, canine tooth, molars, and premolars on the ipsilateral mandibular arcade. This block may also be used for laceration repairs involving the lower lip or skin.

CONTRAINDICATIONS

Skin infection at the puncture site
Bleeding diathesis
Peripheral neuropathy

CLINICAL ANATOMY

The inferior alveolar nerve originates in the mandibular nerve on the lateral aspect of the medial pterygoid muscle (**Fig. 8**). The mandibular nerve divides into 2 branches (lingual nerve and inferior alveolar nerve) between the pterygoid medial and lateral muscles.

The lingual nerve is sensory to the rostral two-thirds of the tongue and conveys tactile, noxious, and thermal sensations as well as taste. It is a large nerve that crosses the pterygoid muscles and gives off branches to the buccal mucosa of the isthmus of

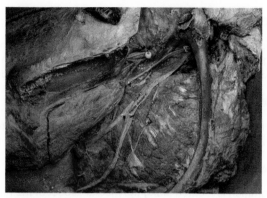

Fig. 8. Dissection of the trigeminal nerve (mandibular branch). Note that the mandible has been partially removed.

the fauces. At the base of the tongue, the lingual nerve gives off the sublingual nerve, which innervates the sublingual mucosa.

The buccal nerve (or branch) of the mandibular nerve (not to be confused with the buccal branch of the facial nerve), passes between the lateral pterygoid head, migrating from medial to the mandibular ramus to lateral, crossing over the anterior ridge of ramus.

The inferior alveolar nerve has both motor and sensory fibers. It supplies the motor function to the muscles that move the mandible, such as masseter, temporalis, medial and lateral pterygoids, rostral digastricus, and mylohyoideus muscles.

The inferior alveolar nerve, before entering the mandibular foramen on the medial side of the ramus, gives out the mylohyoid nerve. The mylohyoid nerve may either present as a branch of the inferior alveolar nerve or may arise separately from the mandibular nerve. It runs medial to the ramus of the mandible and gives off a muscular branch to the rostral belly of the digastricus muscle and some cutaneous branches that supply a cutaneous area of the inferior lip and cheek, caudal to the cutaneous area of the mental branches and cutaneous area of the intermandibular region. The mylohyoid nerve supplies the mylohyoideus muscle, which raises the floor of the oral cavity and pulls the basihyoid rostrally.

EXPECTED DISTRIBUTION OF ANESTHESIA

The inferior alveolar nerve block results in desensitization of the mandible and mandibular teeth. Via the mental branch, it desensitizes the labial soft tissues from the premolars to midline. It also desensitizes the soft tissues of the chin and lower lip.

Tip

In order to desensitize the lingual gingiva of the mandible and the floor of the mouth, the lingual branch needs to be additionally blocked. Following a lingual nerve block, the rostral two-thirds of the tongue are also anesthetized. The buccal nerve (division of the mandibular branch) provides sensory innervation to the soft tissues of the buccal aspect of the mucosa of the first, second, and third molars as well as the skin over the cheek and therefore needs to be anesthetized in order to obtain a complete block.

Additional minor innervation originating in C1 and C2 is also present in some individuals. Therefore, in some instances, a buccal submucosal infiltration of the mandible and/or periodontal infiltration may be necessary for complete desensitization.

LOCAL ANESTHETIC: DOSE AND VOLUME

Bupivacaine or ropivacaine are typically used for the inferior alveolar nerve block for an expected prolonged procedure time. Alternatively, mepivacaine can also be used. A volume of approximately 20 mL of local anesthetic is recommended.

PATIENT PREPARATION AND POSITIONING

With the sedated horse in the stocks, the puncture site should be surgically prepared. Local infiltration with 1% buffered lidocaine increases patient tolerance to the procedure.

SURFACE ANATOMY AND LANDMARKS TO BE USED

The mandibular foramen is located along the medial aspect of the mandibular ramus. Its projection can be found at the intersection of 2 lines: (1) horizontal line from commissure and parallel to the facial crest, (2) vertical line from 2 to 3 cm caudal to the vascular notch (at the angle of the mandible) to the lateral canthus of the eye. The basihyoid bone should be palpated in the intermandibular area. The puncture site is located lateral to the basihyoid bone (the ramus of the mandible diverges, so a strict vertical needle insertion would miss the nerve).

NEEDLE INSERTION TECHNIQUE

With the electrolocator set at 1 mA, 0.1 milliseconds, and 1 Hz, the needle should be advanced until contact is made with the bone plate of the medial aspect of ramus (**Fig. 9**). The needle should be redirected following the medial aspect of ramus in a

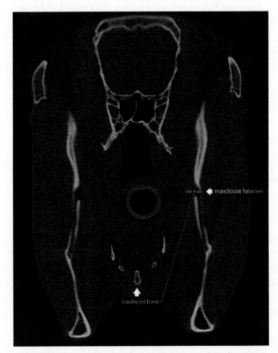

Fig. 9. CT at the level of the mandibular foramen. Note the direction of the stimulating needle.

dorsal direction. Mylohyoid muscle and digastricus muscle response may be elicited (caused by stimulation of the mylohyoid nerve) as the needle is approaching the nerve. Further dorsal needle advancement for another 2 to 3 cm should be performed until a masticatory response is obtained (note that the mandibular branch of the trigeminal nerve contains motor fibers).

In adult horses, the final needle position is approximately 110 to 120 mm from the puncture site (vertical distance from the ventral edge of the mandible).

Expected Motor Responses from Nerve Stimulation

The mandibular nerve is both sensory and motor. It supplies the motor function to the masseter, temporalis, medial and lateral pterygoids, rostral digastricus, and mylohyoideus muscles. Electrostimulation results in lateral movement of the mandible.

Negative blood aspiration must be ensured before injection. No resistance to injection should be encountered. Several negative blood aspirations should be verified during injection.

Block Effects and Patient Management

Caution must be taken and patients must be starved/muzzled (prevented from chewing) until function is regained postoperatively.

Potential Complications

- Vascular laceration.
- Intravascular injection. To avoid this complication, the local anesthetic solution should be injected slowly, with frequent aspirations to verify correct needle placement.
- Direct nerve contact (neuropraxia).
- Horses should be muzzled to prevent choking from improper chewing of food as well as accidental laceration of the tongue.

Mental foramen block
Indications
- Extraction of the mandibular canine teeth on the ipsilateral side
- Extraction of the mandibular incisors on the ipsilateral side
- Laceration repair of the lower lip and gingiva

Landmarks
- The horizontal ramus
- Deep to the depressor labii inferioris muscle
- Interdental space

Equipment
- Needle: Tuohy 4 mm (1.5 inch), 22 gauge

Local anesthetic
- Up to 5 mL of local anesthetic

Goal: the needle needs to engage the foramen for approximately 1 cm in a discrete ventromedial direction.
Complexity level: moderate.

WHAT IS ALREADY KNOWN?

Anesthesia to the rostral third of the mandibular region can be provided by using the mental foramen block. This procedure has been described by Skarda[53] (1991), Klugh[45] (2004), as well as multiple other investigators.

The mental foramen block targets the rostral portion of the inferior alveolar nerve as it exits the mental foramen and becomes the mental nerve. Needle direction and orientation have been debated for best efficacy. Tremaine[33] (2007) recommended a rostrocaudal needle direction; Skarda[53] (1991) and Skarda and Tranquilli[54] (2007) recommended angling dorsolateral to ventromedial. Final needle position has also been tested with variable results by Skarda[53] (1991) as well as Klugh[45] (2004). These articles concluded that the infiltration and needle placements should be confirmed as submucosal and therefore supraperiosteal (over the area of the root of the tooth to be addressed). The bevel of the needle should be pointed toward the nerve root.

Reported volume of anesthetic agent for the block can be between 3 mL[33,34] and 10 ml.[53]

The most comprehensive evaluation of the mental foramen block in cadavers and in vivo in equine patients to date was performed by Rawlinson and colleagues[55] (2018). The investigators compared 2 different volumes and 2 different injection techniques in equine cadaver heads and in 3 anesthetized horses. The results showed a moderate success rate (up to 58%) and an unexpected irregular staining pattern with a volume of injectate up to 5 mL that would achieve anesthesia up to the first or second premolar at best. Crean and Powis[56] (1999) found that volumes close to 10 mL may increase the risk of neural ischemia secondary to increasing regional pressure.[56,57]

INDICATIONS FOR THE BLOCK

This block can be used for performing dental extractions of mandibular incisors, canine tooth, and possibly first premolar on the ipsilateral side. This block may also be used for laceration repairs involving the lower lips or skin up to the mental foramen (chin).

CONTRAINDICATIONS

Skin infection at the puncture site
Bleeding diathesis
Peripheral neuropathy
Uncooperative horse

CLINICAL ANATOMY

The inferior alveolar nerve, once it passes through the mandibular foramen, courses rostrally, sending off branches to the alveoli of the mandibular premolars and molars until it emerges from the mental foramen, where it is then referred to as the mental nerve.[56]

EXPECTED DISTRIBUTION OF ANESTHESIA

The mental nerve block results in desensitization of the skin and associated soft tissue of the ipsilateral lip and chin; if the injectate penetrates the mandibular canal and comes into contact with the inferior alveolar nerve, the mandibular incisor, mandibular canine, first premolar, and possibly up to the second premolar may become desensitized.

LOCAL ANESTHETIC: DOSE AND VOLUME

Bupivacaine or ropivacaine is typically used for the maxillary nerve block for an expected prolonged procedure time. Alternatively, mepivacaine can also be used. A volume of up to 5 mL of local anesthetic has been recommended.

PATIENT PREPARATION AND POSITIONING

With the sedated horse in the stocks, the puncture site should be surgically prepared. Benzocaine or lidocaine gel in the buccal mucosa as well as local infiltration with 1% buffered lidocaine increases patient tolerance to the procedure.

SURFACE ANATOMY AND LANDMARKS TO BE USED

The mental foramen opening is located below the commissure of the lips on the lateral aspect of the horizontal portion of the ramus of the mandible. In the middle of interdental space on the horizontal ramus, the foramen can be palpated by elevating the tendon of the depressor labii inferioris muscle.

NEEDLE INSERTION TECHNIQUE

With the tendon elevated, the puncture site should be located approximately 25 mm (1 inch) rostral to the mental foramen and coursing caudally toward the foramen (**Fig. 10**). Rawlinson and colleagues[55] (2018) recommended a ventromedial needle direction with the shaft of the needle 40° lateral to the parasagittal plane of the lateral mandible and 25° dorsal to the dorsal plane of the incisive-premolar interproximal space. The needle is recommended to be inserted into the mandibular canal at a depth of approximately 1 cm.

After ensuring a negative blood aspiration, injection of local anesthetic can be performed. Note that Rawlinson and colleagues[55] (2018) reported high injection pressure (resistance) in 15 out 24 hemiheads. The injection pressure did not seem to be related

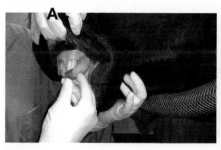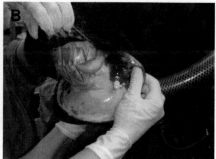

Fig. 10. (A) A Tuohy needle is advanced toward the mental foramen through the buccal mucosa. Observe the index finger or the operator palpating the mental foramen and at the same time elevating the tendon of the depressor labii inferioris muscle. (B) The needle is in its final position, at a depth of approximately 1 cm into the mandibular canal, past the foramen.

to age, the distance traveled by the injectate, the diffusion pattern of the injectate, or the soft tissue area stained.

Block Effects and Patient Management

Caution must be used and patients must be starved/muzzled (prevented from chewing) until function is regained postoperatively.

Potential Complications

Neuropraxia caused by direct needle-to-nerve contact is likely and poorly tolerated. Local infiltration with 1% buffered lidocaine increases patient tolerance to the procedure.

SUMMARY

Regional anesthesia of the head drastically reduces the required level of sedation and augments the patient's tolerance to otherwise invasive oromaxillofacial surgical procedures and dental extractions. The appropriate use of regional anesthesia is paramount to providing a cooperative and pain-free patient as well as providing postprocedural analgesia. Becoming familiar with the techniques discussed in this article is key in decreasing complications and failures.

DISCLOSURE

The authors have no relationship with any commercial company that has a direct financial interest in the subject matter or materials discussed in this article or with any company making a competing product.

REFERENCES

1. Wohlfender FD, Doherr MG, Driessen B, et al. International online survey to assess current practice in equine anaesthesia. Equine Vet J 2015;47(1):65–71.
2. Seddighi R, Doherty TJ. Anesthesia of the geriatric equine. Vet Med (Auckland, N.Z.) 2012;3:53–64.
3. Dugdale AH, Polly PM, Taylor M. Equine anaesthesia-associated mortality: where are we now? Vet Anaesth Analg 2016;43(3):242–55.
4. Young SS, Taylor PM. Factors influencing the outcome of equine anaesthesia: a review of 1,314 cases. Equine Vet J 1993;25(2):147–51.
5. Johnston GM, Eastment JK, Wood J, et al. The confidential enquiry into perioperative equine fatalities (CEPEF): mortality results of Phases 1 and 2. Vet Anaesth Analg 2002;29(4):159–70.
6. Bidwell LA, Bramlage LR, Rood WA. Equine perioperative fatalities associated with general anaesthesia at a private practice–a retrospective case series. Vet Anaesth Analg 2007;34(1):23–30.
7. Daunt DA, Dunlop CI, Chapman PL, et al. Cardiopulmonary and behavioral responses to computer-driven infusion of detomidine in standing horses. Am J Vet Res 1993;54(12):2075–82.
8. Wertz EM, Dunlop CI, Wagner AE et al. (1994) Three chemical restraint techniques for mares undergoing standing colpotomy surgery. Proceedings of the 5th International Congress of Veterinary Anesthesia. The American College of Veterinary Anaesthesiologists, Guelph, Canada. Aug 21-25, 1994. pp. 133 (abstract).

9. Bettschart-Wolfensberger R, Bettschart RW, Vainio O, et al. Cardiopulmonary effects of a two hour medetomidine infusion and its antagonism by atipamezole in horses and ponies. J Vet Anaesth and Analg 1999a;26(1):8–12.

10. Bettschart-Wolfensberger R, Clarke KW, Vainio O, et al. Pharmacokinetics of medetomidine in ponies and elaboration of a medetomidine infusion regime which provides a constant level of sedation. Res Vet Sci 1999;67(1):41–6.

11. Wilson DV, Bohart GV, Evans AT, et al. Retrospective analysis of detomidine infusion for standing chemical restraint in 51 horses. Vet Anaesth Analg 2002; 29(1):54–7.

12. van Dijk P, Lankveld DP, Rijkenhuizen AB, et al. Hormonal, metabolic and physiological effects of laparoscopic surgery using a detomidine-buprenorphine combination in standing horses. Vet Anaesth Analg 2003;30(2):72–80.

13. Aguiar AJA, Medeiros LQ, Dessen MR et al. (2009) Hemodynamic and sedative effects of constant rate infusions of detomidine associated with butorphanol, and detomidine alone in conscious horses. Proceedings of the 10th World Congress of Veterinary Anaesthesia. Association for Veterinary Anaesthetists, Glasgow, UK. Aug 31-Sep 4, 2009. pp. 169 (abstract).

14. Solano AM, Valverde A, Desrochers A, et al. Behavioural and cardiorespiratory effects of a constant rate infusion of medetomidine and morphine for sedation during standing laparoscopy in horses. Equine Vet J 2009;41(2):153–9.

15. Goodrich L, Ludders J. How to attain effective and consistent sedation for standing procedures in the horse using constant rate infusion. Proc Am Ass Equine Practitioners 2004;50.

16. England GC, Clarke KW, Goossens L. A comparison of the sedative effects of three alpha 2-adrenoceptor agonists (romifidine, detomidine and xylazine) in the horse. J Vet Pharmacol Ther 1992;15(2):194–201.

17. Ringer SK, Portier KG, Fourel I, et al. Development of a Romifidine Constant Rate Infusion with or without Butorphanol for Standing Sedation of Horses. Vet Anaesth Analg 2012;39(1):12–20.

18. Ringer SK, Portier KG, Fourel I, et al. Development of a xylazine constant rate infusion with or without butorphanol for standing sedation of horses. Vet Anaesth Analg 2012b;39(1):1–11.

19. Hamm D, Turchi P, Jochle W. Sedative and analgesic effects of detomidine and romifidine in horses. Vet Rec 1995;136(13):324–7.

20. Clarke KW, England GCW, Goossens L. Sedative and cardiovascular effects of romifidine, alone and in combination with butorphanol, in the horse. J Vet Anaesth 1991;18(1):25–9.

21. Kohler I, Armbruster S, Lanz F, et al. Analgetische Wirkung von Romifidin kombiniert mit Butorphanol oder Levomethadon beim Pferd. Tierarztl Prax Ausg G 2004;32(06):345–9.

22. Holopherne D, Faucher C, Desfontis J-C et al. (2005) Comparison of three sedative protocols for use in the horse: romifidine vs romifidine/morphine vs romifidine/butorphanol. Proceedings of the AVA Fall Meeting. Association for Veterinary Anaesthetists, Newmarket, UK. September 20, 2005. pp. 52 (abstract).

23. DeRossi R, Jorge TP, Ossuna MR, et al. Sedation and pain management with intravenous romifidine–butorphanol in standing horses. J Equine Vet Sci 2009; 29(2):75–81.

24. Marly C, Bettschart-Wolfensberger R, Nussbaumer P, et al. Evaluation of a romifidine constant rate infusion protocol with or without butorphanol for dentistry and ophthalmologic procedures in standing horses. Vet Anaesth Analg 2014;41(5): 491–7.

25. Browning AP, Collins JA. Sedation of horses with romifidine and butorphanol. Vet Rec 1994;134(4):90–1.

26. Knych HK, Casbeer HC, McKemie DS, et al. Pharmacokinetics and pharmacodynamics of butorphanol following intravenous administration to the horse. J Vet Pharmacol Ther 2013;36(1):21–30.

27. Müller TM, Hopster K, Bienert-Zeit A, et al. Effect of butorphanol, midazolam or ketamine on romifidine based sedation in horses during standing cheek tooth removal. BMC Vet Res 2017;13:381.

28. Frank ER. Nerve blocking for upper cheek teeth. In: Veterinary surgery notes, Revised edition, Burgess (MN): Burgess Publishing company; 1947. p. 120.

29. Newton SA, Knottenbelt DC, Eldridge PR. Headshaking in horses: possible aetiopathogenesis suggested by the results of diagnostic tests and several treatment regimes used in 20 cases. Equine Vet J 2000;32(3):208–16.

30. Fletcher BW. How to perform effective dental nerve blocks. Proc Am Ass Equine Practnrs 2004;50:233–9.

31. Stephenson R. Oral extraction of equine cheek teeth. UK Vet 2004;9:11–7.

32. Schumacher J. Anaesthesia of the head and penis. In: Doherty T, Valverde A, editors. Manual of equine anesthesia and analgesia. Oxford (UK): Blackwell; 2006. p. 282–6.

33. Tremaine WH. Local analgesic techniques for the equine head. Equine Vet Educ 2007;19(9):495–503.

34. Rice MK. Regional nerve blocks for equine dentistry. J Vet Dent 2017;34(2): 106–9.

35. Bardell D, Iff I, Mosing M. A Cadaver Study Comparing Two Approaches to Perform a Maxillary Nerve Block in the Horse. Equine Vet J 2010;42(8):721–5.

36. Staszyk C, Bienert A, Bäumer W, et al. Simulation of local anaesthetic nerve block of the infraorbital nerve within the pterygopalatine fossa: anatomical landmarks defined by computed tomography. Res Vet Sci 2008;85(3):399–406.

37. O'neill HD, Garcia-Pereira FL, Mohankumar PS. Ultrasound-guided injection of the maxillary nerve in the horse. Equine Vet J 2013;46(2):180–4.

38. Stauffer S, Cordner B, Dixon J, et al. Maxillary Nerve Blocks in Horses: an Experimental Comparison of Surface Landmark and Ultrasound-Guided Techniques. Vet Anaesth Analg 2017;44(4):951–8.

39. Nannarone S, Bini G, Vuerich M, et al. Retrograde Maxillary Nerve Perineural Injection: A Tomographic and Anatomical Evaluation of the Infraorbital Canal and Evaluation of Needle Type and Size in Equine Cadavers. Vet J 2016;217:33–9.

40. Caruso M, Schumacher J, Henry R. Perineural Injection of the Ethmoidal Nerve of Horses. Vet Surg 2016;45(4):494–8.

41. Tanner RB, Hubbell JAE. A Retrospective Study of the Incidence and Management of Complications Associated With Regional Nerve Blocks in Equine Dental Patients. J Vet Dent 2019;36(1):40–5.

42. Wilkins PA. Cyproheptadine: Medical treatment for photic headshakers. Comp Cont Educ Pract Vet 1997;19:98–111.

43. Berg R, Budras KD. Contributions to clinical-functional anatomy, head. In: Anatomy of the horse. 6th edition. Hannover (Germany): Schluetersche; 2011. p. 145–50.

44. Liuti T, Reardon R, Dixon PM. Computed tomographic assessment of equine maxillary cheek teeth anatomical relationships, and paranasal sinus volumes. Vet Rec 2017;181(17):452.

45. Klugh DO. Infiltration anesthesia in equine dentistry. Compend Contin Educ Vet 2004;26:631–3.

46. Coomer RP, Fowke GS, McKane S. Repulsion of Maxillary and Mandibular Cheek Teeth in Standing Horses. Vet Surg 2011;40(5):590–5.
47. Doherty T. Chapter 15- Dental restraint and Anesthesia. In: Schumacher J, editor. Equine dentistry. 3rd edition. Edinburgh, NY: Saunders Ltd; 2011. p. 241–4.
48. Doherty T, Schumacher J. Dental restraint and anesthesia. In: Easley J, Dixon PM, Schumacher J, editors. Equine dentistry. 3rd edition. WB Saunders; 2011. p. 241–4.
49. Fletcher BW. How to perform effective equine dental nerve blocks. Horse Dentistry & Bitting Journal 2005;6:18–20.
50. Weber S, Ohlerth S, Mosing M, et al. Ex Vivo Evaluation of the Distribution of a Mixture of Mepivacaine 2% and Iopromide Following Local Infiltration of the Infraorbital Nerve via the Infraorbital Foramen (2019). Equine Vet Educ 2019; 32(S11):65–70. https://doi.org/10.1111/eve.13108.
51. Henry T, Pusterla N, Guedes AG, et al. Evaluation and clinical use of an intraoral inferior alveolar nerve block in the horse. Equine Vet J 2014;46(6):706–10.
52. Harding Pg, Smith RL, Barakzai SZ. Comparison of two approaches to performing an inferior alveolar nerve block in the horse. Aust Vet J 2012;90(4):146–50.
53. Skarda RT. Local anesthetics and local anesthetic techniques in horses. In: Muir WW, Hubbell JAE, editors. Equine anesthesia: monitoring and emergency therapy. 1st edition. St. Louis, Mo: Mosby Year Book; 1991. p. 199–246.
54. Skarda RT, Tranquilli WJ. Local and regional anesthetic and analgesic techniques: horses. In: Tranquilli WJ, Thurmon JC, Grimm KA, editors. Lumb & Jones' veterinary anesthesia and analgesia. 4th edition. Ames, Iowa: Blackwell Publishing; 2007. p. 608.
55. Rawlinson JE, Bass L, Campoy L, et al. Anatomic analysis of the equine mental foramen and rostral mandibular canal using computed tomography. Vet Anaesth Analg 2018;45(3):357–65.
56. Crean SJ, Powis A. Neurological complications of local anaesthetics in dentistry. Dent Update 1999;26(8):344–9.
57. Diesem C. Organ of vision. In: Sisson S, Grossman JD, editors. Sisson and Grossman's. the anatomy of domestic animals. 5th edition. Philadelphia: W.B. Saunders Co.; 1975. p. 703–18.

Equine Dental Floating (Crown Osontoplasty)

Edward T. Earley, DVM[a],*, Jeffrey D. Reiswig, DVM, MS, PhD[b]

KEYWORDS

- Equine • Tooth • Dental • Malocclusion • Odontoplasty • Float • Enamel Point

KEY POINTS

- A quality oral examination should be the most important and frequent dental procedure performed in the horse.
- With normal attrition, the equine dentition is designed to last between 18 and 25 years of life.
- Oral endoscopy is the gold standard for a comprehensive oral examination.
- Even though dental floating has been practiced for hundreds of years, there is minimal to no scientific-based evidence to support this procedure.
- Enamel points/ridges, cingula, and transverse ridges most likely improve mastication by functioning to tear, shred, and grind forage.

DEFINITIONS

Floating: The process of smoothing down the sharp buccal or lingual enamel points on the cheek teeth of horses. The act of using rasps to remove sharp edges from teeth.[1]

Occlusion: Surface-to-surface contact between opposing teeth.[1]

Malocclusion: Any deviation from normal occlusion.[2]

Odontoplasty: The removal and shaping of a tooth crown to decrease interference with another tooth or to eliminate soft tissue trauma.

Triadan tooth numbering system: The dentition is divided into four quadrants. The right maxillary is the 100-quadrant, the left maxillary is the 200-quadrant, the left mandibular is the 300-quadrant, and the right mandibular is the 400-quadrant. Each tooth in a quadrant is given a number 1 for the first incisor through 11 for the third molar. For example, the upper right fourth premolar is the 108-tooth. The incisors are always 1 through 3, canine teeth are always 4s, and the first molars are always 9s.[3]

---

[a] Large Animal Dentistry, Equine Farm Animal Hospital, Cornell University, Ithaca, NY 14853, USA; [b] Equine Veterinary Dental Services, LLC, PO Box 333, Granville, OH 43023, USA
* Corresponding author.
E-mail address: ete9@cornell.edu

Vet Clin Equine 36 (2020) 501–526
https://doi.org/10.1016/j.cveq.2020.08.011
0749-0739/20/© 2020 Elsevier Inc. All rights reserved.
vetequine.theclinics.com

The equine skull and dentition in its current anatomic form of the Equidae phylogeny has been present for more than 20 million years. Literature describing dental disease in the horse was first published around 1855 by E. Mayhew. Dental floating, enamel point reduction, tooth odontoplasty, and dental equilibration are all terms for corrective dental procedures that have been performed on the horse for hundreds of years. Although floating is likely the most common treatment performed on horse teeth since the nineteenth century, its merit is debated among veterinarians and there is scant evidence-based medical literature to support it.

In normal centric occlusion the upper incisors are in contact and level with the lower incisors, and the midlines of each should oppose each other. As in all domestic species there is anisognathia, with the upper jaw being wider than the lower. This is observed in the horse by pulling the cheek laterally, and with a bright headlamp looking down the cheek tooth arcade to observe three premolars and 3 M in each arcade (collectively called cheek teeth). The upper cheek teeth sit outside the lower teeth and are not in contact, creating a free space (**Fig. 1**). The upper and lower cheek teeth should be aligned mesially/distally and abutted to each other with no gaps in the interproximal space. The cheek teeth have a physiologic occlusal angle that averages 15° to 20° dorsopalatal-ventrobuccal and that increases rostral (06) to caudal (11).[4] The physiologic occlusal angle varies because of skull anatomy and asymmetry.[5] With the cheek retracted the mandible is moved laterally side to side to observe the cheek teeth coming into occlusal contact. This measurement of lateral excursion to molar contact has been previously defined and characterized in normal horses and those with malocclusions.[6] Inappropriate odontoplasty also affects premolar/molar

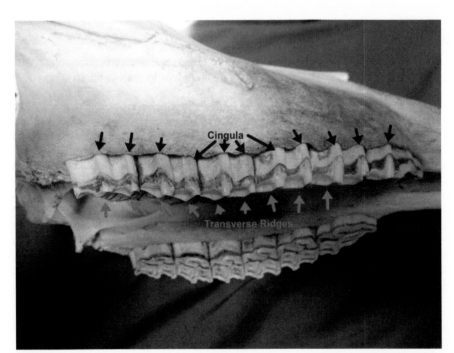

Fig. 1. An equine skull with the cingula that form the sharp enamel points identified with *blue arrows* and the transverse ridges that form on the occlusal surface identified with *red arrows*.

contact.[5] When the cheek teeth make occlusal contact the upper and lower incisors move apart. This approximates the end of the chewing cycle, which has been well documented through video studies.[7] The amount of lateral excursion to molar contact increases when eating hay as compared with eating grain, and more of the occlusal surface is used during mastication of hay diets.[7] Normal occlusion, occlusal angle, and anisognathia and physiologic attrition lead to the formation of sharp enamel points on the buccal surface of the upper cheek teeth and lingual surface of the mandibular cheek teeth.[3]

The equine cheek tooth is an anelodont tooth (forms a true root 1–2 years poster-uption) in a hypsodont form (radicular hypsodont tooth with an extensive reserve crown).[3] The three dental hard tissues are (1) dentin, (2) enamel, and (3) cementum. The density of these three materials are different, with cementum being the least calcified and enamel being the most calcified. As the occlusal surface wears with mastication, there is a difference in attrition of these three materials. Cementum being the softest wears first, leaving dentin with elevated regions of enamel called transverse ridges (typically two per cheek tooth) (see **Fig. 1**). This varied attrition process creates an irregular occlusal surface with transverse enamel ridges that is superior for the shredding and grinding of course forage.[3] The normal attrition rate of the equine cheek tooth averages 2 to 3 mm per year. The average reserve crown length of cheek teeth varies among the three premolars and the 3 M. The shortest reserve crown length of 3.3 cm is noted with the second premolar, and the longest reserve crown is reported with the fourth premolar at 5.1 cm. The second molar has the longest reserve crown of the 3 M averaging 5.0 cm.[8] When comparing average attrition rates (2.5 mm/y) with average reserve crown lengths (3.3 cm for second premolar and 5.1 cm for fourth premolars), the life expectancy of a normal cheek tooth posteruption ranges between 13.2 years (second premolar) and 20.4 years (fourth premolar). Given that all permanent equine dentition is present around 5 years of age, it is estimated that the equine dentition has a life span ranging between 18.2 years (second premolar) and 25.4 years (fourth premolar). With the current modern-day horses capable of living well into their early 30s,[9] it is apparent that the horse has the potential to outlive the functional longevity of their dentition. Unnecessary annual or biannual odontoplastic procedures could significantly reduce the functional longevity of the cheek teeth.

Cingula, transverse ridges, and enamel points serve a function for mastication in the Equidae and other herbivore species (see **Fig. 1**). The two cingula along the buccal surface of each maxillary cheek tooth act as pillars that strengthen the tooth and increase the area of the occlusal surface. Transverse ridges also act to increase the total occlusal area and have a tearing/mincing effect on forage. Enamel points may have a greater effect on shredding forage. In geriatric horses with significant reduction in functional occlusal surface area (nearly expired reserve crowns), floating of enamel points and odontoplasty of tooth elongations may result in even further inability to effectively chew forages (**Fig. 2**). This stresses the importance and need for a comprehensive oral examination coupled with conservative odontoplasty focused on specific dental pathology.

The continuously erupting radicular hypsodont teeth, under normal circumstances, balances the attrition that occurs during mastication. However, any malocclusion, crown fracture, or tooth malformation may result in tooth elongations. These dental overgrowths interfere with proper movement of the jaws, cause soft tissue lacerations of the oral cavity, and effect occlusal forces that cause teeth to move creating pathologic diastemata. Food stagnates in the diastema, initiating periodontal disease (**Fig. 3**).

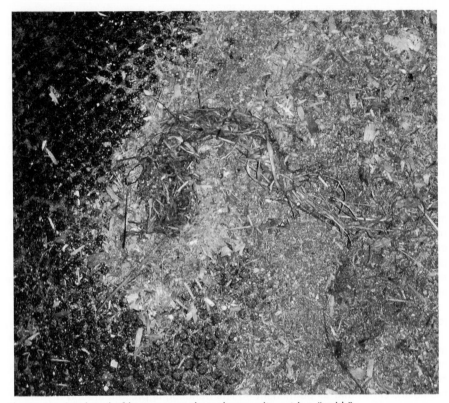

Fig. 2. A twisted wad of hay or grass that a horse spits out is a "quid."

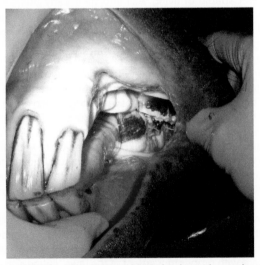

Fig. 3. A rostral to caudal view of the 200 and 300 cheek tooth arcades demonstrating anisognathia and a malocclusion in which the 306 is misaligned mesial with respect to tooth 206 causing a ramp on tooth 306, which has erupted into the palate. Feed material is seen packing within the diastema between teeth 306 and 307.

Recently, dental floating principles have been correlated with orthodontic forces, dental movement, and bone remodeling secondary to malocclusions.[5] Malocclusions are classified into five categories (**Table 1**). Class I malocclusions, which may have resulted in abnormal movement of teeth, are commonly addressed with odontoplasty. Six types of tooth movements are described: (1) extrusion, (2) tipping, (3) radicular, (4) rotation, (5) translation, and (6) intrusion (**Table 2**). When performing an oral examination, it is important to consider how masticatory forces affect tooth movement along with the opposing arcade and/or tooth. The primary dental pathology is often with the opposing dentition. Significant reduction of orthodontic force is achieved with conservative odontoplasty. Typically, 1 to 2 mm of crown reduction take a tooth out of occlusion and remove the undesired orthodontic force.

A few cases illustrate some important points. The first case is an 8-year-old Morgan mare that has a tipped left maxillary third molar (211) (**Fig. 4**). Timothy grass is trapped between the tooth and the buccal mucosa. There is a small buccal ulcer evident at the mesial enamel point (just below the grass). If the dental examination consisted of simply palpating enamel points, the perceived treatment would be to reduce the enamel points and cingula of 211 and unknowingly risk pulp exposure of the tooth caused by the buccal tipping. With oral endoscopy, the initial impression is that the mesial enamel point of 211 is only creating a minor ulcer and that the tooth is extremely tipped in a buccal direction and trapping food. A thorough oral examination should be performed to determine the primary cause of the malocclusion and what orthodontic forces are involved.

A class I malocclusion is often found in the opposing arcade, in this case the left mandibular arcade. Examination of the left mandibular second and third molars (310 and 311) is indicated to evaluate the occlusal force placed on tooth 211. Oral endoscopy shows that the clinical crowns of 310 and 311 are normal (**Figs. 5** and **6**). The next step is to consider the contralateral side of the skull. Examination of the right maxillary arcade reveals a severe overlong tooth right maxillary third premolar (107) (**Fig. 7**). The opposing tooth, right mandibular third premolar (407) has not erupted and is evident just below the gingiva. The right mandibular second premolar (406) is tipped distally over a portion of the unerupted 407 crown (**Fig. 8**). A ventral oblique radiograph shows that the unerupted 407 crown has continued to develop, with the reserve crown and roots extending through the ventral aspect of the right mandible (**Fig. 9**). An off-set mandible dorsoventral radiograph shows extensive bone remodeling along the medial

Table 1 Classifications of occlusion	
Orthodontic Classification	Orthodontic Description
Class 0	Normal occlusion relative to the species and breed.
Class I	Neutroclusion where the mandible and maxilla are normal length. Teeth are in a normal mesiodistal location. Teeth are displaced in a buccal, lingual, or palatal orientation. Rotated or crowded teeth.
Class II	Distoclusion where either the mandible is short or the maxilla is long.
Class III	Mesioclusion where either the mandible is long or the maxilla is short.
Class IV	Mesiodistoclusion is a special classification where one jaw is in mesioclusion and the other is in distoclusion.

From Earley ET. How to diagnose class I malocclusions in the horse. AAEP Proceedings 2016; 62:55-62; with permission.

Table 2
Six types of tooth movement (listed in order from easiest to the most difficult)

Tooth Movement	Description
Extrusion	Movement of the tooth out of the alveolus. Easiest type of tooth movement.
Tipping	Crown tipping. Tooth movement of mostly crown, the roots move slightly in the opposite direction. Center of rotation occurs at the junction of the middle and apical thirds of the tooth. Most common type of tooth movement.
Radicular (root)	Root tipping. Tooth movement of mostly root. Center of rotation occurs at the junction of the coronal and middle thirds of the tooth.
Rotation	Rotation around the long axis of the tooth. All periodontal ligaments are stretched in the same spiral direction. Ligament recoil is common.
Translation	Bodily movement of the entire tooth (crown and root) in the same direction.
Intrusion	Movement of the tooth into the alveolus. Most difficult type of movement. Force is applied in the same direction as occlusal forces. The periodontal ligament attachments are designed to resist this movement. Compressive forces may compromise vascular supply to the apex of the tooth.

From Earley ET. How to Diagnose class I malocclusions in the horse. AAEP Proceedings 2016; 62:55-62; with permission.

aspect of the right mandible (**Fig. 10**). Computed tomography in a coronal view of the right mandible demonstrates pathologic fractures of the lateral and medial mandibular cortices (**Fig. 11**). In this situation, mastication is most likely shifting to the left side to avoid pain from the pathologic fractures of the right mandible. As a result, orthodontic forces are shifted predominately to the left side, causing excessive tipping of tooth 211 and trapping feed material along the buccal aspect. The best option in this case is to treat the primary cause by addressing the unerupted 407 and reducing the overlong

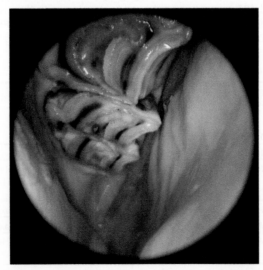

Fig. 4. An oral endoscopic image of tooth 211 showing that it is tipped buccally in relation to tooth 210, lacerating the buccal mucosa and trapping grass during mastication.

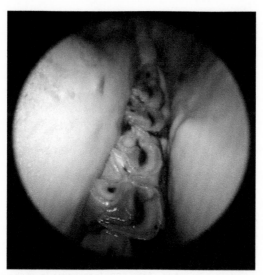

Fig. 5. The oral endoscope image comes from the same horse as **Fig. 4** and shows the normal opposing arcade. Teeth 310 and 311 are visible with a buccal laceration caused by the enamel points of the tipped tooth 211 from **Fig. 4**.

107, to allow healing of the pathologic fracture. This case demonstrates the importance of a complete oral examination to find the primary cause and treat it as opposed to the secondary and tertiary effects.

Another clinical case is a 27-year-old Appaloosa mare (**Fig. 12**). The mare was floated one time in her life at age 5. The mare has lived in the same turnout pasture and wooded lot her whole life where hay is available continuously. At 27 years of age she is in a positive nutritional plane with a body grade of seven to eight on a scale

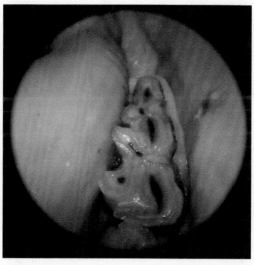

Fig. 6. A closeup of 311 and the buccal laceration first observed in **Fig. 5**.

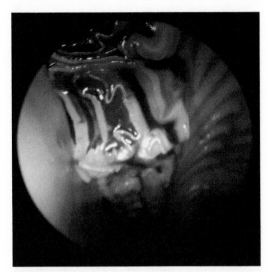

Fig. 7. This is an oral endoscopic image of the 100-dental arcade of the same horse as **Figs. 4–6**. Tooth 107 has a severe dental overgrowth (step).

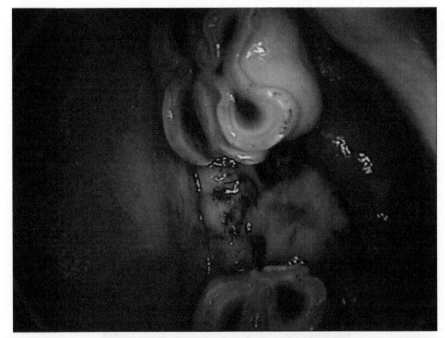

Fig. 8. An oral endoscopic image of the 400-dental arcade from the same horse as **Figs. 4–7**. Tooth 407 has not erupted. The crown is observed just below the gingival margin. Tooth 406 is tipped distally, whereas tooth 408 is tipped mesially entrapping tooth 407.

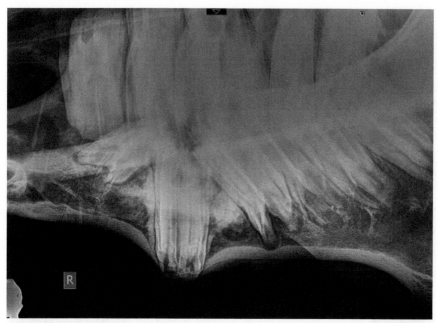

Fig. 9. A left 45° ventral right dorsal oblique radiograph of the horse from **Fig. 8**. Tooth 407 has developed but has not erupted. Tooth 406 is severely tipped distally and tooth 408 is tipped mesially and seems to entrap tooth 407.

of nine (see **Fig. 12**).[1] Oral examination reveals enamel points present along the buccal aspect of the maxillary cheek teeth 3 to 5 mm long (**Figs. 13** and **14**). The mandibular cheek teeth have enamel ridges along the lingual aspect at 2 to 3 mm in height (**Fig. 15**). Associated with the enamel points of the right and left maxillary third molars (111, 211) are minor buccal lacerations or mucosal calluses. Despite a 22-year span of nonintervention, this horse has maintained a normal occlusion. This clinical example suggests that if normal occlusion exists annual or biannual enamel point reduction may not be needed.

This case correlates with a research study that compares "Thoroughbred type" horses raised on free-range grass with horses that are stabled and fed high-concentrate diets. The results show that the stabled horses have greater numbers of dental overgrowths (exaggerated transverse ridges and ramps) than the free-range horses.[10] Considering that horses fed high-concentrate diets have decreased lateral excursion,[7] it may be that diet and decreased lateral excursion also contribute to dental overgrowths. Additionally, it could be argued that exaggerated transverse ridges may be a normal variation observed without any pathologic consequence (and possible benefit of improved mastication).

The primary signs of disease requiring odontoplasty include evidence of trauma to the oral soft tissues, pain during mastication or riding, and malocclusions producing dental overgrowths. Soft tissue trauma is often seen as acute or chronic buccal or lingual mucosal lacerations. These are corrected by floating the sharp points associated with the lacerations, although the authors know of no research to prove this. Pain is observed as an avoidance reaction while palpating the cheeks over the teeth arcade before sedation. There are several presentations of horse performance problems, such as difficulty with the bit, resistance to the bit, not giving to the bit, not being on

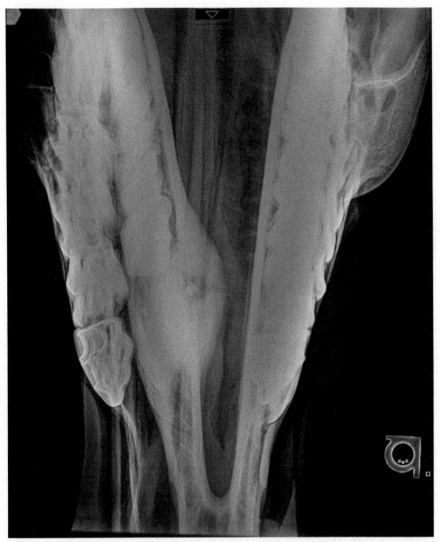

Fig. 10. A dorsoventral view with the mandible offset to the left from the same horse as **Fig. 9**. A mandibular fracture with extensive bone remodeling is observed at the sight of the unerupted tooth 407.

the bit, and tossing the head. Although the signs may be vague, the rider complaints are often eliminated after reducing sharp enamel points and tooth overgrowths. Malocclusions may generate forces that move teeth and cause gaps between the interproximal spaces forming pathologic diastemata. The diastema collects food that stagnates and initiates periodontal disease (see **Fig. 3**).

Disease prevention is important to oral health. Reducing overgrowths before they move teeth or cause soft tissue trauma or pain is preventive medicine. Dental disease can lead to abnormal chewing patterns or quidding, which leaves twisted wads of hay or grass on the stall floor (see **Fig. 2**). Quidding may correlate with dental disease and/

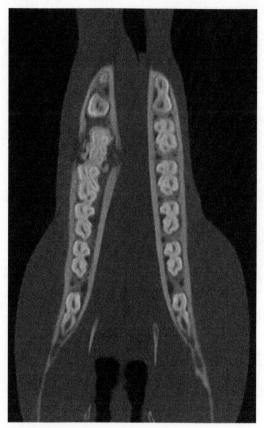

Fig. 11. The coronal view of a computed tomography image of the horse mandible from **Figs. 4–10**. Cortical fractures of the medial and lateral wall of the right mandible are seen.

or missing dentition. Prevention of all these clinical signs of disease should be considered during the annual examination.

To illustrate prevention of periodontal disease, consider a clinical case where the maxillary cheek teeth arcades are a centimeter rostral to the mandibular premolars and molars. This class I malocclusion would result in the formation of tooth elongations on the mesial aspect of the maxillary second premolars (106, 206) and the distal aspect of the mandibular third molars (311, 411) (**Figs. 16** and **17**). With each masticatory cycle the forces generated tend to push the 106 and 206 mesial and the 311 and 411 distally, potentially creating pathologic diastema. This illustrates the current working hypothesis of using odontoplasty to reduce the overgrowths to prevent abnormal forces along the occlusal surface. If left untreated, these overgrowths may also elongate into the soft tissue of the lower mandible mesial to the 306 and 406 and the palate distal to 111 and 211, creating soft tissue lacerations or ulcers (**Fig. 18**). When evaluating the distal portion of the third mandibular molars (311/411), careful oral endoscopic examination helps to distinguish a true overlong tooth from a tooth following the alveolar ridge along the curvature of Spee. If the tooth is following the curvature of Spee, the distance from the occlusal surface to the gingival margin is the same along all aspects of the tooth (see **Fig. 6**).

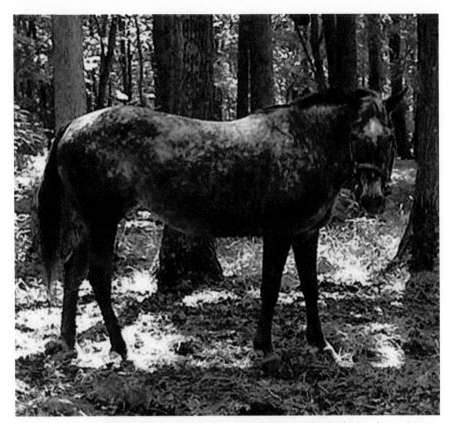

Fig. 12. A 27-year-old Appaloosa mare with a BCS of 7 to 8. BCS, Body Condition Score.

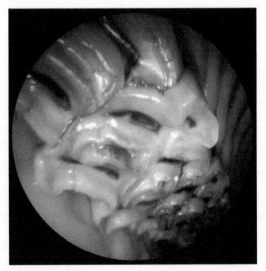

Fig. 13. An endoscopic image of the 100-tooth arcade (107) of the horse in **Fig. 12** showing the varied attrition of the three dental hard tissues: peripheral and infundibular enamel, dentin, and cementum. The normal wear pattern of the occlusal surface of equine teeth creates the transverse ridges and the enamel points of the cingula.

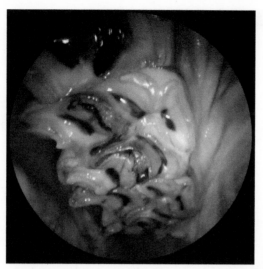

Fig. 14. An endoscopic image of teeth 110 and 111 from the horse in **Fig. 12**. Observe the enamel points extending from the mesial and distal cingula of tooth 111 and creating buccal lacerations.

Although removal of sharp enamel points and crown reduction are frequent treatments, they are performed with minimal evidence-based research. A current literature search through January 2020 for scientific articles on the topics of equine, horse, dental float, equilibration, correction, odontoplasty, routine dentistry, digestibility, rideability, and fecal fiber length revealed several articles[11–27] published in peer-reviewed journals evaluating the benefit of dental floating. In looking at the level of evidence with these articles (where grade I evidence is the highest level and grade IV

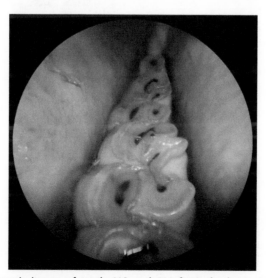

Fig. 15. An endoscopic image of teeth 410 and 411 from the horse in **Fig. 12** showing normal transverse ridges and enamel points.

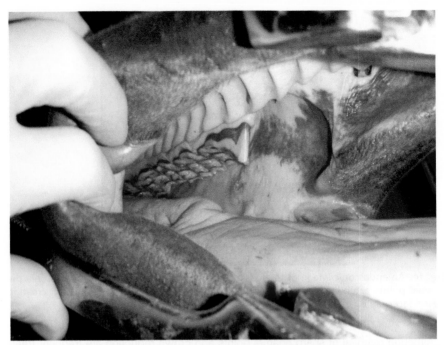

Fig. 16. An overgrowth on tooth 206 (hook) with an oral buccal laceration. This overgrowth occurred because the upper tooth arcade sits rostral to the lower arcade.

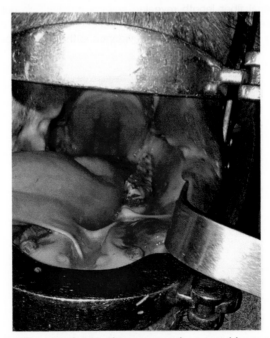

Fig. 17. An overgrowth on tooth 311. This overgrowth occurred because the upper tooth arcade sits rostral to the lower arcade.

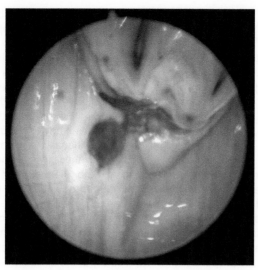

Fig. 18. An endoscopic image of a laceration distal to tooth 211 from the overgrowth seen in **Fig. 17**.

evidence is the lowest, **Table 3**) only three articles[11,14,20] have grade I evidence. These three articles concluded that dental floating improved rostral caudal mobility of the mandible but did not affect parameters, such as weight gain, feed digestibility, fecal particle size, body condition, or rideability. Six articles are grade III evidence. These studies were not randomized and the treatment and control groups were with the

Table 3 Levels of evidence[5]	
Grade I evidence	Highest level of evidence. Randomized control clinical study. Target species with naturally occurring clinical condition.
Grade II evidence	Randomized controlled clinical study in a laboratory setting. Target species with naturally occurring clinical condition in a laboratory setting.
Grade III evidence	Peer-reviewed journals. Clinical study without randomization. Cohort or case-controlled analytical study. Disease simulations in target species. Case series.
Grade IV evidence	Lowest level of evidence. Peer and nonpeer reviewed journals. Opinion based clinical experience documented in textbooks, proceedings, and so forth. Descriptive studies. Studies in other species. Reports from expert committees.

From the Center for Evidence Based Medicine Website. Available at: www.cebm.net; and *From* Earley ET. How to Diagnose class I malocclusions in the horse. AAEP Proceedings 2016; 62:55-62; with permission.

same animals. There were variable results with fecal fiber length and digestibility.[12,16,18,21,24,27] The remaining five articles are case reports and expert opinion.[17,19,22,25,26]

During examination, the presence of buccal or lingual lacerations in the location of a sharp enamel point seems to imply an association. Even though this is commonly discussed in expert opinion papers and books, little actual peer-reviewed research documentation exists. A retrospective observational study discussed the association of buccal lacerations with sharp enamel points in 55% of horses presented for dental examination.[28,29] No statistics were presented with this study to document the conclusions made with respect to age and breed. Additionally, a study has shown an increase in acute buccal ulceration opposite the maxillary second premolar teeth and lip commissures in horses being ridden with a bridle and bit.[30] This study found an increase in these lesions regardless of floating; however, the timing of floating was not examined in relation to the lacerations.

Various hand instruments and power equipment are available for odontoplasty. The variety can make it difficult for veterinarians to decide which equipment is a good investment. Instrument selection is largely by personal preference. The equipment should provide for the proper treatment and safety of the clinician. Some practitioners prefer to use odontoplasty instruments while monitoring the reduction with digital palpation. Others prefer visual dentistry and the ergonomics of power equipment. With direct visualization crown reductions are more precise. All equipment should be used with a proper understanding of tooth anatomy to avoid injury to the teeth or gums.

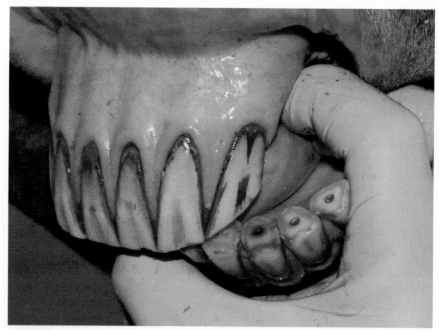

Fig. 19. Pulp horn defects observed in all three left mandibular incisors of a 17-year-old appendix quarter horse gelding after the crowns had been amputated by a lay floater the previous year.

Excessive filing 106, 206, 306 and 406

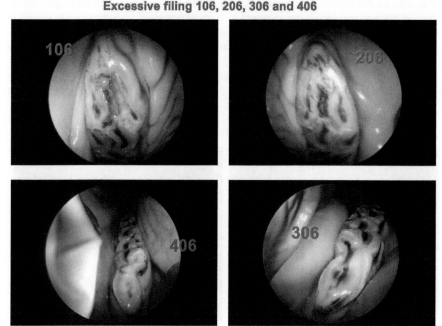

Fig. 20. Endoscopic images of teeth 106, 206, 306, and 406 in a 19-year-old Arabian gelding. All of the second premolars (which have the least amount of reserve crown) are overfiled to the point that normal pulp horn anatomy is barely recognizable. Teeth 306 and 406 are expired down to the furcation of the remaining root tips.

The tooth is a living structure with arteries, veins, nerves, and lymphatics within the pulp cavity; therefore, any excision of tooth material is surgery. The surface anatomy of an upper cheek tooth has peripheral cementum surrounding undulating white enamel that circumscribes a cream-colored primary dentin. Central to the primary dentin is secondary dentin, which is less calcified than primary dentin and is stained brown in color from forage tannins. Secondary dentin is produced by odontoblasts in the coronal aspect of the pulp horns in response to normal attrition, thus preventing pulp exposure to the oral cavity. This is recognizable as the dental star in incisors.[3] Teeth 07 through 10 have five areas of secondary dentin on the occlusal aspect of the five pulp horns. The 06 teeth have six pulp horns and six areas of secondary dentin staining, and the 11s have six or seven pulp horns. Learning where these pulp horns are located and what they look like is important to avoid pulp exposures during odontoplasty. A scanning electron microscopy study of the tooth surface after odontoplasty (using two types of hand rasps and a motorized rotary disk) showed that odontoblastic processes were exposed and amputated during the procedures. The carbide chip motorized disk float produced a smoother surface and maintained a smear layer (an adherent layer of organic and inorganic tooth material) that may help protect the tooth.[31]

How much tooth can be removed at one time, and how is thermal damage prevented during therapy?[28,32–34] Several studies have investigated the amount of dentin between the occlusal surface and the pulp.[35–37] The depth of subocclusal dentin in cheek teeth ranges from 2 to 33 mm.[37] The depth of subocclusal dentin has poor correlation to the age of the tooth or the length of the crown. Removal of as little as 2 mm of secondary dentin could result in pulp exposure.[36,37] Subocclusal dentin is thinner in overlong teeth than adjacent cheek teeth within the same arcade. If an overlong tooth is reduced to the level of the normal arcade, it has been reported that there is a 58% chance of exposing pulp.[36]

Incisor subocclusal dentin is more variable than cheek teeth (**Fig. 19**). Maxillary incisor subocclusal dentin ranges from 1.5 to 11.7 mm and in mandibular incisors

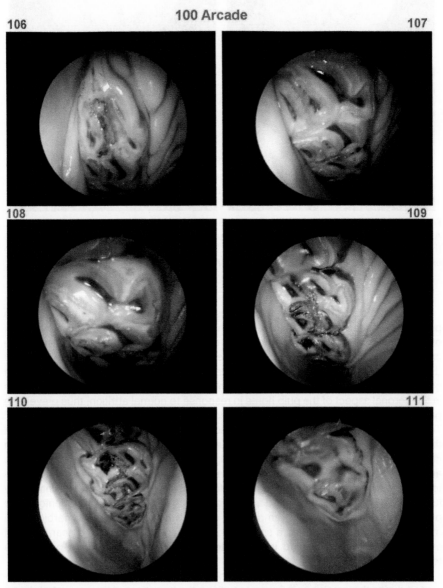

100 Arcade

Fig. 21. Endoscopic images of each cheek tooth in the 100-arcade of the same horse as **Fig. 20** showing that the cingula along the right maxillary arcade have been leveled and removed to the level of the gingiva (observed in tooth 111).

from 0.7 to 6.7 mm. These depths tend to decrease with age.[35] Even if the pulp is not exposed during an odontoplasty procedure, the possibility of thermal damage exists.[28,32–34] The best way to prevent thermal damage is with continuous water irrigation. If water is not used during the procedure, the reduction should be limited to less than 20 seconds or immediate water irrigation should be used following the procedure. A quick rinse cools the tooth rapidly.[34]

DAMAGE CAUSED BY AGGRESSIVE FLOATING

With legalized equine lay dentistry in New York, aggressive grinding, filing, and floating procedures are being performed regularly. As a result, numerous horses have the life expectancy of their dentition drastically reduced. **Figs. 20–23** show the effects of chronic aggressive grinding in an older horse (19-year-old Arabian gelding). The changes include severe resorption, hypercementosis, apical disease, root blunting, and a reduced functional life of the teeth.

Aggressive overfiling in a young horse is demonstrated with a 6-year-old Warmblood gelding. The horse was presented for a fractured tooth 309. Oral endoscopy revealed only a small fragmented portion remaining of the clinical crown (**Fig. 24**). In this image, overfiling is evident in teeth 308, 310, and 311. This is alarming because the teeth are young with recent eruption in the last 1 to 2 years. In the same horse, there was complete cingula removal down to the gingiva of teeth 208 (**Fig. 25**) and 209 (**Fig. 26**). In the endoscopic image of 209 (see **Fig. 26**) complete removal of

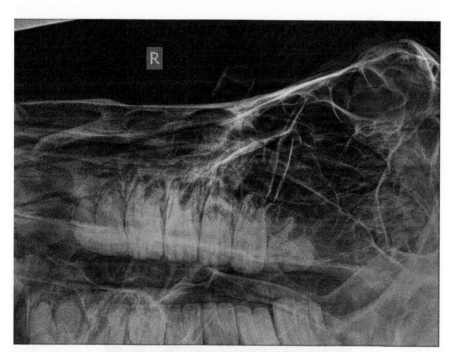

Fig. 22. A radiograph of the 100-arcade, corresponding to the images in **Fig. 21**, showing extensive root resorption (particularly noticeable with teeth 106 and 111), and reactive cementum (hypercementosis) of tooth 106. Additionally, apical pathology is observed involving the roots of teeth 107 and 108.

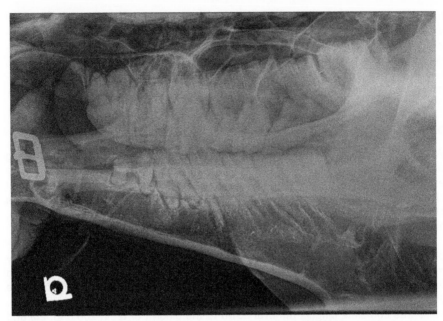

Fig. 23. A radiograph of the 300-arcade of the same horse as **Fig. 20** shows extreme resorption and blunting of tooth 306 roots along with apical changes involving teeth 307 and 308.

peripheral cementum along with most of the enamel is evident along the entire buccal aspect of the tooth. A developing clinical crown defect/fracture is evident at the distal infundibulum. In the same horse there is aggressive profiling of tooth 206 that has removed all dental hard tissue surrounding the mesial pulp horn (number 6) down to

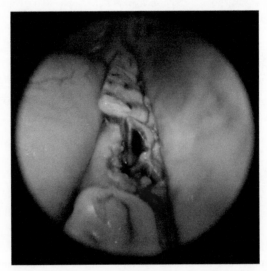

Fig. 24. An endoscopic image of a 6-year-old Warmblood gelding presenting for evaluation of a fractured tooth 309. Only a small fragmented portion remains of the clinical crown. Overfiling is evident in teeth 308, 310, and 311.

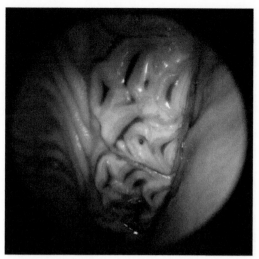

Fig. 25. An endoscopic image of tooth 208 in the same horse in **Fig. 21** shows complete removal of the cementum and enamel of the mesial and distal cingula. The excessive odontoplasty extends into the primary dentin of pulp horns number 1 and number 2 and apically to the gingiva.

the gingiva. Additionally, complete enamel point and cingula reduction has been performed down to the gingiva exposing the two buccal pulp horns (number 1 and 2) (**Fig. 27**). This case example demonstrates the damage that is created with aggressive filing. These procedures reduce the function and longevity of the tooth and can lead to dental fracture and/or apical abscessation that require tooth extraction.

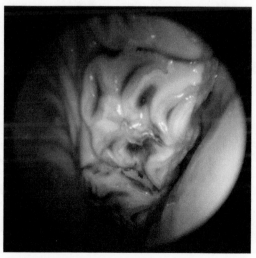

Fig. 26. An endoscopic image of 209 in the same horse in **Fig. 21** shows complete removal of cementum and most of the enamel along the distobuccal pulp horn (number 2). A developing clinical crown defect/fracture is evident at the distal infundibulum.

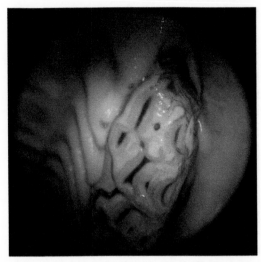

Fig. 27. An endoscopic image of 206 in the same horse in **Fig. 21** shows aggressive profiling of tooth 206 that has removed all dental hard tissue surrounding the mesial pulp horn (number 6) down to the gingiva. Additionally, complete enamel point and cingula reduction has been performed down to the gingiva exposing the secondary dentin of pulp horns number 1 and number 2.

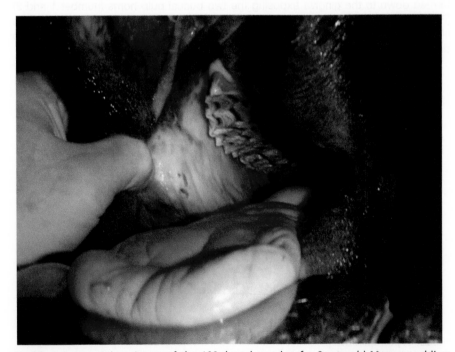

Fig. 28. A preoperative picture of the 100-dental arcade of a 9-year-old Morgan gelding currently in work. A 3-mm 106 hook (2 mm of this hook involves secondary dentin) is present with sharp enamel points and a buccal laceration in the location of a 106 enamel point.

ASSESSMENT

After emphasizing the importance of making a specific diagnosis for formulation of a treatment plan, it is illogical to say how one should treat a typical horse. Enamel points that create buccal or lingual lacerations may cause discomfort. If sharp enamel points are reduced, it should be done conservatively to preserve the occlusal surface (**Figs. 28** and **29**). The point is gently rounded along the cingula. An overgrowth may be reduced to the coronal level of the transverse ridge. In geriatric patients with severe attrition (cupped and/or expired teeth), odontoplasty is not indicated.

As illustrated in the previous case examples, the dentition of an aged equine (27 years of age) with no odontoplasty procedures performed in the last 22 years of her life is better than the dentition of a young (6 year old) horse with aggressive dentistry. With a normal functioning dentition having the average potential of 18 to 25 years of life, this 27-year-old has exceeded the range by at least 2 years with no rasping intervention. Enamel points, cingula, transverse ridges, and arcade curvature (wave) are viewed as normal anatomy in the equine dentition that may even serve a purpose for healthy mastication. The practice of equine dentistry has evolved from a recommended routine annual float (more recently upgraded to the ambiguous term "occlusal equilibration") to an examination process emphasizing oral endoscopy. Dentin, enamel, and cementum are evaluated on individual teeth assessing clinical findings, such as occlusal fissures, cemental cracks and decay (peripheral and internal), mineralization of pulp horns, enamel health, tooth resorption, and so forth. If

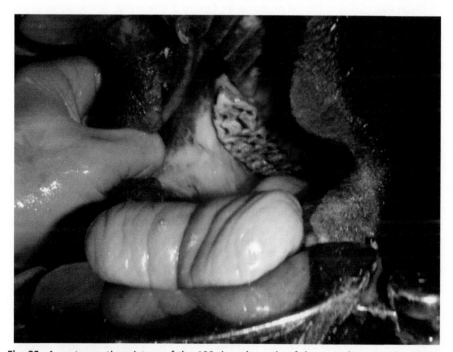

Fig. 29. A postoperative picture of the 100-dental arcade of the same horse as **Fig. 28**. The 106 hook has been reduced and a light brown coloring of the secondary dentin of the sixth pulp horn is observed. The points have been reduced to the level of the peripheral enamel of the occlusal surface and 2 to 3 mm along the buccal surface of the cingula.

odontoplasty is performed, it should be conservative, as determined by careful clinical evaluation, formulation of a diagnosis, and always in a manner that "does no harm."

SUMMARY

Odontoplasty (floating and occlusal equilibration) is currently the most commonly performed procedure in equine dentistry. Many monetary and business models of the equine practitioner are based on numbers of dental floats performed. From an anatomic perspective, an irregular occlusal surface, prominent cingula, transverse ridges, and enamel points all contribute to the function, form, and longevity of the equine cheek tooth. With limited reserve crown available and an average functional life range between 18 and 25 years, removal of tooth structure should be conservative. The authors consider a quality oral examination to be the most important dental procedure performed in the horse. Individual tooth evaluation should lead to a specific diagnosis and treatment plan. If tooth odontoplasty is part of the dental treatment plan it should be site-specific.

REFERENCES

1. Easley J, Dixon PM, Schumacher J. Equine dentistry. 3rd edition. Philadelphia: Saunders/Elsevier; 2010. p. 188.
2. Lobprise HB. Occlusion and orthodontics. In: Lobprise HB, Dodd JR, editors. Wigg's veterinary dentistry. 2nd edition. Hoboken (NJ): John Wiley & Sons, Inc; 2019. p. 413.
3. Dixon PM, duToit n. Dental anatomy. In: Easley J, Dixon PM, Schumacher J, editors. Equine dentistry. 3rd edition. Philadelphia: Saunders/Elsevier; 2010. p. 51–76.
4. Listmann L, Schrock P, Failing K, et al. Occlusal angles of equine cheek teeth. Livestock Sci 2016;186:78–84.
5. Earley ET. How to diagnose class I malocclusions in the horse. AAEP Proc 2016; 62:55–62.
6. Klugh DO. Dental examination. In: Klugh DO, editor. Principles of equine dentistry. Boca Raton (FL): LRC Press LLC; 2010. p. 14.
7. Bonin SJ, Clayton HM, Lanovaz JL, et al. Comparison of mandibular motion in horses chewing hay and pellets. Equine Vet J 2007;39(3):258–62.
8. Liuti T, Reardon R, Dixon PM. Computed tomographic assessment of equine maxillary cheek teeth anatomical relationships and paranasal sinus volumes. Vet Rec 2017. https://doi.org/10.1136/vr.104185.
9. Welsh CE, Duz M, Parkin TDH, et al. Prevalence, survival analysis and multimorbidity of chronic diseases in the general veterinarian-attended horse population of the UK. Prev Vet Med 2016;131:137–45.
10. Masey O'Neill HV, Keen J, Dumbell L. A comparison of the occurrence of common dental abnormalities in stabled and free-grazing horses. Animal 2010;4: 1607–701.
11. Carmalt JL, Allen AL. Effect of rostro-caudal mobility of the mandible on feed digestibility and fecal particle size in horses. J Am Vet Assoc 2006;229:1275–8.
12. Carmalt JL, Carmalt KP, Barber SM. The effect of occlusal equilibration on sport horse performance. J Vet Dent 2006;23(4):226–30.
13. Carmalt JL, Townsend HGG, Allen AL. Effect of dental floating on the rostro-caudal mobility of the mandible of horses. J Am Vet Assoc 2003;223:666–9.

14. Carmalt JL, Townsend HGG, Janzen ED, et al. Effect of dental floating on weight gain, body condition score, feed digestibility and fecal particle size in pregnant mares. J Am Vet Assoc 2004;225:1889–93.
15. Cockcroft PD, Holmes MA. In: Handbook of evidence-based veterinary medicine. Blackwell Publishing; 2003. p. 3.
16. Di Filippo PA, Vieira V, Rondon DA, et al. Effect of dental correction on fecal fiber length in horses. J Equine Vet Sci 2018;64:77–80.
17. Earley ET, Rawlinson JT. A new understanding of oral and dental disorders of the equine incisor and canine teeth. Vet Clin North Am Equine Pract 2013;29(2): 273–300, v.
18. Johnson C, Williams J, Phillips C. Effect of routine dentistry on fecal fiber length in donkeys. J Equine Vet Sci 2017;57:41–5.
19. Klugh DO. Acrylic bite plane for treatment of malocclusion in a young horse. J Vet Dent 2004;21(2):84–7.
20. Moine S, Flammer SA, Maia-Nussbaumer P, et al. Evaluation of the effects of performance dentistry on equine rideability: a randomized, blinded, controlled trial. Vet Q 2017;37:195–9.
21. Ralston SL, Foster DL, Divers T, et al. Effect of dental correction on feed digestibility in horses. Equine Vet J 2001;33(4):390–3.
22. Rawlinson JT, Earley E. Advances in the treatment of diseased equine incisor and canine teeth. Vet Clin North Am Equine Pract 2013;29(2):411–40, vi-vii.
23. Rice MK. Odontoplasty: beyond enamel point reduction. AAEP Proc 2019;65: 443–7.
24. Rodrigues JB, Ferreira LM, Bastos E. Influence of dental correction on nociceptive test responses, fecal appearance, body condition score and apparent digestibility coefficient for dry matter of Zamorano-leones donkeys (Equus asinus). J Anim Sci 2013;91:4765–71.
25. Tremaine H. Advances in the treatment of diseased equine cheek teeth. Vet Clin North Am Equine Pract 2013;29(2):441–65, vii.
26. Wagner AE, Mama KR, Contino EK, et al. Evaluation of sedation and analgesia in standing horses after administration of xylazine, butorphanol and subanesthetic doses of ketamine. J Am Vet Med Assoc 2011;238(12):1629–33.
27. Zwirglmaier S, Remler HP, Senckenberg JF, et al. Effect of dental correction on voluntary hay intake, apparent digestibility of feed and faecal particle size in horse. J Anim Physiol Nutr (Berl) 2011;97(1):72–9.
28. Allen ML, Baker GJ, Freeman DE, et al. In vitro study of heat production during power reduction of equine mandibular teeth. J Am Vet Med Assoc 2004;224: 1128–32.
29. Allen TE. Incidence and severity of abrasions on the buccal mucosa adjacent to the cheek teeth in 199 horses. AAEP Proceedings 2004;50:31–6.
30. Tell A, Egenvall A, Lundstrom T, et al. The prevalence of oral ulceration in Swedish horses when ridden with bit and bridle and when unridden. Vet J 2008;178: 405–10.
31. Kempson SA, Davidson MEB, Dacre IT. The effect of three types of rasps on the occlusal surface of the equine cheek teeth: a scanning electron microscopic study. J Vet Dent 2003;20:19–27.
32. Haeusslers S, Luepke M, Seifert H, et al. Intra-pulpar temperature increase of equine cheek teeth during treatment with motorized grinding systems; influence of grinding head position and rotational speed. BMC Vet Res 2014;10:47. Available at: http://www.biomedcentral.com/1746-6148/10/47.

33. O'Leary JM, Barnett TP, Parkin TDH, et al. Pulpar temperature changes during mechanical reduction of equine cheek teeth: comparison of different motorized dental instruments, duration of treatments and use of water cooling. Equine Vet J 2013;45:355–60.
34. Wilson GJ, Walsh LJ. Temperature changes in dental pulp associated with the use of power grinding equipment on equine teeth. Aust Vet J 2005;83:75–7.
35. Englisch LM, Rott P, Lupke M, et al. Anatomy of equine incisors: pulp horns and sub-occlusal dentine thickness. Equine Vet J 2018;50:854–60.
36. Marshall R, Shaw DJ, Dixon PM. A study of sub-occlusal secondary dentine thickness in overgrown equine cheek teeth. Vet J 2012;193:53–7.
37. White C, Dixon PM. A study of the thickness of cheek teeth sub-occlusal secondary dentine in horses of different ages. Equine Vet J 2010;41:119–23.

Equine Imaging
Computed Tomography Interpretation

Erin Epperly, DVM[a],*, Justin A. Whitty, DVM[b]

KEYWORDS

- Equine • Sinonasal • Hounsfield units • Periodontal disease
- Computed tomography

KEY POINTS

- Computed tomography (CT) allows for exceptional spatial resolution, bony detail, and soft tissue contrast in evaluation of the equine head.
- Dental disease and primary sinusitis are common, but challenging, diseases to discriminate in equine practice. CT has increased sensitivity and specificity compared with radiography.
- Osseous lesions that are challenging to image with radiographs (fracture, congenital malformation, and infraorbital canal) can be elucidated clearly with CT, which allows reconstruction in multiple planes and 3-dimensional modeling.
- The improved soft tissue contrast of CT and ability to measure x-ray attenuation (Hounsfield units) can aid in differentiation of mass lesions (sinus cysts, melanomas, ethmoid hematomas, and other neoplasms). The administration of iodinated contrast medium can further augment the conspicuity of soft tissue lesions.

INTRODUCTION

Diseases of the paranasal sinuses and dental arches are common in the horse and encompass traumatic, developmental, inflammatory, infectious, and neoplastic etiologies.[1] Computed tomography (CT) has revolutionized the veterinarian's ability to image the equine skull and led to improved diagnostic accuracy and clarity for surgical planning.[2–4] Because of the complex anatomy of the equine head and the inherent limitations of radiography rendering a 2-dimensional image of a 3-dimensional (3-D) object, the cross-sectional nature of CT allows the interpreter to much more confidently place a lesion in the correct anatomic location than with radiographs.[5] As with any novel modality, however, new interpretation skills must be developed. This article reviews the normal CT appearance of the equine skull and presents examples and key

[a] Cornell University College of Veterinary Medicine, 930 Campus Road, Box 25, Ithaca, NY 14853, USA; [b] Department of Clinical Sciences, Cornell University College of Veterinary Medicine, 930 Campus Road, Box 25, Ithaca, NY 14853, USA
* Corresponding author.
E-mail address: eee36@cornell.edu

Vet Clin Equine 36 (2020) 527–543
https://doi.org/10.1016/j.cveq.2020.08.007
vetequine.theclinics.com

features of several common diseases (tooth fracture, tooth resorption, dental associated sinusitis, sinus disease, neoplasia, and fracture).

TECHNIQUE

It is important to briefly discuss the various types of CT scanners currently available for imaging the equine head. The images provided in this article come from the authors' institution, which has a 16-slice multidetector CT scanner. Multidetector CT of at least 16 slices allows for isotropic reconstruction, which means that multiplanar reconstruction can be performed with high fidelity in any orientation (**Fig. 1**). Conventional CT scanners also generate excellent soft tissue contrast, which can be detected on visual inspection, subjectively (gas, fat, fluid, soft tissue, mineral, and metal) or objectively quantified using Hounsfield units (HUs) (**Table 1**). Iodinated contrast material can be administered both intravenously and intra-arterially to further characterize soft tissue lesions; however, there are limited references to dosage and technique.[6–9] At the authors' institution, 500 mL of 350 mgI/mL iohexol (2 mgI/kg) is administered rapidly intravenously via bilateral jugular catheters followed immediately by initiation of the

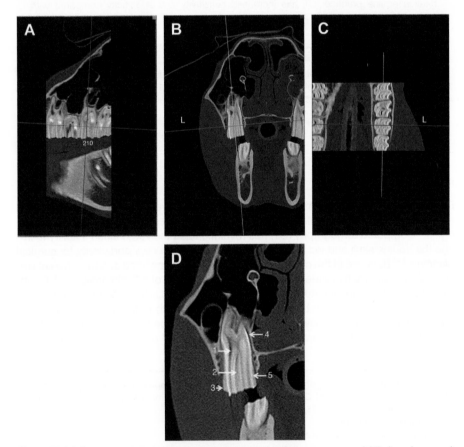

Fig. 1. Multiplanar reconstructions in the (*A*) sagittal, (*B*) transverse, and (*C*) dorsal coronal planes. (*D*) Enlarged transverse image: pulp horn (1), cementum-filled infundibulum (2), peripheral cementum of the clinical crown (3), periodontal ligament space (4), and enamel (5).

Table 1
Hounsfield units of various tissue types

Tissue	Hounsfield Units	Tissue	Hounsfield Units
Gas	−1000		
Fat	−100	Dental pulp	−1000 to +700
Water	0	Dentin	1300–2600
Purulent material	0–40	Cementum	1500–2400
Soft tissue	30–60	Enamel	2000–3700
Hemorrhage	60–100		
Melanin	100	Bone	1000
Soft tissue post–iodinated contrast	100–300	Metal	>2000

CT scan. Contrast material accumulates in blood vessels and within tissues with increased vascularity. As such, many neoplastic and inflammatory lesions become hyperattenuating (whiter) to surrounding normal tissue, whereas necrotic tissue and abscesses are hypoattenuating (darker) (**Fig. 2**). Currently, a majority of equine head CT examinations are performed recumbent under general anesthesia. A few institutions, however, have modified similar multidetector systems to perform standing, sedated CT of the equine head, the details of which have been published.[10] Additionally, cone beam CT is being developed to image the head of standing horses, and, although there currently are substantial disadvantages (motion artifact, scatter, and

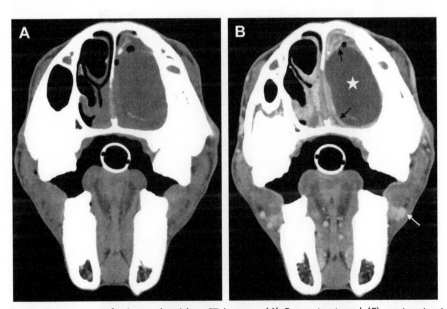

Fig. 2. Transverse, soft tissue algorithm CT images. (*A*) Precontrast and (*B*) postcontrast administration. (*A*) There is a soft tissue attenuating mass filling the left paranasal sinuses. (*B*) Absent contrast enhancement centrally (*star*) with a thin, peripheral rim of contrast enhancement (*black arrows*). Blood vessels are seen as many, round, hyperattenuating structures (*white arrow*).

poor soft tissue contrast), technologic improvements likely will increase the availability of this modality[11] (**Fig. 3**).

DENTAL DISEASE

In cases of supernumerary teeth, complex congenital anomalies, and malocclusion, multiplanar reconstruction and 3-D model generation can aid in surgical planning (**Fig. 4**). Additionally, CT allows for better definition of the relationship between fracture margins and alveolar bone and dental structures (**Fig. 5**). Although the majority of the cases described focus on the cheek teeth, CT also can be used to evaluate the incisors (**Fig. 6**). CT interpretation in cases of dental disease (with or without sinus disease) can be relatively straightforward (**Fig. 7**) or require close scrutiny (**Fig. 8**). The main CT findings seen in cases of alveolitis are gas within pulp cavities (<1000 HUs), widening of pulp cavities, periapical lysis or gas, root blunting or fracture, widened periodontal space, and tooth fracture.[12,13] A nondetectable lamina denta dura has been described as a sign of alveolitis; however, the thin nature of this structure means it not always is identified on CT and should not be used as the sole sign of apical infection.[14] The first maxillary molars (109 and 209) are the most commonly affected teeth, followed by the adjacent premolars and molars.[13,15] Infundibular gas is seen commonly and is easy to misinterpret as pulp gas for the novice (**Fig. 9**). Although infundibular gas usually is incidental, infundibular caries can lead to alveolitis; however, some controversy exists around this topic.[16–18] Secondary sinusitis is common given the intimate association between the maxillary tooth roots and the maxillary sinuses.[19,20] Discriminating dental origin sinusitis and primary sinusitis can

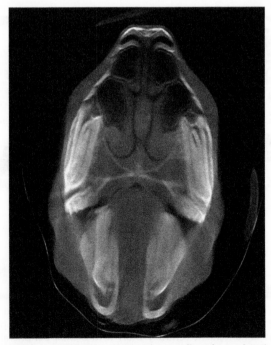

Fig. 3. Transverse cone beam CT image. Notice the excellent bony detail, marked streaking artifact, and lack of soft tissue contrast.

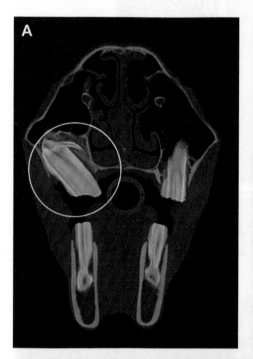
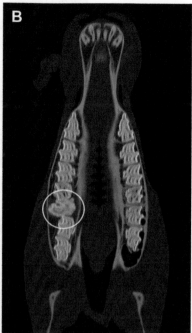

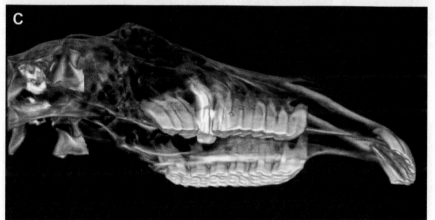

Fig. 4. Supernumerary tooth. (*A*) Transverse slice (bone window) centered on the supernumerary tooth between 109 and 110 and corresponding (*B*) dorsal plane. The circle denotes the malpositioned supernumerary tooth causing focal malocclusion. (*C*) A 3-D rendered model of the right maxillary arch.

be challenging on CT, particularly when concurrent dental lesions and sinopathy exist, which were almost a third of cases in 1 study[21] (**Fig. 10**).

SINUS DISEASE

Sinus disease in the horse can be divided into primary-acute, primary-chronic, dental, traumatic, sinus cyst, sinus neoplasia, mycotic, and ethmoid hematoma.[21]

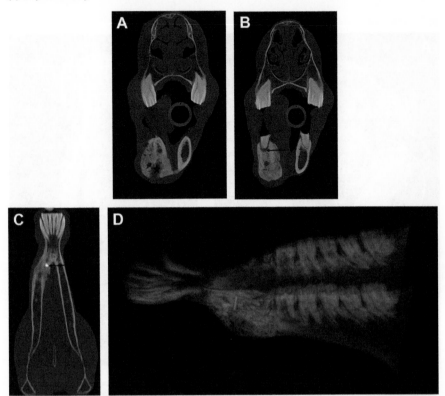

Fig. 5. Healed, right mandibular fracture and osteomyelitis. (*A*) Transverse image at the level of the interdental space revealing a large diameter draining tract (*star*). (*B*) Transverse image at the level of 407 revealing a moderately sized periapical lucency (*arrow*). (*C*) Dorsal plane of the healed right mandibular fracture with retained screw fragment (*arrow*). (*D*) A 3-D volume-rendered image.

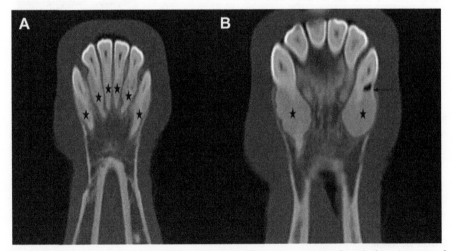

Fig. 6. Equine odontoclastic tooth resorption and hypercementosis: dorsal plane images of the mandibular incisors at differing levels. (*A*) Stars denote regions of moderate hypercementosis. (*B*) The arrow delineates a region of crown resorption.

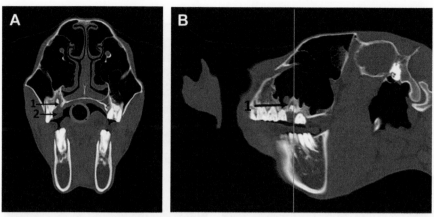

Fig. 7. (A) Crown-root fracture of the right maxillary second molar (110). (1) Mesial tooth root fracture. (2) Sagittal crown fracture. Transverse, bone window. (B) Mild right rostral maxillary sinusitis secondary to fracture of 110. The vertical line depicts the approximate location of the transverse image in (A). Small accumulation of sinus fluid/thick mucosa (1) in the right rostral maxillary sinus.

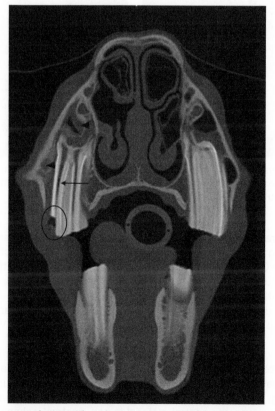

Fig. 8. Crown fracture of 108 with pulpitis, rostral maxillary sinusitis, and mild maxillary osteitis. Pulp gas (*arrow*), fluid within the rostral maxillary sinus with overlying maxillary osteitis (*arrowheads*), and crown fracture involving the pulp horn (*circle*).

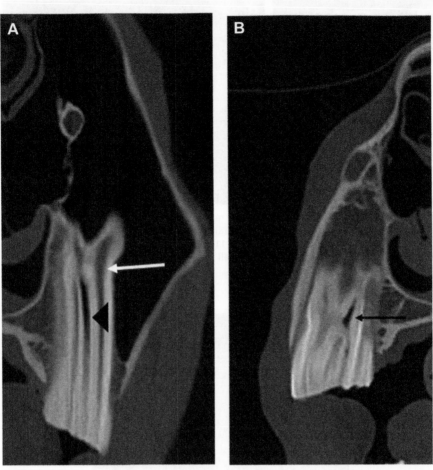

Fig. 9. (*A*) Transverse image at the level of the right maxillary fourth premolar (108). Infundibular gas (*arrowhead*) and normal pulp (*arrow*). (*B*) Left maxillary first molar (209) from a different horse; pulp gas (*arrow*).

Although radiography can be useful for sinus disease, CT is more sensitive and specific for localizing the paranasal sinuses affected.[21,22] The defining characteristics of sinus disease on CT include thick mucosa and fluid–to–soft tissue attenuating material within the sinus (**Fig. 11**). Descriptions of primary-acute sinusitis on CT are lacking in the literature, which likely is due to case selection and the efficacy of radiographs for diagnosis. Additional CT findings can help differentiate the types of sinus disease and are discussed later; dental origin signs were discussed previously.

Primary-chronic sinusitis affects all paranasal sinuses, with the caudal and rostral maxillary the most commonly affected.[21] Inspissated purulent material can have increased attenuation (see **Table 1**) and heterogeneous granular texture due to admixture with gas (**Fig. 12**). This tissue may display peripheral contrast enhancement due to thick mucosa; however, the central material is non–contrast enhancing. The ventral conchal sinus most commonly contains inspissated material.[21] Additionally, disease extension to the ventral and dorsal conchal bullae recently has been identified as a

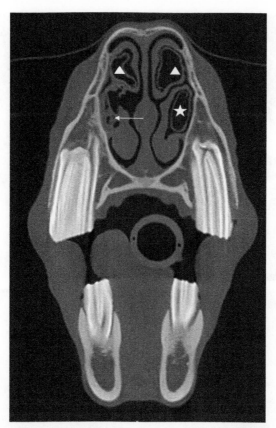

Fig. 10. Transverse image at the level of the right maxillary third premolar (107) revealing collapse and moderate thickening of the right ventral conchal bulla (*arrow*) secondary to dental associated (108) sinusitis. The left ventral conchal bulla (*star*) and dorsal conchal bulla (*arrowhead*)s are normal.

cause of sinusitis treatment failures.[23,24] Although primary fungal sinusitis of the conchal bullae is reported, a majority of the cases are secondary to dental disease (see **Fig. 10**). Traumatic sinusitis is characterized by concurrent skull fracture (**Fig. 13**). Upon evaluation of the soft tissue window, the HUs of the sinus material may be hyperattenuating, indicating acute hemorrhage. Sinus cysts are the most common paranasal sinus mass and have characteristic CT signs.[1,15,21,25] Sinus cysts are round-to-ovoid, fluid-attenuating, non–contrast enhancing, expansile masses that typically lead to thinning and distortion of the surrounding cortical bone. These lesions affect all of the paranasal sinuses, including the sphenopalatine sinus, as shown in **Fig. 14**. The anatomy of the sphenopalatine sinus has been reviewed.[26] Sinus neoplasia is a less common cause of equine sinonasal disease.[22,27] Common CT findings included erosion of the cribiform plate, invasion of the cranial cavity, and aggressive osteolysis. A majority of the masses were soft tissue attenuating and hypoattenuating to the masseter muscle; those that received intravenous contrast material displayed moderate enhancement (approximate increased 40 HUs).[22] No CT signs to discriminate between types of neoplasia (sarcoma, carcinoma, fibroma, and myxoma), however, were identified; biopsy is necessary for definitive diagnosis

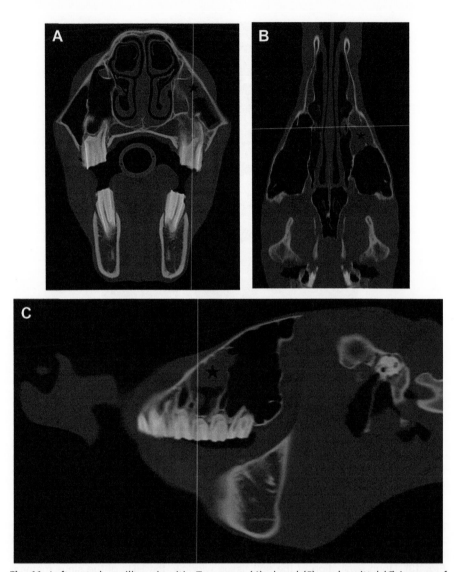

Fig. 11. Left rostral maxillary sinusitis. Transverse (*A*), dorsal (*B*), and sagittal (*C*) images of the left rostral maxillary sinus. Dependent fluid within the rostral maxillary sinus (*star*). The references lines in the dorsal and sagittal reconstructed images depict the approximate location of the transverse plane.

(**Fig. 15**). Ethmoid hematomas share CT characteristics with the aforementioned space occupying lesions of the paranasal sinuses; however, they also have criteria that allow for prioritized diagnosis. Typically, these masses arise from the ethmoturbinates and extend into the caudal maxillary sinus; however, reported cases involved all paranasal sinus (including sphenopalatine) and nasal cavities.[28] All masses were isoattenuating to hyperattenuating (average 101.6 HUs) compared with masseter muscle, and many displayed a hyperdense, swirling pattern[28] (**Fig. 16**). These masses commonly recur and can be bilateral.

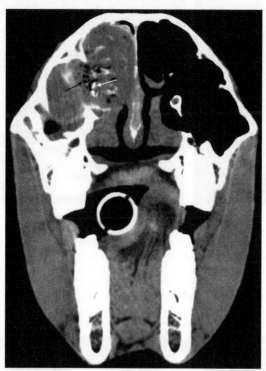

Fig. 12. The right frontal and maxillary sinus is filled with heterogeneous, partially inspissated material characterized by soft tissue attenuation admixed with gas (*black arrow*) and mineral (*white arrow*) foci.

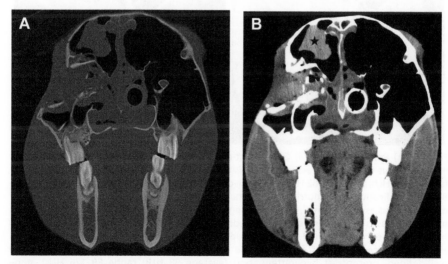

Fig. 13. Transverse CT images in bone (*A*) and soft tissue (*B*) algorithms. Severe right skull fractures from being kicked in the face. Hemorrhage within the right cochofrontal sinus is visible as hyperattenuating material (*star*).

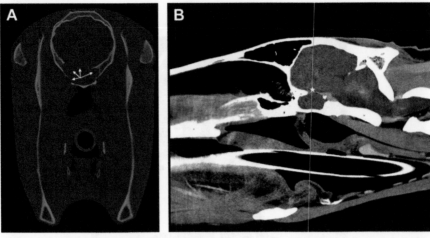

Fig. 14. Sphenopalatine cyst. (*A*) Transverse bone window; (*B*) sagittal soft tissue window. The sphenopalatine sinus contains a large (4.5-cm × 4.5-cm × 3.0 cm), fluid-attenuating (18 HUs), non–contrast-enhancing (21 HUs) mass. The mass causes severe, asymmetric expansion (right side > left side) of the sphenoidal portion of the sinus characterized by marked, focal thinning of the rostral floor of the cranium (*arrows*) and effacement of the normal topography of the right optic canal, both alar canals, and the right cavernous sinus (*arrows*). Dorsally, the mass (*star*) bulges into the cranial cavity causing mild, right, dorsal deviation of the rostral aspect of the cerebrum and pituitary gland (*arrowhead*). A thin, faintly mineralized rim of tissue separates the mass and the brain tissue.

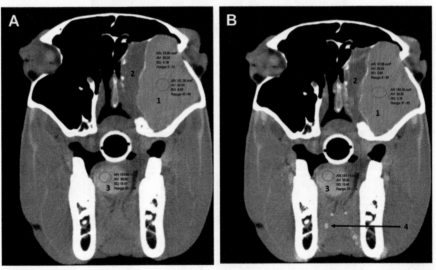

Fig. 15. (*A*) Precontrast and (*B*) CT contrast-enhanced scans of a horse with a left caudal maxillary sinus fibroma and associated sinusitis. The (1) fibroma is mildly hyperattenuating (average 62 HUs; range 43–82 HUs) and non–contrast enhancing (average 66 HUs; range 47–83 HUs), indicative of hemorrhage. The mass causes moderate expansion of the caudal maxillary sinus as well as small, multifocal regions of lysis of the left maxilla. The left rostral maxillary sinus is moderately displaced medially and contains a (2) large accumulation of non–contrast-enhancing fluid–to–soft tissue attenuation (average 23 HUs; range: 6–43 HUs). (3) The caudal aspect of the tongue contains a large (5.3-cm × 4.1-cm × 3.5-cm) well-defined, precontrast hyperattenuating (average 98 HUs; range 89–126 HUs), non–contrast-enhancing (average 92 HUs; range 67–113 HUs) mass; consistent with an incidental melanoma. (4) A normal hyperattenuating lingual vein indicates the image is post–contrast material administration.

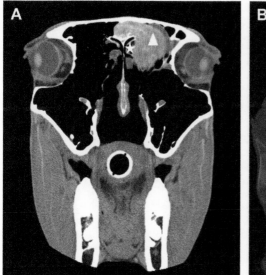
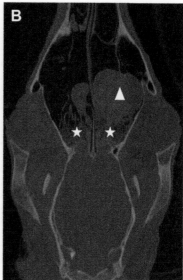

Fig. 16. Ethmoid hematoma. (*A*) Transverse (soft tissue window) at the rostral extent of the ethmoidal labyrinth. (*B*) Dorsal plane (bone window) at the level of the ethmoidal labyrinth. In both (*A*) and (*B*), the stars indicate the region of the ethmoidal conchae and the arrowhead is placed over the hematoma. Note in the soft tissue window how the hematoma is heterogeneous, characterized by regions of hyperattenuation and hypoattenuation consistent with different ages of hemorrhage (hyperattenuation, more acute; hypoattenuation, more chronic).

CASE EXAMPLES

To highlight the clinical relevance of CT, 2 cases are presented with initial radiographs and comparison CT scan. The first case discusses a 20-year-old Thoroughbred mare with chronic right nasal discharge (**Figs. 17** and **18**). In this case, the radiographic findings were subtle, and additional imaging (oral and nasal endoscopy as well as CT) was

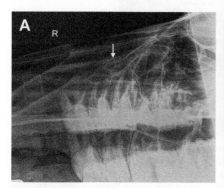
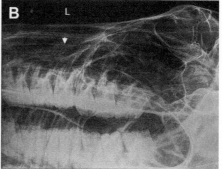

Fig. 17. Radiographs of a 20-year-old Thoroughbred mare with chronic right nasal discharge. (*A*) Right oblique radiograph of the maxillary arch and sinuses. Arrow indicates an ill-defined, granular soft tissue opacity at the level of the ventral conchal sinus; 109 has a crown fracture. No tooth root lesion is detected. (*B*) Left oblique radiograph of the maxillary arch and sinuses; the arrowhead indicates normal comparison of the ventral conchal sinus. CT was obtained to better characterize the cause of the sinusitis.

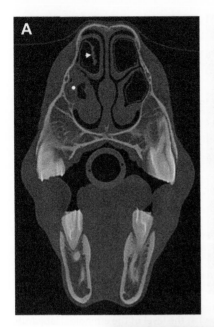
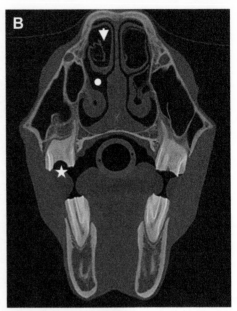
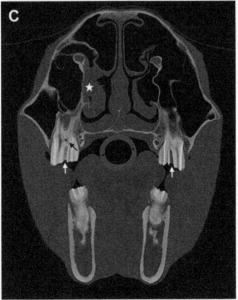

Fig. 18. Representative transverse CT slices (bone algorithm). (*A*) Level of granular material on radiograph (distal 107). Circle indicates collapse of the right ventral conchal bulla with thick fungal plaques. Arrowhead indicates mild thickening and fungal plaques of the right dorsal conchal bulla. The left side is normal. (*B*) Level of 109 crown fracture (*star*). No root lesion or communication with the sinuses is detected. The circle shows absence of the right ventral conchal bulla but no sinusitis. The arrowhead indicates slight collapse of the right dorsal conchal bulla. (*C*) Level of 110. Wide infundibula are present bilaterally (*white arrows*) with gas on the right (*black arrow*). The star indicates ventral conchal sinusitis, which was due to the fungal sinonasal disease, not dental origin.

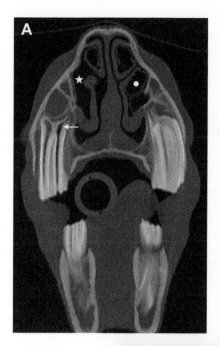
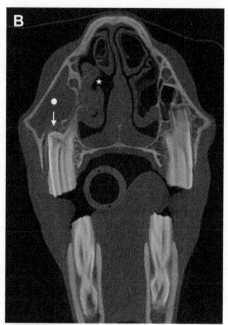
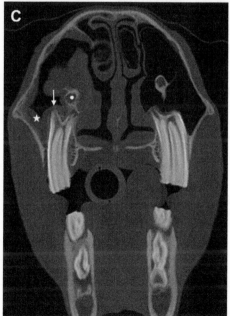

Fig. 19. Representative transverse CT slices (bone algorithm). (*A*) Level of 108. Arrow indicates gas within the pulp. Star indicates absence (collapse) of the right ventral conchal bulla. Circle indicates normal left ventral conchal bulla. (*B*) Level of 109. The right rostral maxillary sinus is filled with fluid-attenuating material (*circle*). There is a fistula between the right ventral conchal sinus and nasal cavity (*star*). At this level there is periapical lysis of 109 (*arrow*). (*C*) Level of 110. The caudal maxillary sinus has thick mucosa (*star*) and a small amount of fluid. There is periapical lysis of 110 (*arrow*). The infraorbital canal is displaced (*circle*) with mild periosteal reaction and surrounding fluid-attenuating content.

necessary to make a diagnosis of primary fungal sinusitis. The second case discusses a 7-year-old gray mare with dental origin sinusitis and extension into the ventral conchal bulla (**Fig. 19**).

SUMMARY

CT has an important role as a diagnostic tool for equine dental and sinonasal disease. The cross-sectional nature of the modality allows for more accurate anatomic localization of abnormal soft tissue opacity within the equine skull, thereby leading to appropriately targeted medical and surgical interventions. In particular, differentiating between primary sinusitis and dental-origin sinusitis is a diagnostic dilemma where radiographs often cannot elucidate a clear answer. The high spatial resolution of CT allows the visualization of pulp gas and subtle alveolar bone loss, thereby aiding the identification of dental disease that may not visible on radiographs. Although CT remains relatively expensive, the added diagnostic information that guides proper case management is invaluable. As technology continues to improve, more and more horses will have access to this diagnostic tool and it is important for the equine clinician to become comfortable with basic CT interpretation.

REFERENCES

1. Boulton CH. Equine nasal cavity and paranasal sinus disease: a review of 85 cases. J Equine Vet Sci 1985;5(5):268–75.
2. Manso-Díaz G, García-López JM, Maranda L, et al. The role of head computed tomography in equine practice. Equine Vet Educ 2015;27(3):136–45.
3. Selberg K, Easley JT. Advanced imaging in equine dental disease. Vet Clin North Am Equine Pract 2013;29(2):397–409.
4. Tucker RL, Farrell E. Computed tomography and magnetic resonance imaging of the equine head. The Veterinary Clinics of North America. Equine Practice, 2001;17(1). https://doi.org/10.1016/S0749-0739(17)30079-2.
5. Probst A, Henninger W, Willmann M. Communications of normal nasal and paranasal cavities in computed tomography of horses. Vet Radiol Ultrasound 2005; 46(1):44–8.
6. Puchalski SM. Advances in equine computed tomography and use of contrast media. Vet Clin North Am Equine Pract 2012;28(3):563–81.
7. Carmalt JL, Montgomery J. Intraarterial injection of iodinated contrast medium for contrast enhanced computed tomography of the equine head. Vet Radiol Ultrasound 2015;56(4):384–90.
8. Lacombe VA, Sogaro-Robinson C, Reed SM. Diagnostic utility of computed tomography imaging in equine intracranial conditions. Equine Vet J 2010;42(5): 393–9.
9. Kinns J, Pease A. Computed tomography in the evaluation of the equine head. Equine Vet Educ 2009;21(6):291–4.
10. Dakin SG, Lam R, Rees E, et al. Technical set-up and radiation exposure for standing computed tomography of the equine head. Equine Vet Educ 2014; 26(4):208–15.
11. Bregger MDK, Koch C, Zimmermann R, et al. Cone-beam computed tomography of the head in standing equids. BMC Vet Res 2019;15(1):289.
12. Liuti T, Smith S, Dixon PM. Radiographic, computed tomographic, gross pathological and histological findings with suspected apical infection in 32 equine maxillary cheek teeth (2012–2015). Equine Vet J 2018;50(1):41–7.

13. Henninger W. CT features of alveolitis and sinusitis in horses. Vet Radiol Ultrasound 2003;44(3):269–76.
14. Bühler M, Fürst A, Lewis FI, et al. Computed tomographic features of apical infection of equine maxillary cheek teeth: a retrospective study of 49 horses. Equine Vet J 2014;46(4):468–73.
15. Tremaine WH, Dixon PM. A long-term study of 277 cases of equine sinonasal disease. Part 1: details of horses, historical, clinical and ancillary diagnostic findings. Equine Vet J 2010;33(3):274–82.
16. Windley Z, Weller R, Tremaine WH, et al. Two- and three-dimensional computed tomographic anatomy of the enamel, infundibulae and pulp of 126 equine cheek teeth. Part 1: findings in teeth without macroscopic occlusal or computed tomographic lesions. Equine Vet J 2009;41(5):433–40.
17. Kopke S, Angrisani N, Staszyk C. The dental cavities of equine cheek teeth: three-dimensional reconstructions based on high resolution micro-computed tomography. 2012. Available at: http://www.biomedcentral.com/1746-6148/8/173. Accessed January 5, 2020.
18. Veraa S, Voorhout G, Klein WR. Computed tomography of the upper cheek teeth in horses with infundibular changes and apical infection. Equine Vet J 2009;41(9):872–6.
19. Brinkschulte M, Bienert-Zeit A, Lüpke M, et al. Using semi-automated segmentation of computed tomography datasets for three-dimensional visualization and volume measurements of equine paranasal sinuses. Vet Radiol Ultrasound 2013;54(6):582–90.
20. Barakzai SZ, Barnett TP. Computed tomography and scintigraphy for evaluation of dental disease in the horse. Equine Vet Educ 2015;27(6):323–31.
21. Dixon PM, Parkin TD, Collins N, et al. Equine paranasal sinus disease: a long-term study of 200 cases (1997-2009): ancillary diagnostic findings and involvement of the various sinus compartments. Equine Vet J 2012;44(3):267–71.
22. Cissell DD, Wisner ER, Textor J, et al. Computed tomographic appearance of equine sinonasal neoplasia. Vet Radiol Ultrasound 2012;53(3):245–51.
23. Liuti T, Reardon R, Smith S, et al. An anatomical study of the dorsal and ventral nasal conchal bullae in normal horses: computed tomographic anatomical and morphometric findings. Equine Vet J 2016;48(6):749–55.
24. Dixon PM, Froydenlund T, Liuti T, et al. Empyema of the nasal conchal bulla as a cause of chronic unilateral nasal discharge in the horse: 10 cases (2013-2014). Equine Vet J 2015;47(4):445–9.
25. Annear MJ, Gemensky-Metzler AJ, Elce YA, et al. Exophthalmus secondary to a sinonasal cyst in a horse. J Am Vet Med Assoc 2008;233(2):285–8.
26. Tucker R, Windley ZE, Abernethy AD, et al. Radiographic, computed tomographic and surgical anatomy of the equine sphenopalatine sinus in normal and diseased horses. Equine Vet J 2016;48(5):578–84.
27. Head KW, Dixon PM. Equine nasal and paranasal sinus tumours. Part 1: review of the literature and tumour classification. Vet J 1999;157(3):261–79.
28. Textor JA, Puchalski SM, Affolter VK, et al. Results of computed tomography in horses ethomoid hematoma. J Am Vet Med Assoc 2012;240(11):1338–44.

Equine Oral Extraction Techniques

Jon M. Gieche, DVM, Fellow AVD EQ

KEYWORDS

- Equine • Extraction • Oral • Spreader • Dentistry • Forceps • Luxation • Elevation

KEY POINTS

- Luxation is any process that breaks down the soft tissue attachment (Periodontal ligaments – PDL) to loosen a tooth from its alveolus.
- Elevation refers to the removal of the tooth from the alveolus. It is achieved with minimal force following complete luxation.
- Oral extraction of cheek teeth commonly utilize spreaders, forceps, fulcrums and local levers.
- Tipping, rotation and vertical forces are used for disruption of the PDL.
- Procedural steps of oral extraction include soft tissue elevation, interproximal spreading, placement of forceps on the clinical crown, utilizing a fulcrum, local luxation, tooth elevation and alveolar protection.

Video content accompanies this article at http://www.vetequine.theclinics.com.

INTRODUCTION

Oral extraction of equine cheek teeth (premolars and molars) is well within the capability of the primary care veterinarian with proper case selection and preparation. Comprehensive patient examination and diagnostic evaluation should be performed before development and execution of the treatment plan. Clinicians should consider numerous factors before proceeding with an oral extraction, including degree of bone attachment (periodontal disease status),[1] clinical crown integrity, and root morphology. Before an extraction procedure, case difficulty, equipment (diagnostic and treatment), experience, and availability of specialty consultation should be considered. Clients should be informed of the potential for complications before, during, and after the procedure. Should complications arise, a referral to

Kettle Moraine Equine Hospital & Regional Equine Dental Center, N8818 HWY 67, Whitewater, WI 53190, USA
E-mail address: kmehredc@gmail.com

Vet Clin Equine 36 (2020) 545–564
https://doi.org/10.1016/j.cveq.2020.08.010
0749-0739/20/© 2020 Elsevier Inc. All rights reserved.

an equine veterinary dental specialist or advanced veterinary care facility may be indicated.

All extraction techniques discussed in this article can be performed in the standing sedated patient. Specific sedative protocols, as well as local and regional anesthetic techniques used during extractions, vary depending on dentist preference. Descriptions may be found in the Luis Campoy and Samantha R. Sedgwick's article, "Standing Sedation and Analgesia in Equine Dental Surgery," elsewhere in this issue. Extraction of cheek teeth is based on disrupting the periodontal ligament and its attachment to alveolar bone. The periodontal ligament is oriented in multiple planes[2] to accommodate the forces of mastication. The extraction process uses instrumentation for mechanical leverage of force along the similar planes to break down the ligament attachments. Forces used for disruption of the periodontal ligament include tipping (mesiodistal and buccal-lingual/palatal), rotation around the axis of the tooth, vertical along the axis of the tooth and local cutting/tearing of the ligament.

INDICATIONS

Indications for exodontia include severe periodontal disease, untreatable dental disease (eg, dental fracture/cavity, endodontic, resorptive), interception of orthodontic disease, pain relief and extension of disease to other teeth, and regional tissue/anatomy. All reasonable attempts to save the teeth should be undertaken. If this fails, extraction is the alternative to the advancement of disease and/or an unnecessary painful existence for the patient. Clinical case examples would include the following:

- Nonvital teeth that are no longer functional and increase the risk of disease advancement to proximal dentition or other juxtaposed tissue.
- Dental pathology associated with a clinical crown fracture involving pulp horn(s) and extending into the reserve crown/root(s).
- Clinical crown fractures that do not involve the pulp horn(s) but are associated with periodontal disease or endodontic disease due to periodontal extension through the root(s) (periodontic – endodontic disease processes).[3,4]
- Painful malocclusions or periodontal disease processes that fail to respond to other treatments resulting in the need for extraction.

EQUIPMENT/SUPPLIES

Proper examination of the dentition and surrounding tissues before and throughout the extraction procedure is critical to a successful outcome. Instrument placement must be monitored during the extraction procedure with an intraoral mirror or oral endoscope. Alveolar contents and packing materials are evaluated during and post extraction. Minimum extraction instrumentation should include gingival elevators, molar spreaders, molar extraction forceps, fragment/root forceps, and extraction fulcrums, along with an assortment of right-angled and straight elevators and luxators. Required ancillary equipment should include a full mouth speculum, bright light source, mirror and/or oral endoscope, and radiographic equipment. When available, advanced imaging equipment such as computed tomography may be helpful but is not usually necessary for the standard nonsurgical extraction.

Gingival Elevators

Gingival elevators are used to separate/dissect the attached gingiva from the crown of the tooth and surrounding marginal bone. They are usually on "T" handles and face either buccally or lingual/palatal. The working edge of the gingival elevator should be sharp with an acute edge. It is not meant to be a cutting tool with a knife edge (**Fig. 1**).

Molar Spreaders

Molar spreaders are designed to apply controlled force to maxillary and mandibular premolars and molars in a mesiodistal direction resulting in a tipping motion that gradually fatigues and ruptures the periodontal ligament fibers. They are wedged in the interproximal space on either side of the tooth being luxated, sequentially forcing it to tip mesially and distally. Intraoral imaging/viewing is necessary for precise blade engagement between the 2 teeth. As the tooth loosens and the proximal teeth are slightly displaced, the thickness of the spreader blades is increased. There are many molar spreader designs available (**Fig. 2**). Types that can be disarticulated at the hinge allow for multiple variations in spreader blade size combinations (**Fig. 3**). This type may also be assembled with a spreader on one side and forceps on the other side, allowing for even greater flexibility in technique when needed (**Fig. 4**).

Molar Extraction Forceps

Molar extraction forceps are available in a multitude of configurations using different working heads, shafts, and handles. Forceps are designed to fit the tooth with maximum purchase of the of the working head to the clinical crown. This allows

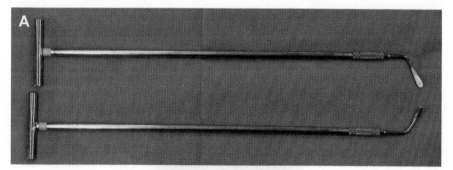

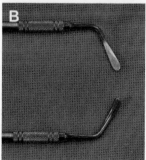

Fig. 1. Gingival elevators. (A) T-handled gingival elevators, acute adage (*top*), blunt edge (*bottom*). (B) Expanded view of (A).

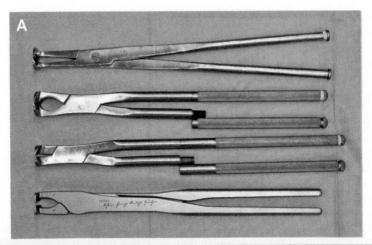

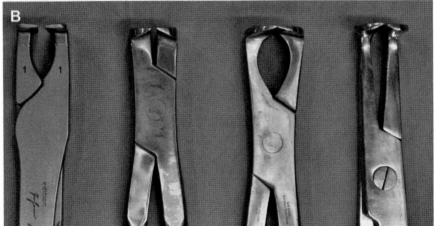

Fig. 2. Molar spreaders. (*A*) Common spreader types. Note the different jaw and handle types as well as blade thicknesses. (*B*) Expanded view of spreader joints and jaws in (*A*).

mechanical forces to be transmitted directly to the tooth without slippage or damage to the crown. General categories of extraction forceps include maxillary, mandibular, reverse fulcrum, root tip/fragment, left and right 3 pronged, and 4 pronged (**Fig. 5**). Proper purchase of forceps will require more than 1 size to accommodate the differences in clinical crown shape of mandibular and maxillary teeth as well as breed difference and individual patient variation (**Fig. 6**). When 2-pronged forceps are applied to the tooth, each prong contact surface should apply pressure to the tooth evenly across its entire contact surface. This reduces the risk of fracture due to increased point pressure on one area of the tooth. As the integrity of the clinical crown deteriorates, the purchase capability of a 2-pronged forceps is reduced. Three-pronged forceps are designed to "straddle" the roots of maxillary cheek teeth when there is minimal clinical and reserve crown present. The 2-pronged side of the forceps straddles the palatal root while the one-pronged side rests in the furcation between the mesial and distal buccal roots (**Fig. 7**). This increases the contact surface area, decreasing the risk of fracture due to excessive point pressure on the

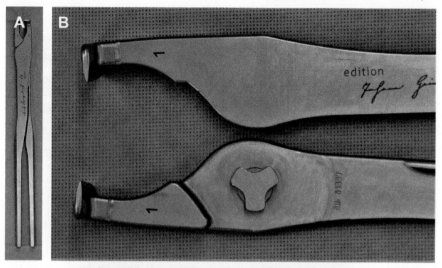

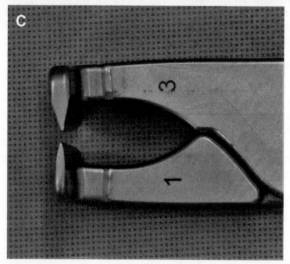

Fig. 3. Interchangeable handled spreader. (*A*) Assembled spreader. (*B*) Expanded view of disassembled spreader joint and jaws. (*C*) Expanded view of reassembled spreader with a thin and thick spreader blade combination.

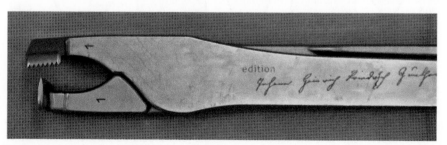

Fig. 4. Interchangeable handled spreader/forceps with forceps on one side and a spreader on the other.

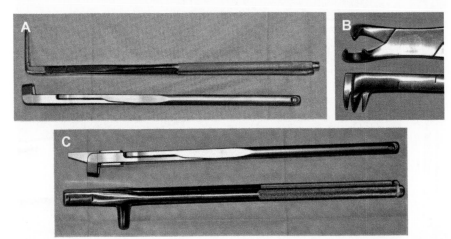

Fig. 5. Molar (premolar and molar) forceps examples. (*A*) Root tip forceps with thin extended prongs for reaching deep into the alveolus to retrieve root tips (*top*) and standard 2-pronged maxillary/mandibular forceps for grasping the exposed crown during manipulation and delivery of the tooth into the oral cavity (*bottom*). (*B*) Maxillary molar 3-pronged forceps. (*C*) Reverse fulcrum molar forceps with detachable fulcrum extension (*top*) and permanent fulcrum extension (*bottom*).

tooth. Four-pronged forceps are used to increase contact with certain dysplastic teeth and in aged patients with severely blunted root tips. Reverse fulcrum forceps have an extension attached to the distal end of the working head. They are advantageous when the target tooth does not have a mesial tooth. In addition, they are useful for creating a vertical extraction force (along the long axis of the tooth) in a slightly caudal direction (see **Fig. 5**C).

Extraction Fulcrums

Fulcrums are used in conjunction with extraction forceps to create a vertical mechanical force along the long axis of the tooth. They may be placed in a "normal rostral"

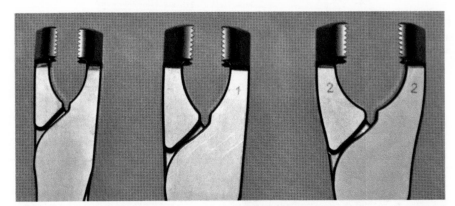

Fig. 6. Molar forceps sizes. Miniature horse/pony, mandibular, and maxillary molar sizes, left to right respectively. Note the contact area of the jaws should be parallel to each other when applied if they fit the tooth perfectly. This decreases excessive point pressure that may fracture the tooth.

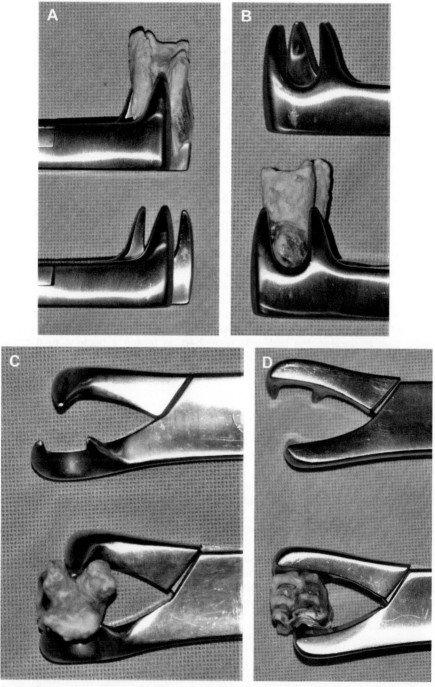

Fig. 7. Three-pronged molar forceps demonstrating proper application on a preserved extracted maxillary molar. (*A*) Buccal view illustrating the single prong between the mesial and distal buccal roots. (*B*) Palatal view illustrating 2 prongs straddling the palatal root. (*C*) Apical view illustrating both (*A*) and (*B*). (*D*) Occlusal view.

position (on the side of the tooth nearest the forceps handles) or a "reverse caudal" position (on the side of the tooth opposite the forceps handles) when used with reverse fulcrum forceps. Choice of fulcrum position will depend on the tooth being extracted and the eruption pathway of the tooth. Fulcrums come in a variety of sizes, shapes, and materials designed to achieve the desired mechanical advantage while maintaining their desired position (**Fig. 8**).

Dental Luxators and Elevators

Luxators are instruments with a very sharp and thin blade designed to locally incise the periodontal ligament. They are inserted into the periodontal ligament (PDL) space and advanced cautiously in an apical direction. Then they are withdrawn, repositioned, and worked circumferentially around the tooth, incising as much of the PDL as possible to loosen the tooth/tooth fragments.

Elevators are sharp instruments that are designed to be inserted into the PDL space between tooth and marginal alveolar bone (**Fig. 9**). They are carefully torqued axially to break down the PDL fibers and expanding marginal bone. An increasing constant force (15–40 seconds) will fatigue the PDL fibers to the point of failure.

Elevators and luxators are often used to loosen fragmented cheek teeth, cementomas, and sequestra. Occasionally they are used with other luxation techniques to achieve breakdown of the PDL with intact teeth or large tooth fragments. Primary breakdown of the PDL in these cases is more commonly accomplished with spreaders, molar forceps, and fulcrums. Elevation technique has been described using a "dental pick" with fractured cheek teeth. Although the true definition of a dental pick is unclear, the pick was described as having a blade 4 to 8 cm in length that worked as an elevator. Successful oral extraction was reported at 87% when using an oral endoscope for site-specific elevation along the axis of the reserve crown.[5]

METHOD

Before any attempt of an extraction procedure, a comprehensive patient evaluation should be performed entailing a minimum of a physical, oral, and radiographic examination. To reduce patient risk, concomitant systemic disease processes are managed before executing the extraction. Extraction procedures described here are performed in the standing, sedated patient, with appropriate local and regional anesthesia administered. See the Luis Campoy and Samantha R. Sedgwick's article, "Standing Sedation and Analgesia in Equine Dental Surgery," elsewhere in this issue.

Preprocedural imaging is required to aid planning and help assess the potential risk of complications. It is imperative that the clinician be aware of potential complicating factors before attempting the extraction. Complicating factors are assessed systemically (eg, Cushing disease, insulin resistance, chronic weight

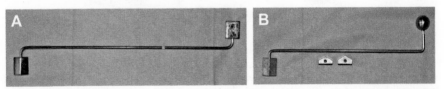

Fig. 8. Fulcrum examples. (*A*) Double-ended fixed fulcrum. (*B*) Fulcrum handle with interchangeable, variably sized fulcrums.

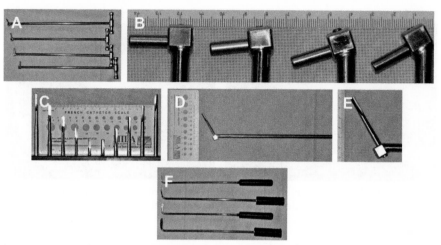

Fig. 9. Examples of elevators. (*A*) T-handles for interchangeable variable length elevators. 0, 8, 18, and 30-degree working angulation from bottom to top, respectively. (*B*) Expanded view of angled heads in (*A*) with blanks inserted and held in place with set screws. (*C*) Interchangeable 4-mm and 5-mm elevators for use in T-handles shown in (*A*) and (*B*). (*D*) 30-degree T-handle with 70-mm-long × 5-mm wide elevator inserted. (*E*) Expanded view of (*D*). (*F*) Examples of fixed, 90° bent end elevators, with smooth and knurled rubber handles.

loss, laminitis), regionally (head trauma, facial swelling, sinus disease) and locally (eg, root morphology, oral soft tissue trauma, tooth/bone fracture). Following the patient evaluation and complication assessment, the best treatment/extraction plan is determined. An alternative extraction plan is established should the primary plan fail to extract the tooth. If both plans fail at oral extraction, a surgical extraction plan is identified that may require referral to a specialist. The patient evaluation, complication assessment, and extraction plans are discussed with the client (and referring veterinarian if indicated) before executing the extraction procedure.

With the patient properly examined and prepped for the extraction procedure, the following are the procedural steps of oral extraction for both maxillary and mandibular cheek teeth:

1. Soft tissue elevation (gingival and mucosal) to the level of the alveolar margin.
2. Use of spreaders to luxate the target tooth along the alveolar margin in a distal and mesial direction
3. Attaching molar forceps to further luxate the tooth and distort alveolar bone. A mechanical lever is created to apply rotational forces around the axis of the tooth along with tipping in a buccal and lingual/palatal direction.
4. Additional luxation using a fulcrum in conjunction with molar forceps to create a mechanical leverage force in a vertical direction along the axis of the tooth.
5. Optional local site-specific luxation with levers that cut (luxator) or tear (elevator) the PDL. It may be necessary to cycle back to steps 2, 3, and 4 for additional loosening of the tooth.
6. Elevation of the tooth from the alveolus.
7. Protection of the alveolus/alveolar contents.
8. Develop a post extraction plan for aftercare and follow-up.

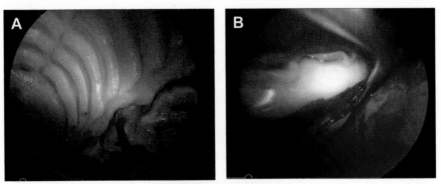

Fig. 10. (*A, B*) Gingival elevation. (*A*) Gingival elevator entering the gingival sulcus of a maxillary molar. (*B*) Gingival elevation of a mandibular molar.

Specific techniques and time spent performing each of the procedural steps will vary greatly depending on age, clinical crown integrity, degree of PDL attachment, and reserve crown/root morphology.

Soft Tissue Elevation

The goal of gingival elevation is to incise the gingival attachments from the tooth to allow for instrumentation around the tooth while minimizing trauma to the gingival soft tissues. The gingival elevator's face should be directed toward the tooth with the toe of the instrument entering the gingival sulcus (**Fig. 10**, Video 1A, B). Firm pressure is applied in an apical direction while maintaining contact with the tooth surface to gently drive the gingival elevator toe along the surface of the tooth toward the alveolar crestal bone. Once the toe of the gingival elevator contacts the crestal bone, the elevator is withdrawn occlusally and the process is repeated along the buccal and palatal/lingual surface of the tooth to completely dissect the attached gingiva from the tooth (**Fig. 11**). A gentle mesiodistal force may also be used to dissect the gingiva

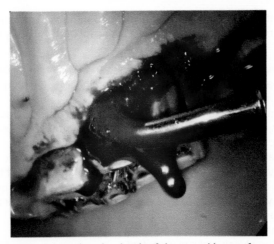

Fig. 11. Gingival elevator inserted to the depth of the crestal bone of a maxillary molar during gingival elevation.

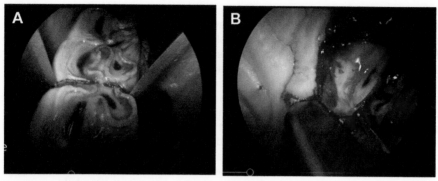

Fig. 12. (*A, B*) Spreader placement. (*A*) Oral endoscopic visual inspection to ensure proper spreader placement in an interproximal space within the mandibular arcade. (*B*) Oral endoscopic visual inspection to ensure proper spreader placement in an interproximal space within the maxillary arcade.

from the tooth. Careful attention should be exercised in the area of the interproximal space so as not to dissect gingiva from the adjacent teeth. Aggressive use of this instrument may cause tissue damage resulting in soft tissue pocketing, infection, greater palatine artery laceration, or instrument failure/breakage.

Molar Luxation with Spreading

Spreading applies mesiodistal tipping force to the tooth using the principal of a wedge (or 2 inclined planes) on the clinical crown. Spreaders are positioned directly into the interproximal spaces between the tooth to be extracted and the proximal tooth, contacting as much of each tooth as possible to the depth of the crestal bone while avoiding injury to the gingiva. Inappropriate engagement results in injury to teeth, bone, or soft tissues. Positioning should be aided by a mirror or an oral endoscope (**Fig. 12**, Video 2A, B). By design, spreading may unintentionally move multiple teeth. Location of the target tooth, spreader design (angle, thickness, and size of the blades), and force applied will affect the amount of movement between the target and anchor tooth., Significant mechanical advantage is achieved with spreaders, and tooth

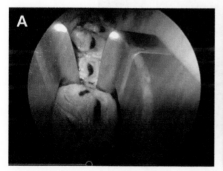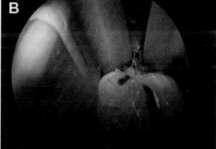

Fig. 13. (*A, B*) Tipping caused by sequential spreading of the molars. (*A*) Figure and video of a closed initial (thinnest) spreader with the resulting occlusal interproximal gap caused by the tipping of the tooth. (*B*) Figure and video of a closed final (thickest) spreader with the resulting occlusal gap. Note the increase in gap width from (*A*) to (*B*).

fracture is a complication of excessive force application. Generally, the initial spreader will use the thinnest blade for applying an even force to the target tooth and the proximal tooth (**Fig. 13**, Video 3A, B). Each application of the spreader may last from 5 to 10 minutes. Once the initial spreading has been completed on either the mesial or distal side of the target tooth and the spreader may be closed, the spreader is slowly removed and placed on the opposite side of the target tooth. Using the same technique, the tooth is tipped back toward the side of original spreader placement. This process continues back and forth on each side of the target tooth until there is little or no resistance to the current spreader. At this point, the next spreader of increasing thickness is applied in the same manner and the sequential process is continued to the point tooth movement is significant (indicating advancing failure of the PDL) or the thickest spreader blade size has been used, whichever results first. Force may be applied through the spreader handles by hand, or, to prevent clinician fatigue, clamps or rubber innertube material may be used (**Fig. 14**). In specific cases in which a large diastema prevents effective standard spreader use, the largest spreader may be placed interproximally in the closed position and its toe tipped mesially and distally by raising and lowering the handles vertically to achieve spreading. Extreme care should be exercised when using this technique, as the force from the spreader is concentrated over smaller areas of the teeth, increasing the risk of fracture (both target and anchor tooth). In addition, this technique may bend spreaders if excessive force is applied in a direction for which the spreader was not intended.

When considering whether the mesial or distal side of the tooth should be spread first, it is important to consider the rest of the arcade and the architecture of the tooth being spread. When the target tooth is the second cheek tooth, spreading between the first and second cheek teeth may move the first cheek tooth primarily. This is due to the anchor tooth (first cheek tooth) lacking structural bone support and a proximal supporting tooth along the rostral aspect. For this reason, it is generally preferable to first spread on the side of the target tooth that has the greater number of teeth sequentially proximal to it. This provides a more substantial base from which to apply the force for tipping of the desired tooth. Dilacerated curved roots should also be considered when spreading. Spreading initially on the convex aspect of the eruption path curvature is preferred. Generally, this applies less stress to root tips compared with spreading on the concave curvature of the eruption path. Clinicians should fully

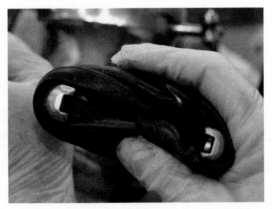

Fig. 14. Rubber bicycle innertube applied to forceps handles helping decrease operator fatigue.

contemplate the effects of forces they will be applying to all teeth before the extraction.

Molar Luxation with Forceps

Molar forceps are applied after spreading has been performed. Regardless of the style of forceps chosen, they must be able to achieve certain criteria for any tooth to which they will be applied. Some forceps will be more applicable than others, but all must fit the tooth well to prevent damaging the tooth and slippage when forces are applied to loosen and extract the tooth. If spreading does not loosen the tooth to the point it can be elevated from the alveolus (and it usually does not), additional forces will need to be applied to continue luxation. Transmitting forces applied through the handles of the forceps to the tooth efficiently, and with minimal damage to the tooth, requires a firm attachment without slippage. If slippage occurs, it will limit the ability to loosen the tooth and cause crown fragmentation that prevents adequate purchase of the crown with forceps (**Fig. 15**).

Once the appropriate forceps have been chosen and correctly applied (contacting as much tooth surface as possible), the application of force commences. Once the leverage of the forceps is engaged with the tooth, there are 2 primary forces applied for further luxation. Rotation around the long axis of the tooth, and tipping of the tooth in a linguobuccal/buccolingual direction. Rotation is achieved by applying force in the plane perpendicular to the average long axis of the tooth. The long axis of first cheek tooth tends to tip slightly in a caudal direction, whereas the fifth and sixth cheek teeth tip rostrally.[6–9] It may be beneficial to raise or lower the forceps handles to achieve an angle more perpendicular to the long axis of the tooth in these cases. In addition, a specialty forceps with an angled working head will accommodate the axial tipping

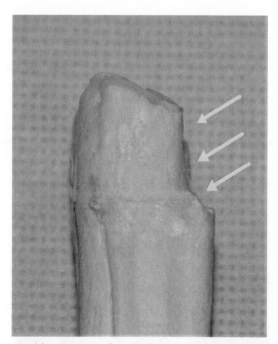

Fig. 15. Damage caused by slippage of molar forceps. Damage to the buccal aspect of a mandibular molar (*yellow arrows*) due to inadequate application of the molar forceps.

of the tooth while orienting the handles parallel to the occlusal line of the arcade. Application of rotational force is achieved with clockwise and counter-clockwise application of a constant force around the axis of the tooth resulting in a rotational stress to break down the PDL. Because alveolar bone is somewhat malleable, this force may also slightly modify 3-dimensional bony architectural impedances, thus aiding extraction (Video 4). Time frame of the "hold" phase of force application will vary depending on the individual case and the current point of elevation achieved. Initially firm but not aggressive force is applied for longer periods (2–3 minutes) in each direction. As the PDL fails (you may hear this as a "crinkling" sound or "feel" it through the forceps handles) and bone conformation changes, the tooth becomes loose in the alveolus. Even when loose, the tooth may not be ready for elevation due to alveolar and dental anatomy, and it may be necessary to use vertical force (fulcrum) or local periodontal ligament release (luxator or elevator) for additional luxation of the tooth (Video 5).

Tipping of the tooth buccally and lingually is executed to further break down the PDL and reshape malleable bone similar to using rotational force. The force is applied by rolling the handles of the forceps right and left relative to the long axis of the handles. Roll and hold the handles to transmit the tipping forces to the tooth (Videos 6 and 7). Methods and results are similar to those described in rotational forces previously. The exception being the force is applied along a different vector, resulting in tipping rather than rotation of the tooth. Frequently, "sloshing" sounds and "frothy blood" may be noted during manipulation when significant rupture of the PDL has occurred (**Fig. 16**).

Additional Luxation with Fulcrums

Vertical extrusional force is applied to loosen the tooth from the alveolus. Fulcrums are placed as close to the tooth to be extracted as possible. Extrusional force is applied along the longitudinal axis of the tooth's eruption path. Careful attention to the direction of this path is essential to decrease the likelihood of complications, especially tooth fracture during elevation from the alveolus. Frequently eruption paths are not straight. They may be curvilinear in one or more directions. This will factor in on the choice of extraction forceps to be applied, the direction of force application, choice of standard or reverse fulcruming, style of fulcrum, and thickness of fulcrum used. Size and conformation of the tooth also will play a role in proper extraction technique. Short, aged teeth, with very short eruption paths remaining, will usually luxate well with the force applied perpendicular to the occlusal plane of the premolar/molar arcade. Long, young to middle age teeth, with eruption angles acute or obtuse to the occlusal

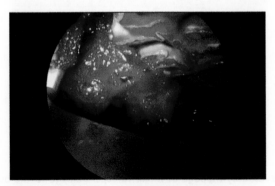

Fig. 16. Oral endoscopy: frothy blood associated with elevation.

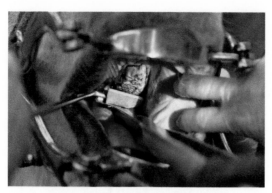

Fig. 17. Fulcrum placement during delivery of a maxillary molar.

plane of the arcade will fare better if extraction forces accommodate these angles (**Fig. 17**). Force is applied to the forceps handles either toward or away from the occlusal surface of the proximal tooth depending on whether standard or reverse fulcrum forceps are used, respectively. Progressively thicker fulcrums may be used sequentially in the extraction process of long teeth. Alternatively, the forceps head can be moved apically along the reserve crown to use the same fulcrum.

Optional Local Luxation (Luxators and Elevators)

Appropriately loosened teeth elevate from the alveolus with minimal force. In the event greater force is needed, complications should be expected, and reevaluation of the patient and technique are indicated. Occasionally, local luxation will aid in the extraction process in conjunction with the use of spreaders, forceps, and fulcrums. More commonly, local luxation is used with reserve crown and root fragments following an incomplete extraction (**Fig. 18**, Video 8). Placement of these instruments should be assisted with a mirror or oral endoscope. The blade is placed in the PDL space tearing/shearing around the fragment to the point the loose fragment may be grasped with root tip forceps, fragment forceps, or teased from the alveolus (**Fig. 19**). If these fail, more advanced techniques may be indicated (see Travis Henry and Ian Bishop's article, "Adjunct Extraction Techniques in Equine Dentistry"; and Edward T. Earley and

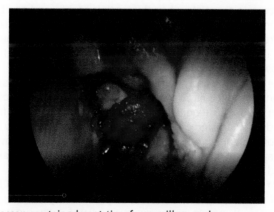

Fig. 18. Oral endoscopy: retained root tip of a maxillary molar.

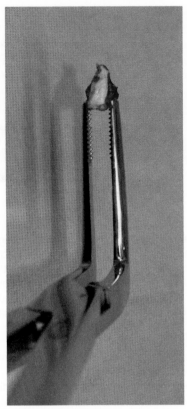

Fig. 19. Video oroscopy: root tip/fragment forceps holding an extracted maxillary molar root tip.

Stephen S. Galloway's article, "Equine Standing Surgical Extraction Techniques"; and John Pigott's article, "Equine Sinus Surgery," elsewhere in this issue).

Elevation

The luxation process is complete when the tooth is mobile and can be elevated with minimal force. On occasion it may be necessary to "roll" a tooth lingually/palatally as it is elevated from the alveolus to provide a clear extraction path between the proximal teeth or the opposing arcade. Excessively long teeth may need to be sectioned with burrs to allow passage into the oral cavity (**Fig. 20**).

Sclerosis of the bone surrounding a tooth will decrease bone malleability, potentially making extraction more difficult. Dilaceration of roots may result in root fractures of the tooth, even when proper luxation has fully relieved attachments. All forces described should be applied with care and caution, as aggressive pressure may result in fracture of dentition or bone. Sequestration of alveolar bone may result from damage during elevation. Clinicians should be prepared with a second or even tertiary backup treatment plan should complications occur.

On elevation of the tooth from the alveolus, radiographs are used to confirm complete removal of the tooth and absence of any potentially complicating pathology. Necrotic granulation tissue is removed via curettage (**Fig. 21**). Overexuberant

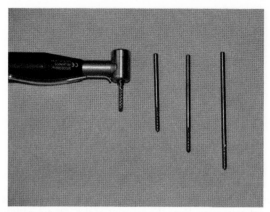

Fig. 20. Rotary system with burs used to section molars when they are too long to be delivered from the alveolus in one piece.

curettage of alveoli may result in a fistula. Excessive curettage of mandibular alveoli may result in damage to the mandibular canal and its contents.

Protection of the Alveolus/Alveolar Contents

Following alveolar debridement, a blood clot is allowed to form in the apical two-thirds of the alveolus over which a packing material is placed to protect the clot during healing (**Fig. 22**). Packing materials may include dental impression material (Vinyl Polysiloxane [VPS]), sterile gauze, iodophor gauze, dental wax, bone cements, and cold-curing dental acrylics.[10,11] When using VPS, if the packing extends too far apically, it can be removed and trimmed to allow for apical blood clot formation (**Fig. 23**). Depending on individual case requirement, material chosen, and healing progress, repacking interval ranges between days and a few weeks until the alveolus has filled

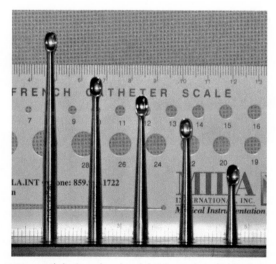

Fig. 21. Spoon curettes used during alveolar debridement. Individual curettes are placed in the T-handle illustrated in **Figs. 9**A, B.

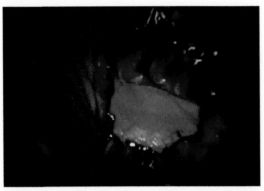

Fig. 22. Oral endoscopy: VPS impression material placed in the coronal two-thirds of a maxillary alveolus post extraction. Note the margins of the VPS are within the gingival margins, not overlapping them. This aids retention of the VPS during healing.

appropriately with granulation tissue. Local debridement, sequestra removal, and curettage may be necessary to stimulate complete healing (**Fig. 24**). Once the alveolus has filled with granulation tissue there is no need for continued packing.

POST EXTRACTION PLAN

Pain is managed according to patient need and clinician preference. Usually a nonsteroidal anti-inflammatory drug is administered for 3 to 7 days. Antimicrobial therapy and diet will vary depending on case specifics. Patients are examined at 3 and 6 months postoperatively with radiographs recommended at 6 months. Six months after extraction, examinations are scheduled with routine annual dental care. Radiographs are repeated at 12 to 18 months postoperatively and then as the case indicates at the time of routine annual dental care.

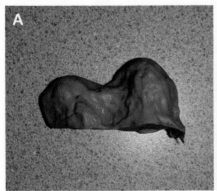
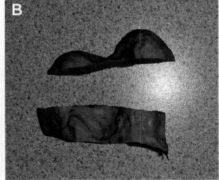

Fig. 23. (A, B) Forming and sectioning the VPS impression material. (A) VPS plug after initial placement within a mandibular cheek tooth extraction site over a partial blood clot filling less than two-thirds of the alveoli. (B) The same VPS plug as in (A) after sectioning to allow room for a larger blood clot to fill two-thirds of the alveoli. The coronal portion of this plug was replanted in the alveoli over the larger clot. Apical portion of plug (*top*). Coronal portion of plug (*bottom*).

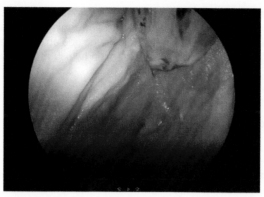

Fig. 24. Granulation tissue 4 weeks post extraction of a mandibular molar.

COMPLICATIONS

Complications related to intraoral extraction of premolars and molars are varied. Complete discussion of complications and their treatment is beyond the scope of this article. Examples of complications include oronasal/oroantral fistulas, sequestration of alveolar bone, tooth fracture with retained reserve crown/root, cementoma formation, fracture of the supporting bone, iatrogenic damage to proximal dentition, and incomplete extraction of ankylosed teeth. Further discussion of complications may be found in the Stephen S. Galloway and Edward T. Earley's article, "Minimizing Equine Tooth Extraction Complications," elsewhere in this issue.

SUMMARY

Intraoral extraction of premolars and molars is within the capability of the general veterinary practitioner provided they receive appropriate training and invest in appropriate equipment. Practitioners should expect to have a moderate investment in a reasonable armamentarium of diagnostic and extraction equipment before attempting these procedures. Availability of radiographic equipment is imperative to proper treatment planning as well as procedural and post-procedural patient evaluation and follow-up.

Careful assessment of individual teeth and surrounding structures are paramount for appropriate case selection, treatment planning, and predicting the likelihood of complications and/or the need for specific equipment. Referral should be considered if the risk of complications is high, or potentially severe. Specialized equipment and advanced procedures may be necessary to achieve a favorable outcome in more complex cases. When client expectations, clinician knowledge and ability, and individual patient specifics are considered, proper case selection is achieved and good success can be expected when performing oral extractions of equine cheek teeth.

CLINICS CARE POINTS

- The intra oral extraction techniques of equine premolars and molars described are well within the capability of the primary care veterinarian.
- A moderate investment in diagnostic, monitoring and extraction instrumentation is necessary prior to attempting intra oral extractions of premolars and molars.

- Case Difficulty, equipment availability, practitioner experience and specialist consultation should be considered prior to performing an extraction.
- Treatment planning for an extraction should include an alternate extraction technique and a final option of surgical extraction (which may include a referral to a specialist).

DISCLOSURE

The author has no conflicts of interest to report.

SUPPLEMENTARY DATA

Supplementary data related to this article can be found online at https://doi.org/10.1016/j.cveq.2020.08.010.

REFERENCES

1. Duncanson GR. A case study of 125 horses presented to a general practice in the UK for cheek teeth removal. Equine Vet Educ 2004;6(3):212–6.
2. Cordes V, Gardemin M, Lupke M, et al. Finite element analysis in 3-D models of equine cheek teeth. Vet J 2012;193(2):391–6.
3. Wiggs RB, Lobprise HB. Basic endodontic therapy. In: Wiggs RB, Lobprise HB, editors. Veterinary dentistry: principles and practice. Philadelphia: Lippincott-Raven Publishers; 1997. p. 287–9.
4. Newman MG, Takei HH, Carranza FA, et al. The periodontic-endodontic continuum. In: Cochran DL, Giannobile WV, Kenney EB, et al, editors. Carranzas clinical periodontology. 10th edition. Philadelphia: W.B. Saunders Co; 2006. p. 873–7.
5. Ramzan PHL, Dallas RS, Palmer L. Extraction of fractured cheek teeth under oral endoscopic guidance in standing horses. Vet Surg 2011;40:586–9.
6. Dixon PM, du Toit N. Dental anatomy. In: Easley J, Dixon P, Schumacher J, editors. Equine dentistry. 3rd edition. Saunders Elsevier; 2011. p. 66.
7. Floyd MR. The modified Triadan system nomenclature for veterinary dentistry. J Vet Dent 1991;(8):18–20.
8. Gieche JM. How to assess equine oral health. In: American Association of Equine Practitioners 53rd annual convention proceedings, vol. 53. Lexington (KY): American Association of Equine Practitioners; 2007. p. 499.
9. Gieche JM. Oral examination of equidae. In: American Association of Equine Practitioners 360 degree approach to learning equine dentistry. . Lexington (KY): American Association of Equine Practitioners; 2010. Section 2.1.
10. Dixon PM. Dental extraction and endodontic techniques in horses. Compend Contin Educ Pract Vet 1997;19:628–37.
11. Easley J, Dixon P, Schumacher J. Exodontia. In: Easley J, Dixon P, Schumacher J, editors. Equine dentistry. 3rd edition. Saunders/Elsevier; 2011. p. 328.

Adjunct Extraction Techniques in Equine Dentistry

Travis Henry, DVM[a],*, Ian Bishop, DVM[b]

KEYWORDS

- Equine dentistry • Extraction • Buccotomy
- Partial coronectomy commissurotomy sectioning

KEY POINTS

- Standard oral extraction carries the lowest risk of complications compared with other extraction techniques.
- Adjunct extraction techniques usually are preceded by standard intraoral extraction techniques.
- Partial coronectomy and tooth sectioning change the shape of the target tooth and divide the target tooth into separate pieces, respectively. Both techniques facilitate luxation and elevation of the tooth or tooth fragments.
- Minimally invasive buccotomy and commissurotomy provide alternative access to the target tooth, when a patient's conformation or the crown shape prevents use of standard oral extraction instruments.

INTRODUCTION

Standard oral extraction has become the preferred method for extracting teeth in the horse, due to its comparatively low rate of complications.[1,2] Variations in the shape and integrity of target teeth and limited access to the oral cavity may necessitate adjunct extraction techniques. Oral extraction techniques with molar spreaders, forceps, and fulcrums create luxation forces on both the target tooth and proximal teeth. A target tooth without enough clinical crown to be grasped or spread against, or that lacks the crown integrity to sustain extraction forces, requires an adjunct technique. All clinical situations utilize nonsurgical extraction techniques to some extent, particularly in breaking down the periodontal attachment. There are few exceptions within this article that do not employ adjunct techniques without a veterinarian having first begun with standard oral extraction.

a University of Wisconsin, Madison, WI, USA; b 988 Portage Road, Kirkfield, Ontario K0M 2B0, Canada
* Corresponding author. Midwest Veterinary Dental Services, PO Box 466, Elkhorn, WI 53121.
E-mail address: midwestequine@me.com

Vet Clin Equine 36 (2020) 565–574
https://doi.org/10.1016/j.cveq.2020.08.002
0749-0739/20/© 2020 Elsevier Inc. All rights reserved.
vetequine.theclinics.com

It is incumbent on the veterinarian to have a thorough knowledge of the anatomy of the head and to prevent iatrogenic trauma. The local anatomy is densely populated with large nerves and blood vessels and other important structures, such as the parotid salivary duct. The veterinarian should understand the anatomy of all of the pertinent structures, including the paranasal sinuses, foramina and canals, arteries, nerves, and veins related to the oral cavity. These structures are mentioned because they relate to each technique, but it is beyond the scope of this article to discuss the anatomy of the head in detail.

The veterinarian should be prepared for the many complications that can occur with oral surgery. Hemorrhage, transection of the parotid duct, and fracture of the alveolar plate[3–6] are only a few examples. The use of cutting burs in the mouth or accessing the oral cavity through the cheek comes with the inherent risk of damage to the surrounding structures It is prudent to consider and discuss with clients how they will proceed if there is a failure to extract the tooth (or complete tooth) via standard oral techniques. Communication should include if the primary veterinarian is able to perform adjunct extraction techniques versus referral to a specialist.

As with any surgical procedure, dental and oral surgeries require a significant investment in instrumentation, equipment, and clinical training. Special instrumentation generally is necessary when performing the techniques discussed in this article. Any veterinarian considering expanding their skill set and available services to include the following procedures also should be cognizant of the necessity to maintain a sufficient caseload to allow the development and maintenance of that skill set.

PARTIAL CORONECTOMY

Partial coronectomy is the removal of tooth material from the crown-reserve crown with a cylindrical rotary burs. Partial coronectomy is used when there has been a failure to increase the mobility of the tooth with standard oral extraction techniques and/or there is a concern that the crown integrity is so compromised that it is expected to fail when grasped with forceps.[4] In the horse, the rostral and caudal angulations of the cheek teeth create very tight interproximal spaces. This tight packing of the cheek teeth increases the difficulty of loosening a tooth through spreading and rotation. The healthy teeth essentially must be forced away from the diseased tooth in order to gain space to achieve mesiodistal and rotational movements. Partial coronectomy creates a space between the target tooth and the adjacent tooth that relieves the crown interlock in the interproximal space and allows for mesiodistal and rotational luxation movements.

Partial coronectomy is preceded by standing sedation, appropriate local and regional anesthesia, and techniques of standard oral extraction aimed at the breakdown of the periodontal attachment. To perform a partial coronectomy, the extraction pathway, interproximal crown to crown contact of the target tooth, and proximal teeth are assessed visually (with dental mirror or oral endoscope) and radiographically. A burs of appropriate length and diameter on a water-cooled instrument is used to remove the distal or mesial side of the target tooth, without damaging the adjacent tooth. This generally is performed with a 3-mm diameter, 52-mm long burs from the occlusal surface to the level of the interproximal alveolar bone. Thus, the tooth-tooth contact has been eliminated on either the mesial or distal aspect of the target tooth. The target tooth now can be spread into the space created without being blocked by the adjacent tooth. Cutting in a lingual to vestibular (buccal) direction reduces the chance of iatrogenic damage to the palate or tongue (**Fig. 1**) The cuts are

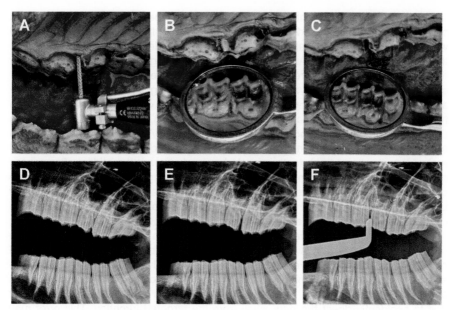

Fig. 1. (*A*) A water-irrigated instrument with a 3 mm tile-cutting burs is positioned to begin the partial coronectomy. (*B*) The initial cut is examined to confirm its proper placement. (*C*) The cut is continued in a palatal-to-buccal direction, removing crown from only the target tooth's distal edge. (*D*) A radiograph is taken to check the placement and trajectory of the cut. (*E*) The cut is extended to the level of interproximal bone and confirmed with radiographs. (*F*) In this image, a spreader has been placed mesial to the target tooth and closure of the space created by the partial coronectomy can be seen.

made removing 2 mm to 4 mm at a time and the area rinsed with water and visualized with an oral endoscope or dental mirror. After every 6 mm to 12 mm of depth, a radiograph should be obtained to be sure that the path of the cut is appropriate. In the authors' experience, the extraction pathway and shape of most cheek teeth are such that a distal partial coronectomy often is more beneficial. Mandibular cheek teeth tend to have distally curving roots and the distal cut allows molar spreaders in the mesial interproximal space to push the tooth toward its more concave side.

Complications of partial coronectomy generally result from misplacement of the burs and are of increased risk in an inadequately sedated or locally anesthetized patient. The adjacent soft tissues (gingiva, cheek, tongue, and palate) or adjacent teeth may be traumatized. A misplaced cut may not eliminate tooth-tooth contact and, therefore, fail to provide an advantage or even further compromise the integrity of the target tooth and predispose to fracture. When performing the partial coronectomy, the mesiodistal angulation of the burs can be difficult to judge, and an inappropriate angle can result in damage to the adjacent tooth or sectioning through the root of the target tooth. Making frequent small cuts with careful endoscopic visualization and radiographic assessment is most helpful in reducing this risk.

TOOTH SECTIONING

Tooth sectioning is preceded by standing sedation, appropriate local and regional anesthesia, and initial techniques of standard oral extraction aimed at the disruption of the periodontal attachment. Sectioning is indicated when the shape and angulation of the roots prevent easy extraction of the entire tooth. It can be particularly helpful with extraction of mandibular cheek teeth of senior patients, which may have long, thin distally angled roots. Additionally, when sectioning caudal mandibular cheek teeth, the anatomic curvature (curve of Spee) of the alveolar ridge is considered for correct burs angulation. Dysplastic teeth may be irregular and enlarged apically and, therefore, require sectioning in order to be elevated orally. Long-standing crown fractures may allow encroachment of adjacent teeth, narrowing the extraction pathway. Strategic sectioning of the fractured tooth may allow oral extraction of the smaller fragments. Sectioning also is useful in geriatric patients when the palatal root of the maxillary cheek teeth is angled severely toward the midline. Divergence of the 3 roots makes the apical portion of the tooth larger than the crown-reserve crown, preventing elevation of the entire tooth without fracturing the roots or alveolar bone. Sectioning these teeth into buccal and palatal portions greatly increases the dentist's ability to elevate the tooth with the roots intact.

Tooth sectioning is practical only when the target tooth has a short enough reserve crown to separate with the available instruments. Cutting burs are available in a limited number of lengths through veterinary suppliers and hardware retail stores. Additionally, there are positioning limitations using long burs below the gingiva in the caudal aspect of a patient's mouth. The longer the tooth that is being sectioned, the easier it is to accidently direct the burs away from the targeted furcation. This error may complicate the extraction further by cutting off a root or weakening the apex of the tooth.

The extraction pathway and shape of the target tooth is assessed radiographically. Critical evaluation is indicated because radiographs may not reveal the true extent of palatal root dilaceration with maxillary cheek teeth. A burs of appropriate length and diameter on a water-cooled instrument is used to section the target tooth, without damaging the adjacent teeth, alveolar bone, or oral soft tissues. In most circumstances, when sectioning teeth of geriatric patients, a 3-mm diameter by 52-mm long burs[a] is appropriate and it is highly recommended to use water spray for irrigation and cooling. A mandibular cheek tooth may be sectioned lingually to vestibularly to separate the mesial and distal roots. A maxillary cheek tooth may be sectioned sagittally along the midline of the tooth, along the infundibula and between the pulp horns, to separate the palatal root from the buccal roots. If necessary, the buccal roots then may be separated by making a cut from palatal to vestibular between the 2 buccal pulp horns. The cut is made in a palatal-to-vestibular direction so that if the instrument slips, the veterinarian is more likely to cause trauma to the buccal mucosa rather than the palate. Often, a partial coronectomy has been performed distally on the maxillary cheek teeth to be sectioned as well. This allows the dentist to have a space to start the sectioning process. It is important to remember that these teeth taper from clinical crown to apex, with the narrowest point in the furcation. When sectioning the tooth mesial to distal, extreme care must be exercised to prevent cutting into the adjacent tooth with the burs. Multiple radiographs are taken to confirm and guide the trajectory of the cuts (**Fig. 2**). When the attachment of the tooth has been divided into single rooted sections, the pieces of the tooth are luxated separately. If the fragments still are attached, then evaluate for areas of incomplete sectioning. Applying force without having the tooth fully sectioned can cause it to fracture in an inappropriate manner.

---

[a] Roto Zip TC4 1/8-in Tile-Cutting Carbide Zip Bit.

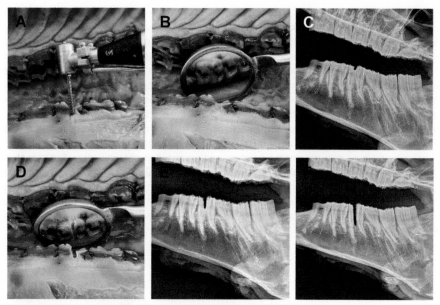

Fig. 2. (*A*) A water-irrigated instrument with a 3 mm tile-cutting burs is positioned to begin the tooth sectioning. (*B*) The initial cut is examine to confirm its proper placement. The cut is continued across the midline of the tooth in a lingual-to-buccal direction, (*C*) and a radiograph is taken to assess the trajectory and placement. (*D*) The cut is extended apically, and (*E*) additional radiographs are taken to assess the trajectory (*F*) until it has been confirmed that the root segments have been separated.

Complications of tooth sectioning are similar to those of partial coronectomy and generally result from misplacement of the burs. Risks are increased with an inadequately sedated or locally anesthetized patient. The adjacent soft tissues (gingiva, cheek, tongue, palate), bone, or proximal teeth may be traumatized. A misplaced cut may not separate rooted sections of crown and, therefore, fail to provide an advantage or even further compromise the integrity of the target tooth and predispose it to fracture. A transverse cut (lingual to buccal) can be assessed for placement and angle with standard radiographic dental views (ie, extraoral maxillary dorsoventral oblique and extraoral mandibular ventrodorsal oblique). These views do not, however, provide helpful information on a sagittal cut made to separate the palatal root of a maxillary cheek tooth. In the authors' experience, an offset dorsoventral skull view is not helpful either. This cut is made with careful planning based on knowledge of the crown length and shape from presurgical radiographs and by cutting in stages, while pausing to examine the tooth and check for independent motion of the segments.

MINIMALLY INVASIVE BUCCOTOMY AND TRANSBUCCAL SCREW EXTRACTION

Minimally invasive buccotomy (MIB) or minimally invasive transbuccal screw extraction is preceded by standing sedation, appropriate local and regional anesthesia, and initial techniques of standard oral extraction aimed at the breakdown of the periodontal attachment. It is used when the crown cannot be grasped or accessed by working through the mouth and an alternative access is required.[5] Specialized instrumentation for minimally invasive transbuccal screw extraction generally include a lateralizing/offset speculum, trocars of different lengths, elevators, luxators, and curettes designed to work through the cannula, drill guides, drill bits of varying diameters with matching taps and screws, and a slotted mallet (see **Fig 4I**).

A 5F to 8F polypropylene catheter, that is, 56 cm[b] or longer, is placed in the parotid duct to allow it to be palpated. The skin is clipped and aseptically prepared. The parotid duct, branches of the facial artery and vein, and branches of the facial nerve are identified and marked with a surgical marker. Markers, such as sterile skin staples, may be placed over the target tooth. The radiographic markers identify the location and extraction pathway of the tooth, allowing for accurate placement of the trocar. Local anesthetic then is placed to desensitize the buccotomy site. A scalpel is used to create an incision through the skin only, to allow the introduction of the trocar. The incision is made in a horizontal fashion to minimize the risk of cutting the facial nerve. The trocar is introduced, the obturator removed, and the cannula is used as straight-line access to instrument the tooth with specialized instruments (**Fig. 3**).

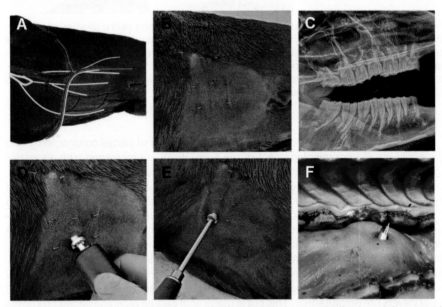

Fig. 3. (*A*) The branches of the facial artery (*red*), vein (*blue*), nerve (*yellow*), and the parotid duct (*white*) are palpated and marked. Significant individual variation may be found from the expected anatomy. (*B*) Staples are placed at the level of the occlusal surface of the mandibular and maxillary cheek teeth and at the level of the apex of the target tooth. (*C*) The staples are visible on the radiographs and aide in planning the location and trajectory of the trocar-cannula. (*D*) The trocar-cannula is placed through a small, horizontal skin incision. (*E*) and (*F*) Straight-line elevators and luxators may be used through the cannula.

---

[b] Sovereign Polypropylene Catheter, 5F × 56 CM, Cardinal Health.

The offset speculum[c] is essential by allowing the mandible to be deviated for better access. The mandible is moved laterally to the maxilla to allow access to a mandibular cheek tooth or medially to improve access to a maxillary cheek tooth. The first 4 maxillary cheek teeth are accessed by placing the trocar rostral to the parotid duct. The last maxillary cheek tooth (and sometimes the second to last) are accessed by placing the trocar caudal to the parotid duct, through the masseter. The first 4 mandibular cheek teeth are accessed by placing the trocar rostral to the parotid duct. The last 2 mandibular cheek teeth generally cannot be accessed via an MIB due to anatomic restrictions.

Mobility of the tooth is achieved with instrumented luxation through the trocar. Next, a drill guide and drill bit are introduced through the cannula and a hole is drilled parallel to the long axis of the tooth, centered just buccally to the midline of the tooth. A series of radiographs are taken to confirm the trajectory of the drill bit and to ensure that the hole is drilled to an appropriate depth and not beyond that into the periapical structures. The goal is to guide the drill into the furcation of the tooth and not up into a root. If the drill is guided into a root, it often causes the root to fracture when extraction is attempted. When working with a fractured crown, the veterinarian must use judgment for the safest and most advantageous location to drill into the tooth. In some cases, it may be helpful to contour the fractured crown to create a flatter surface for the drill guide or to drill first with a 3-mm burs to create a starting point for the drill bit.

The drill bit is removed and the hole is lavaged and tapped to create threads within the hole. The number of turns of the tap is noted so that the threaded extraction rod then can be placed with the same number of turns. The depth of the hole is noted by placing a small Steinmann pin through the cannula and into the drilled hole and marking at the occlusal surface. The marked measurement on the Steinmann pin is transferred to the correct thread depth of the extraction rod, preventing over insertion into the apical tissues. The extraction rod is turned into the threaded hole according to previous measurement. The screw's purchase on the tooth can be checked by carefully moving the extraction rod horizontally (rostro-caudally or laterally). It may be helpful to break down the periodontal attachment further. The slotted mallet then is used to tap against the extraction rod along the long axis of the tooth in the direction opposite of the apex, to elevate the tooth into the mouth (**Fig. 4**).

The alveolus then is inspected visually, and radiographs are taken to demonstrate a vacated alveolus. The cannula is removed and the skin is closed with either sterile staples or an appropriate suture. Only the skin is closed. To eliminate the risk of ligating a nerve, vessel or the parotid duct, the mucosa and subcutaneous tissues are left to heal by second intention.

Proper placement of the trocar greatly reduces the risk of complications associated with inadvertent transection or trauma to the pertinent structures of the cheek. When placing the trocar, potential complications include trauma to the parotid duct, branches of the facial artery and vein, and branches of the facial nerve. When drilling into the target tooth, care must be taken to avoid drilling too far because doing so may enter the paranasal sinuses, nasal passages, hard palate, or mandibular canal. The angle of the drill must be accurate to prevent exiting the reserve crown before reaching the apex. Also, if the hole is not drilled parallel to the eruption path of the tooth, the forces applied by the slotted mallet will not be aligned optimally and may be predisposed to stripping the threads or fracturing the tooth. If the screw strips the threads or the tooth fractures, additional attempts to

---

[c] Gunther Offset Equine Speculum.

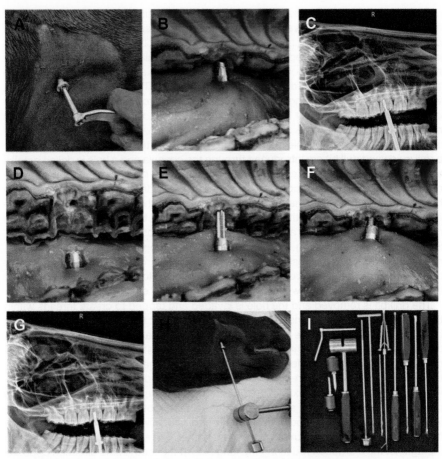

Fig. 4. (*A*) A drill guide is placed through the cannula and is necessary for protection from thermal damage caused by friction of the drill bit. (*B*) It is used to help direct the bit against the target tooth. (*C*) Radiographs are used to confirm the trajectory and depth of the drill. (*D*) The drill hole is flushed between instruments. (*E*) A tap is used to create threads within the hole (*F*) so that a screw/bolt can be placed with secure purchase on the target tooth. (*G*) The depth of the bolt also may be checked radiographically and (*H*) before applying force with the slotted mallet. (*I*) An image of a commercially available buccotomy set.

drill and place a screw may be attempted. If the tooth continues to fragment, it may be extracted in pieces by using elevators, luxators, and fragment forceps through the cannula.

COMMISSUROTOMY

A commissurotomy is the creation of a full-thickness incision through the skin, muscle, and mucosa starting at the lip commissure and extending to the rostral aspect of the masseter muscle. With the mouth opened, the incision is placed midway between the occlusal surfaces of maxillary and mandibular cheek teeth. This procedure allows for greater access to the oral cavity, which is useful for instrumentation in smaller patients.[b] It is used in conjunction with extractions, mass removals, oronasal fistula management, and fracture repairs and can be performed standing or under general anesthesia. The face is clipped and surgically prepped, and appropriate local and regional anesthesia is employed. Commissurotomy is indicated when the size and shape of a patient's head and mouth, and location of the tooth prevents access with appropriate instruments for oral extraction or MIB. It allows access and visualization across the space of the oral cavity rostral to the masseter. Although infrequently performed, the technique occasionally is used in other species with poor oral access for dental and oral surgery.[6] The veterinarian should not perform a commissurotomy with the intention of being able to open the mouth more widely, because the temporomandibular joint and associated structures limit this rather than the lips and cheeks.

The parotid duct, branches of the facial artery and vein, and branches of the facial nerve are identified with a surgical marker. Catheterization with a 56-cm, 5F to 8F

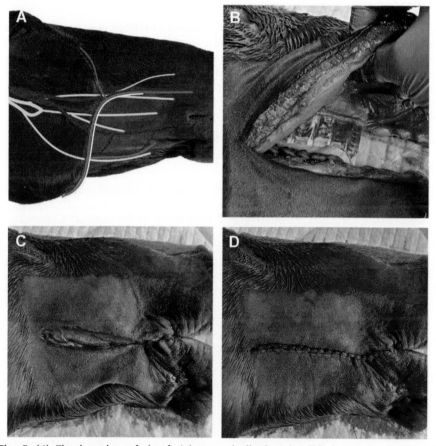

Fig. 5. (*A*) The branches of the facial nerve (*yellow*), veins (*blue*), arteries (*red*), and the parotid duct (*white*) are identified. (*B*) An incision is made through the skin, muscles, and mucosa of the cheek to create access to the oral cavity. (*C*) The muscle and mucosa are closed in 1 layer with an absorbable monofilament suture. (*D*) The skin is closed.

polypropylene catheter[f] facilitates palpation and location of the parotid duct. This may be difficult particularly in smaller patients due to limited oral access. The parotid duct runs caudally from the orifice in a horizontal fashion before curving ventral just before the masseter muscle. While avoiding these structures, a full-thickness incision is made through the skin, subcutaneous tissues, muscle, and buccal mucosa, starting from the commissure of the lips and continuing caudally to just rostral to the masseter. Great care must be taken to not continue the incision too far caudally because the parotid duct and branches of the facial artery and vein course ventrally just rostral to the masseter. Once the oral procedure is completed, the commissurotomy is closed in 2 (buccal mucosa/muscle and skin) or 3 layers (buccal mucosa, muscle, and skin) using an absorbable monofilament suture[g]. Alternatively, the skin may be closed with stainless steel staples (**Fig. 5**).

Complications of commissurotomy include iatrogenic trauma to the parotid duct, branches of the facial artery and vein, and branches of the facial nerve and postoperative infection and dehiscence. It often is expected that swelling at the incision site can cause transient facial nerve paralysis that generally subsides in 48 hours to 72 hours.

SUMMARY

When variation of the shape or integrity of the patient's dentition or access to the oral cavity prevents or complicates standard oral extraction, adjunct extraction techniques can be used to assist in delivery of the tooth orally. With training and special instrumentation, a veterinarian can extract a vast majority of teeth without requiring repulsion and achieve a significantly lower complication rate.

DISCLOSURE

No competing interests have been declared.

REFERENCES

1. Dixon P, Dacre I, Tremaine WH, et al. Standing oral extraction of cheek teeth in 100 horses (1998–2003). Equine Vet J 2005;37(2):105–12.
2. Caramello V, Zarucco L, Foster D, et al. Equine cheek tooth extraction: Comparison of outcomes for five extraction methods. Equine Vet J 2020;52(2):181–6.
3. Earley E. Complications with extractions. AAEP Proceedings 2012;58:289–93.
4. Rice M, Henry T. Standing intraoral extractions of cheek teeth aided by partial crown removal in 165 horses (2010–2016). Equine Vet J 2018;50:48–53.
5. Langeneckert F, Witte T, Schellenberger F, et al. Cheek tooth extraction via a minimally invasive transbuccal approach and intradental screw placement in 54 equids. Vet Surg 2015;44:1012–20.
6. Wilson G. Commissurotomy for Oral Access and Tooth Extraction in a Dwarf Miniature Pony. J Vet Dent 2012;29(4):250–2.

[f] Sovereign Polypropylene Catheter, 5F × 56 CM, Cardinal Health.

[g] Monocryl (poliglecaprone 25) Suture, Ethicon.

Equine Standing Surgical Extraction Techniques

Edward T. Earley, DVM[a],*, Stephen S. Galloway, DVM, AVDC[b]

KEYWORDS

- Equine • Fracture • Surgical extraction • Incisor • Canine • Premolar • Molar
- Cheek tooth

KEY POINTS

- Incisor and canine extractions are approached independently with a single releasing flap or collectively with a large envelope flap.
- Maxillary premolars are approached through the maxilla directly over the apical aspect of the tooth.
- Maxillary molars are approached from within the sinus.
- Mandibular premolars are accessed with a horizontal (or semicurved) soft tissue approach. The fourth premolar may also be accessed with a vertical incision directly over the reserve crown.
- Mandibular molars are accessed with a vertical soft tissue approach through the masseter muscle directly over the reserve crown of the affected tooth.

INTRODUCTION

Surgical extraction procedures that require a soft tissue incision and removal of bone to expose the reserve crown or roots before extraction of a diseased tooth are described in this article. Oral extraction techniques are described in Jon M. Gieche's article, "Equine Oral Extraction Techniques," elsewhere in this issue. Sectioning of teeth without soft tissue and bone removal is described in Travis Henry and Ian Bishop's article, "Adjunct Extraction Techniques in Equine Dentistry," elsewhere in this issue. Most surgical extraction techniques are now routinely performed with the horse standing because of the implementation of improved sedation and analgesic techniques (discussed in Luis Campoy and Samantha R. Sedgwick's article, "Standing Sedation and locoregional Analgesia in Equine Dental Surgery," elsewhere in this issue). Six surgical extraction techniques are described based on the type of tooth and location: (1) incisor, (2) canine, (3) maxillary premolar (excluding premolar 1), (4) maxillary molar, (5) mandibular premolar (excluding premolar 1), and (6) mandibular molar.

[a] Large Animal Dentistry, Equine Farm Animal Hospital, Cornell University, Ithaca, NY 14853, USA; [b] Animal Dental Care Specialist, 8565 Highway 64, Somerville, TN 38068, USA
* Corresponding author.
E-mail address: ete9@cornell.edu

Vet Clin Equine 36 (2020) 575–612
https://doi.org/10.1016/j.cveq.2020.08.008
0749-0739/20/© 2020 Elsevier Inc. All rights reserved.

INDICATIONS FOR SURGICAL EXTRACTION

Surgical extraction is indicated when preoperative clinical and radiographic evaluation reveals tooth morphology or pathology that predisposes nonsurgical techniques to difficulty and/or significant complications. For example, isolated areas of widened reserve crown, curved roots, and apical hypercementosis predispose simple extraction techniques to fractured roots and/or alveolar sequestrum. Additionally, surgery is indicated when nonsurgical techniques fail to extract the diseased tooth as expected because of undiagnosed intraoperative complications, such as dentoalveolar ankylosis or root fracture. Bone and root pathology are underestimated (up to 50%) radiographically.[1–4]

ADVANTAGES AND DISADVANTAGES OF SURGICAL EXTRACTION

Surgical extractions are specialty-level procedures that require surgical and dental instrumentation (**Fig. 1**) to perform. They require a veterinary dentistry team (dentist, anesthesia technician, surgical technician, and dentistry technician), who all have experience in anesthesia, dentistry, and orofacial surgery. The dentist must possess the skills and experience to use a high-speed bone cutting drill in a confined space while making precise cuts often less than 2 mm in thickness. Prerequisite to this precision instrumentation is a detailed understanding of dental anatomy and pathology. Also, the surgical approaches described in this article require a detailed understanding of the regional anatomy of the head to prevent potentially permanent iatrogenic complications.

Although the current use of surgical extractions is limited by the number of veterinary dentists performing these procedures, the outcome is significantly better when compared with repulsion techniques. Surgical extractions allow for direct visualization and access to diseased tissues, which facilitates accurate surgical debridement and minimizes iatrogenic trauma. When performed by a skilled dentist, surgical extractions result in predictable, time-saving procedures and promote rapid, uncomplicated healing. Finally, and contrary to most of the current veterinary literature, surgical extractions do not require general anesthesia. As with other surgical procedures of the head in horses, surgical extraction techniques are routinely performed in the standing

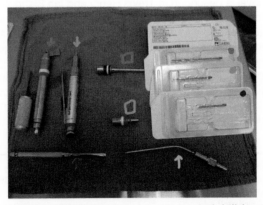

Fig. 1. Pneumatic surgical saw (*red arrow*), pneumatic surgical drill (*green arrow*), gingival periosteal elevator (*blue arrow*), Frazier suction tip (*orange arrow*), extralong bur guard (*red square*), medium bur guard (*green square*), medium oval carbide bur (*blue dot*), long oval carbide bur (*green dot*), and extralong oval carbide bur (*red dot*).

sedated horse with regional anesthesia (discussed in Luis Campoy and Samantha R. Sedgwick's article, "Standing Sedation and locoregional Analgesia in Equine Dental Surgery," elsewhere in this issue).

TREATMENT PLANNING FOR SURGICAL EXTRACTION

Comprehensive preoperative assessment and treatment planning facilitates accurate procedural estimates and scheduling, reduces time under sedation and anesthesia, and prevents unexpected complications. Complete orofacial evaluation and dental radiography are the minimum preoperative assessment requirements for any extraction. Additional diagnostic imaging modalities, such as oral, nasal, and/or sinus endoscopy, along with computed tomography, may be indicated for challenging cases. A surgical extraction is broken down into five phases: (1) surgical approach, (2) osteotomy/alveolectomy, (3) tooth elevation, (4) alveolar debridement, and (5) surgical closure. Each phase of the procedure must be preplanned for a successful outcome. Unplanned extractions may require flap modifications that could compromise the closure and delay healing.

SURGICAL APPROACHES

Surgical approaches for the reserve crown and roots of cheek teeth have been previously described[5–10] and the approaches preferred by the authors are described in this article. Mucoperiosteal flaps are used during the surgical extraction of the incisor and canine teeth but have received limited attention in the equine dentistry literature; therefore, the principles of flap design are discussed. The techniques and examples presented in this article are not intended to represent the definitive solution for extracting a specific tooth. Techniques and instrumentation must be individualized for each specific case.

MUCOPERIOSTEAL FLAP TYPES AND DESIGN PRINCIPLES

Mucoperiosteal flaps are used in surgical exodontia to access and remove the alveolar bone (osteotomy) covering the reserve crown and roots of teeth. Three types of flaps are commonly used in surgical extractions: (1) the envelope flap, (2) the triangular mucogingival flap (single releasing flap), and (3) the pedicle mucogingival lap (double releasing flap). Sharp instruments minimize tearing the flap, and scalpel blades should be changed often because most incisions intentionally contact bone.

An envelope flap is made by incising the sulcular epithelial attachment at the alveolar margin and making a subperiosteal elevation of the attached gingiva to expose the alveolar bone of the target tooth. This flap is commonly used during periodontal surgery and exodontia procedures to gain access to the alveolar bone margin. To increase exposure, the flap design may be extended to include one or more adjacent teeth It is the simplest flap, but has the poorest access to the alveolar bone (see **Figs. 12, 13, 15, 16, 18,** and **19**). If a tooth has severe gingivitis/periodontitis, the dentist may elect to perform an internal (reverse) bevel incision (modified Widman flap)[11] to remove the diseased sulcular epithelium. Instead of inserting the blade into the sulcus to incise the gingival attachment, the diseased portion of free and attached gingiva is incised with the blade directed toward the alveolar bone. To elevate the flap, the periosteal elevator is placed into the incision, under the periosteum, and the healthy gingival margin of the flap is elevated off the marginal bone. The remaining collar of diseased tissue is extracted with the tooth or removed with a sulcular incision before osteotomy.

A triangular mucoperiosteal flap (single releasing flap) is the most commonly used flap for surgical extractions. It consists of an envelope flap with a single vertical releasing incision at one end of the envelope flap (see **Figs. 6**, **7**, and **14**). The releasing incision is made with firm pressure cutting through the gingiva and periosteum in an apical and diverging direction and is continued through the mucogingival line into the oral mucosa in a single stroke. The flap is elevated starting at the corner of the releasing incision carefully working horizontally and apically to ensure the mucosa is not damaged.

A pedicle mucoperiosteal flap (double releasing flap) provides the best exposure for challenging extractions where extensive bone must be removed. The pedicle flap is an extension of the envelope flap with vertical release incisions on each end (**Fig. 2**).

Flap design should include the following principles:

1. The flap should not compromise vital structures, such as mental artery, vein, or nerve.
2. The flap must be large enough to expose the surgical area, without exposing peripheral tissue unnecessarily. Vertical releasing incisions should not be used indiscriminately. When learning flap techniques, veterinarians should and will create large flaps to facilitate visualization and bone exposure. With experience, dentists will minimize flap size.
3. Vertical releasing incisions should be made at the line angle of the tooth being extracted or in an edentulous interdental space ensuring that adjacent teeth have a complete gingival collar when the flap is closed. A vertical releasing incision should not be cut through an interdental gingival papilla (a line angle is a corner where two vertical walls of the tooth meet).
4. The length of the vertical releasing incision into the mucosa should approximate the length of the root requiring exposure.
5. The width of the flap's base should be equal to or larger than the width of the gingival free margin to ensure adequate blood supply (diverging vertical releases). Adequate blood supply is the most critical factor in tissue healing.[12]
6. The flap should be gently handled and manipulated. The use of stay sutures to manipulate flaps that require extensive development minimizes iatrogenic trauma.
7. The edges of the flap should be supported over bone whenever possible to decrease mobility of the incision after closure. The soft tissue access should be larger than the bone window.

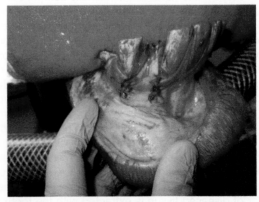

Fig. 2. A pedicle mucoperiosteal (four corner) flap used for surgical extraction of an individual mandibular incisor (402-right mandibular second incisor).

8. The flap closure must be tension-free. A tension-free closure is usually obtained by cutting the periosteum under nonkeratinized vestibular mucosa so that the flap is coronally advanced over the alveolus. Keratinized mucosa (eg, gingiva and palatal mucosa) is inelastic and does not appropriately advance after a periosteal release.

Mucoperiosteal Flaps in Equid

Even when the principles of mucoperiosteal flap design are meticulously followed, flap dehiscence in equine patients is common. Wound immobility is a principle of primary closure that is rarely achieved in horses because of their constant chewing behavior. Also, the extensive elevation of the attached gingiva in the incisive area often compromises the vascularity of this tissue. Although some degree of dehiscence is expected after closure, a mucoperiosteal flap prevents gross contamination of the surgical site and supports alveolar blood clot formation during the initial phase of healing. Areas of dehiscence rapidly granulate and heal by second intention.

ALVEOLECTOMY FOR INCISOR AND CANINE TOOTH EXTRACTION

After surgical exposure is created with a mucoperiosteal flap, the buccal alveolar bone covering the reserve crown and/or roots is removed to facilitate tooth elevation. An end-cutting carbide bur (round, oval, or pear bur) on a water-cooled high-speed handpiece is used to remove the bone by making sweeping "paint brush" strokes across the bone. The prominent jugae outlining the reserve crown of the maxillary incisors are used to guide bone removal; however, cortical bone often masks the reserve crown of other teeth. The safest method of ensuring that excessive bone is not removed, or that adjacent teeth are not damaged, is to start alveolectomy at the alveolar margin of the tooth and work apically while identifying and using the periodontal ligament (PDL) of the reserve crown as the mesial and distal limits of alveolectomy. In most cases, removal of one-third to one-half of the bone covering the reserve crown is sufficient to facilitate elevation of the tooth; however, in teeth with complicating root morphology/pathology or with compromised peripheral bone, greater than 75% of the alveolar bone may need to be removed. Once the buccal alveolar bone is removed, outlining/widening the PDL space around the roots with a small round bur facilitates insertion of the luxator/elevator blade.

TOOTH ELEVATION

After alveolectomy, the PDL is broken down with dental luxators and elevators. Luxators are sharp instruments that are inserted into the PDL with an apically directed force and used to sever the attachment. Elevators are noncutting instruments that are wedged into the PDL space and then used as a lever to further rupture the remaining PDL attachments and displace the tooth. Forceps are used to extract the loosened tooth from the alveolus. Inappropriate or premature use of forceps often results in tooth fracture and prolonged surgical time. Immobility of the tooth after luxation/elevation is an indication for continued alveolectomy. Sectioning of a tooth during or after alveolectomy may facilitate extraction of teeth with complicated morphology or multiple roots.

ALVEOLAR WOUND MANAGEMENT

After tooth extraction, a bone curette is used to remove granulomatous and necrotic tissue from the alveolus; however, stripping the alveolus to the bone should be avoided because PDL remnants provide fibroblast for healing and contribute to angiogenesis and new bone formation. Rough bone margins left after tooth extraction are a source of discomfort and can cause delayed healing secondary to soft tissue abrasion/laceration. Rongeurs may be used to remove irregular or sharp bone spicules. A general-purpose diamond bur[a] on a water-cooled high-speed handpiece is typically used to smooth the alveolar bone margin (alveoloplasty). Before wound closure, the extraction site should be flushed with a physiologic solution to remove loose debris, bacteria, and inflammatory mediators. Chlorhexidine rinsing should be avoided because it is toxic to fibroblasts. A stable blood clot is the foundation for bone healing, and bone augmentation (graft material) is rarely indicated in extraction site alveoli.

SURGICAL CLOSURE

Tension-free apposition of the wound margins is critical to the primary closure of all soft tissue wounds. The closure of a mucoperiosteal flap after tooth extraction presents unique challenges. In preparation for flap closure, the recipient epithelium and flap gingiva are debrided/freshened using a diamond bur or scissors. Healthy keratinized gingiva should not be trimmed from the flap margin because it provides better purchase for suture than nonkeratinized mucosa. The recipient edges of the palatal or mandibular mucosa are slightly elevated to facilitate placement of the suture needle.

Most flaps do not close over the extraction site without tension if returned to their original position; therefore, they must be coronally repositioned. A full-thickness flap consists of the elastic mucosal layer overlying the inelastic periosteum. A periosteal releasing incision is performed to provide the mobility necessary for coronal advancement of the flap. The periosteal release incision is made apical to the mucogingival line with scissors, bluntly dissecting between the periosteum and the mucosa. The flap is positioned and tested to ensure a tension-free closure before suturing. The suture pattern for closure is at the dentist's discretion; however, placement of strategic simple interrupted sutures at the wound corners often facilitates repositioning and redistribution of the flap tissue and produces a more functional and cosmetic result. The flap should be repositioned laterally, whenever possible, to ensure a gingival collar wraps around the teeth on the wound margin. Sutures should not be expected to provide a hermetic seal for the flap; therefore, lacerated vasculature should be ligated to prevent hematoma formation.

Suture type, size, and pattern are routinely debated with a paucity of evidence to support any opinion. The authors typically use a 2–0 absorbable monofilament[b,c] for all closures described in this article. Simple interrupted and continuous suture patterns are appropriate for the closures described, but the authors prefer a continuous interrupted Aberdeen[13,14] suture pattern for most cases.

SURGICAL EXTRACTION OF INCISOR TEETH

Simple oral extraction of an incisor may be feasible when there is poor PDL and bone attachment (**Fig. 3**). The PDL is separated (luxation) and the tooth extracted with elevation (**Figs. 4** and **5**). Surgical extraction of a diseased incisor (eg, nonvital, fractured) may be indicated when there is substantial PDL and bone attachment present. Tooth (and bone) resorption may also be an indication for an incisor surgical extraction.

---

[a] Coarse Multi Use Diamond Surgical Length Round, BencoDental, Pittston, PA.

[b] 2–0 Monocryl, Ethicon, Johnson and Johnson, Bridgewater Township, NJ.

[c] Surgical mallet, Millennium Surgical, Bala Cynwyd, PA.

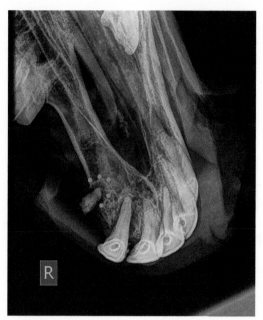

Fig. 3. Note bone loss with reserve crown/root of 102 (right maxillary second incisor) (*red dots*) and the root tip of 103 (right maxillary third incisor) (*green dots*). Simple extraction (nonsurgical) is indicated by straight line luxation followed with elevation.

The surgical approach to the maxillary incisors involves the development a vestibular mucoperiosteal flap. A sulcar incision is made with a scalpel blade (size 15) along the alveolar margin. A releasing incision is made along the mesiobuccal line angle of the incisor to be extracted (**Figs. 6–9**).[15] When all incisors are surgically extracted, a single large envelope flap is created. The long, thin interdental gingival papillae are amputated during the initial incision creating a flap that has a uniform margin. A periosteal elevator[d] is used to create the flap by separating the periosteum, from the underlying bone. Care should be taken during flap elevation to avoid the incisive artery as it passes through the interincisive canal (**Fig. 10**).[16] A submucosal fibrous attachment is present between the first incisors. Careful elevation (or sharp dissection) is required to prevent tearing the oral mucosa in this location.

Alveolectomy during an incisor surgical extraction is best instrumented with an air-driven, high-speed surgical drill and an oval carbide bur[e,f]. An assistant provides saline lavage and suction (Frazier tip[g]) at the surgical site for bur cooling and visualization. Starting coronally and advancing apically, the alveolar bone outlined by the juga of the tooth is removed to expose the reserve crown of the incisor. Interproximal bone is also removed along the mesial and distal aspects of the reserve crown and root to widen the PDL space and facilitate instrument placement (**Fig. 11**). A luxator[h] is

---

[d] Periosteal elevator EX 60, Cislak Manufacturing Inc, Niles, IL.

[e] Hall's surgical drill, Surgairtome, Hall Powered Instruments, Conmed, Utica, NY.

[f] Oval bur medium carbide, Hall Powered Instruments, Conmed.

[g] Frazier tip suction #10, Jarit, Integra Life Sciences, Princeton, NJ.

[h] Long handle luxator, Medco, Hickory Hills, IL.

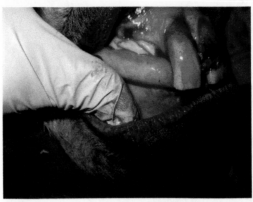

Fig. 4. Appearance of 102 following luxation of soft tissue attachments along the reserve crown/root. Root tip of 103 has been elevated and extracted.

gently inserted into the PDL space and worked circumferentially around the tooth until the tooth is mobile. A thin right-angle spreader[i] is placed interproximal to aid in breakdown of the PDL and elevation of the tooth. Final rotation and extraction of the tooth is achieved with extraction forceps[j]. The alveolus is then debrided with a curette and rongeurs[k] are used to remove any remaining large irregular bone spicules. Alveoloplasty is performed with a water-cooled high-speed diamond bur, and the alveolus is flushed with physiologic saline to ensure all diseased tissue and debris are removed. Postoperative radiographs should be taken to confirm complete extraction of the incisors before the mucoperiosteal flap is closed (**Fig. 12**).

Mandibular incisors are surgically extracted in a similar fashion. The elevation of a mandibular incisive mucoperiosteal flap may require isolation of the rostral branches of the mental vascular bundle, and alveolectomy must be performed more cautiously

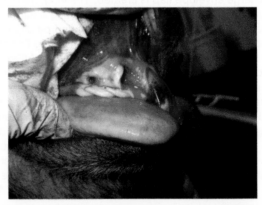

Fig. 5. Simple extraction of 102 without development of a mucogingival flap.

---

[i] Right angle spreader, 3FS Woodward Forceps, Hu-Friedy Mfg. Co, LLC, Chicago, IL.

[j] Right angle extraction Forcep, MD3 Mead Forceps, Serrated, Hu-Friedy Mfg. Co.

[k] Equine compound rongeurs double action, Medco.

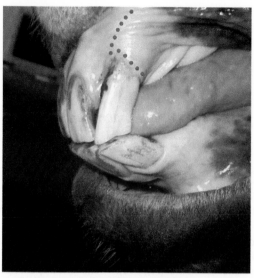

Fig. 6. Outline (*red dots*) of a mucogingival flap for 203 (left maxillary third incisor). The flap starts at the gingival margin and extends into the mucosa along the mesial buccal line angle.

because these teeth usually do not have prominent juga to guide dissection. The weight of the lower lip may contribute to dehiscence; therefore, anchoring of flap to the incisive bone may provide additional immobilization and support during healing.

SURGICAL EXTRACTION OF CANINE TEETH

Simple oral extraction of a canine tooth is rarely feasible because of the long, curved root.[17,18] The mandibular canine tooth is usually surgically approached with a muco-periosteal envelope flap. The flap incision starts in the interproximal mucosa, mesial to

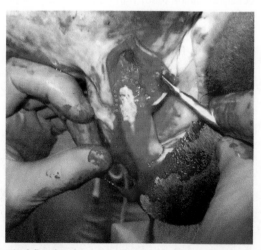

Fig. 7. The mucogingival flap has been elevated. Buccal bone has been removed along the reserve crown (*green dots*).

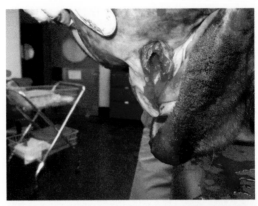

Fig. 8. Remaining 203 alveolus following luxation, elevation, and extraction.

the alveolar ridge of the tooth. The mucoperiosteal incision continues distally and circumferentially through the gingival sulcus of the tooth, and then extends along the dorsobuccal aspect of the mandible (**Fig. 13**).[19] The envelope flap can be extended mesiodistally to increase bone exposure. The preferred surgical approach to the maxillary canine tooth is a vestibular, single releasing mucoperiosteal flap. The envelope flap starts mesial to the crown, and continues distally and circumferentially through the gingival sulcus of the tooth. A releasing incision extends into the mucosa along the distobuccal line angle of the tooth, taking care not to lacerate structures originating from the infraorbital neurovascular bundle (**Fig. 14**). Excessive extension of the flap rostrally could result in the laceration of a branch of the palatine artery that travels through the interproximal space between the third incisor and canine tooth; however, hemostasis of this vessel often occurs without ligation. The mucoperiosteal flap is elevated and retracted apically to expose the underlying bone (**Fig. 15**).

Alveolectomy of a canine tooth is addressed similar as an incisor. However, overlying buccal alveolar bone covering the canine teeth is slightly thicker compared with the incisors. The tooth root often has a slight yellow tint compared to the white alveolar bone, especially in canine teeth with dentoalveolar ankylosis, which is used to guide dissection. Significant (>75%) to complete alveolectomy and definition of

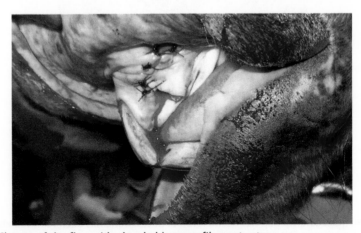

Fig. 9. Closure of the flap with absorbable monofilament suture.

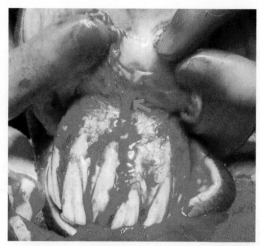

Fig. 10. Creation of a large envelope flap. The incisive artery (*green arrow*) passes through the interincisive canal and branches in three directions into the submucosa.

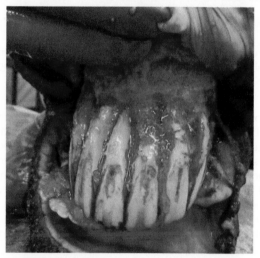

Fig. 11. Buccal and interproximal bone has been removed along all maxillary incisors exposing the reserve crowns and roots.

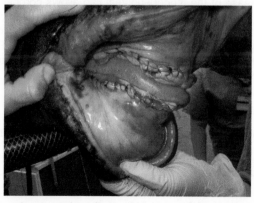

Fig. 12. Closure of two large envelope flaps, which are used for surgical exposure of canines and incisors. A continuous Aberdeen suture pattern is used with an absorbable monofilament.

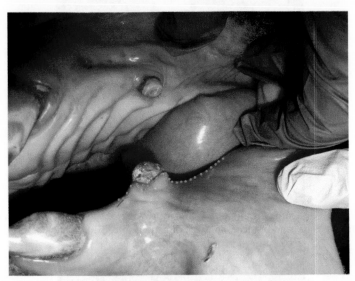

Fig. 13. Outline (*green dots*) of a mucogingival flap for 404 (left mandibular canine). The flap starts on the alveolar ridge just mesial to the crown, extends along the free margin, and continues along the dorsal buccal aspect of the mandible.

the PDL space around the maxillary and mandibular canine teeth may be required to produce tooth mobility (**Figs. 16** and **17**). In some cases, intraoperative removal of the crown of the canine tooth produces improved visualization for continued alveolectomy and luxation. Once the reserve crown/root is clearly defined, luxators and elevators are used to extract the tooth from the alveolus. Careful elevation of the maxillary canine is required to prevent fracture of the thin with palatal bone, causing oronasal fistulation. With the mandibular canine, the cervical portion of the tooth is larger in diameter than the remaining root/reserve crown. When elevating along the lingual aspect of the tooth, follow the curvature of the root to avoid cutting into the body of the mandible. Elevation[l,m,n] (**Fig. 18**) and alveolar debridement are similar to that of an incisor; however, attention to careful alveoloplasty should be exercised to ensure smooth contouring of the dorsal mandible to prevent future implications of bit sensitivity. Periosteal release of the mucoperiosteal flap allows coronal advancement for primary closure of the alveolus (**Fig. 19**). In cases where all of the incisor and canine teeth are to be simultaneously extracted (eg, regional extraction as a treatment of Equine Odontoclastic Tooth Resorption and Hypercementosis [EOTRH]), the envelope flap for the incisors may be extended to include the canine teeth and closed as one continuous flap (see **Fig. 12**).

SURGICAL EXTRACTION OF MAXILLARY PREMOLARS

Successful oral extraction of a premolar or molar may be limited by the integrity of the clinical crown (eg, decayed, fractured) or by the morphology and orientation of the

---

[l] Incisor elevator set, Equine Dental Instruments, Elmwood, WI.

[m] Long elevator set, Equine Blades Direct, Wedmore, Somerset, UK.

[n] Curved bone chisel, 4 Buser Bone Chisel, ProDent USA, East Brunswick, NJ.

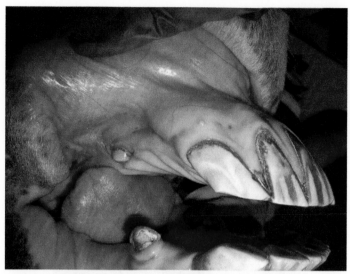

Fig. 14. Outline (*red dots*) of a mucogingival flap for 104 (right maxillary canine). The flap starts slight mesial to the crown, extends along the free margin, and continues into the mucosa along the distal buccal line angle. Avoid extending the flap margin into the rugae of the hard palate mucosa to avoid the palatine artery.

reserve crown/roots (maleruption, impaction, ankylosis, malformation). Repulsion techniques for extraction of equine cheek teeth have been described for decades.[20–22] However, with misdirection of the repulsion force, surgical complications occur creating unanticipated bone damage, such as mandible or hard palate fracture. This extraction technique has a well-established, unacceptably high rate of significant complications.[5,6,23,24]

The surgical approach to the maxillary premolars requires an osteotomy through the rostral maxilla, dorsal to the vestibule of the cheek, ventral to the level of the infraorbital foramen, and directly over the apex of the diseased tooth. Planning for the soft tissue exposure of the maxilla should include final closure over approximately 1 cm of bone after completion of the osteotomy. A sharp straight or ventrally curved incision is made through the skin in a horizontal (rostrocaudal) direction. Subcutaneous blunt dissection is used to identify and isolate the regional neurovascular and salivary structures within the surgical field. Important regional structures include the dorsal branch of the facial nerve; the facial artery and vein; the infraorbital artery, vein, and nerve; and the parotid duct. The dorsal buccal branch of the facial nerve should be isolated° **(Fig. 20)**. If the extraction site is rostral to the infraorbital foramen, the infraorbital artery, vein, and nerve should be retracted dorsally to gain clear access over the tooth roots. This is usually necessary for extraction of the second and third maxillary premolars. The fourth premolar roots/reserve crown is typically ventral to the infraorbital canal/foramen and embedded in the rostral wall of the rostral maxillary sinus. After retracting the important structures, the soft tissue incision is continued through the periosteum to the maxillary bone, and the periosteum is elevated dorsally to expose

---

° Silicone vessel loop, Aspen Surgical Products, Inc, Caledonia, MI.

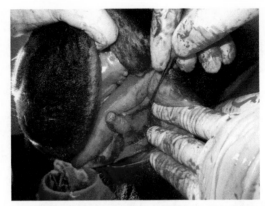

Fig. 15. Elevation of the mucogingival flap for 304 (left mandibular canine).

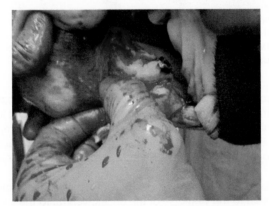

Fig. 16. Buccal bone is removed outlining the root of 404 (right mandibular canine).

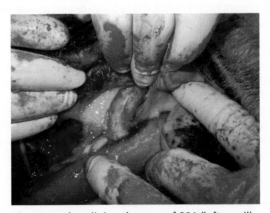

Fig. 17. Buccal bone is removed outlining the root of 204 (left maxillary canine).

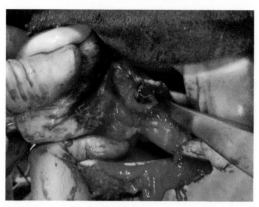

Fig. 18. Elevation (following luxation) of 404 (right mandibular canine).

the osteotomy site. The soft tissue window is maintained with mechanical retraction (eg, Weitlaner, Gelpi, Balfour) (**Fig. 21**).

Both osteotomy and alveolectomy are required to surgically access a maxillary premolar. Access through the maxilla is efficiently achieved with a Galt trephine (15–20 mm diameter)[p]. Once the initial osteotomy is completed additional osseous exposure is customized with a surgical drill and a side-cutting carbide bur[e,f]. Caution must be exercised when cutting through the maxilla in young horses because the developing reserve crowns of the cheek teeth typically lie just beneath the maxillary bone. A more conservative approach using just the surgical drill with gradual expansion of the maxilla bone "window" may be indicated.

Osteotomy through the maxilla provides access to the apical alveolar bone covering the roots of the premolar; however, inflammatory soft tissue (eg, active fistula, abscess) may have to be debrided to visualize the tooth structures. As soon as practical, the location of the osteotomy and the target tooth should be radiographically confirmed using radiopaque markers, such as spinal needles[q] (**Figs. 22** and **23**). After visual and radiographic identification of the diseased tooth, alveolectomy and apicoectomy of the premolar roots is performed with an end-cutting carbide bur to remove curved roots and, more importantly, to provide visualization of the PDL space around the reserve crown, which is used to mark the peripheral limit for tooth resection. With surgical precision, resection of the reserve crown is continued in a coronal direction until an unobstructed extraction pathway is created for the elevation and extraction of the tooth. Continuous saline lavage and suction are required for visualization during drilling. Extralong burs and bur guards (see **Fig. 1**)[r,s,t,u] may be necessary to instrument long reserve crowns (up to 6.6 cm).[25] Periodic intraoperative radiographs with radiopaque markers confirm the correct surgical orientation and prevent drilling into adjacent teeth (**Fig. 24**). The remaining crown is luxated and elevated into the oral cavity or through the osteotomy site (**Fig. 25**). Following extraction, the

---

[p] Trephine 0.75-inch and 1-inch Stainless Steel, Equine Dental Instruments.

[q] Spinal needle, 3.5-inch, 18 gauge, JorVet, Loveland, CO.

[r] Hall's long bur guards, Hall Powered Instruments, Conmed.

[s] Oval bur long carbide, Hall Powered Instruments, Conmed.

[t] Hall's extralong bur guard, Hall Powered Instruments, Conmed.

[u] Oval bur extralong carbide, Hall Powered Instruments, Conmed.

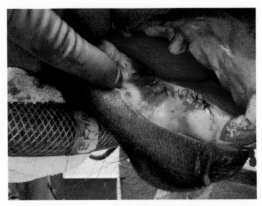

Fig. 19. Closure of the small envelope flap following extraction of 404 (right mandibular canine). A continuous Aberdeen suture pattern is used with a few additional simple interrupted sutures at the rostral aspect of the flap.

alveolus must be thoroughly debrided and flushed with physiologic saline to produce a clean wound. Debridement is visually and radiographically confirmed before closure. A layer of dental packing material[v,w,x,y] is placed into the coronal one-half of the alveolus to form an alveolar plug. Packing the apical part of the alveolus with gauze before placement of the coronal alveolar packing prevents apical advancement of the packing material and promotes laterization into the walls of the alveolus resulting in a better marginal seal. Once the packing material has set, the gauze is removed through the maxillary bone window allowing space for apical blood clot formation. The

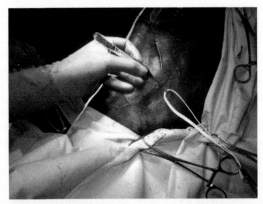

Fig. 20. Soft tissue surgical approach for a maxillary premolar. The dorsal buccal branch of the facial nerve is identified and isolated with a silicone vessel loop.

---

[v] Aquasil Easy Mix Putty STD Mix, BencoDental.

[w] Beveled osteotomes, 5, 10, 20, and 25 mm, Millennium Surgical.

[x] Consil putty, synthetic bone graft, Nutramax Laboratories, Veterinary Science, Inc, Lancaster, SC.

[y] Osteoallograft Periomix, Veterinary Transplant Services, Inc, Kent, WA.

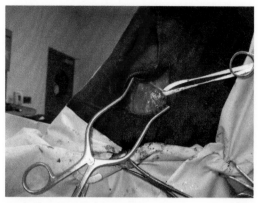

Fig. 21. Soft tissue surgical approach for a maxillary premolar. The periosteum is elevated and a Weitlaner retractor placed for visual access.

subcutaneous tissues with the attached periosteum and the skin are closed in two layers over the osteotomy site.

SURGICAL EXTRACTION OF MAXILLARY MOLARS

The maxillary molars are accessed surgically through the maxillary sinus. The first molar commonly lies within the entire rostral maxillary sinus. The second maxillary molar is positioned at the rostral aspect of the caudal maxillary sinus or just ventral to the maxillary septum. The third molar rests entirely within the caudal maxillary sinus. The bony infraorbital canal passes directly above the second and third maxillary molar with a thin septum of bone commonly extending between the alveolar bone of the second molar and the ventral aspect of the infraorbital canal (**Fig. 26**). The reserve crown and developing roots of "molars in young horses" may extend directly beneath the ventral aspect of the canal (**Fig. 27**), making surgical extraction of the second and third molars challenging. Access to the first and second molar for surgical extraction is typically achieved with a maxillary flap.[21,26,27] A frontonasal flap[26–30] may be indicated for additional exposure for surgical extraction of a third maxillary molar.

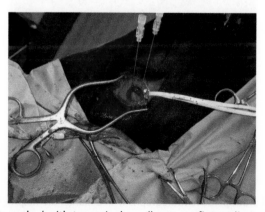

Fig. 22. The root is marked with two spinal needles to confirm radiographic location.

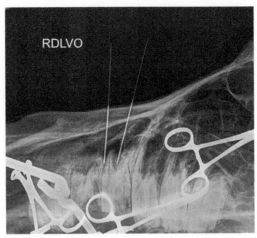

Fig. 23. Intraoperative radiograph showing the osteotomy site and the mesial buccal root of 208 (left maxillary premolar).

The soft tissue landmarks for the maxillary and frontonasal flap are described in John Pigott's article, "Equine Sinus Surgery," in this issue. After surgical access is provided by the appropriate sinus flap, the subsequent four phases of surgical extraction of the maxillary molars are similar to those described for the maxillary premolar surgical extraction.

Surgical extraction of a malformed maxillary first molar (**Fig. 28**) is demonstrated in **Fig. 29**. With the maxillary flap created, the alveolar bone covering the reserve crown and developing roots is removed. Once the fragments are resected, luxated, and elevated from the alveolus the remaining clinical crown is evident at the most coronal extent of the alveolus, which is gently luxated into the oral cavity (**Fig. 30**). Surgical extraction of a fractured first molar is demonstrated in **Fig. 31**. The maxillary flap has been created and a Steinmann pin is being used to radiographically mark the mesial extent of the fractured tooth (**Fig. 32**). Once the fragments of the fractured crown have been removed, the alveolus with healthy bone and the thin bone of the

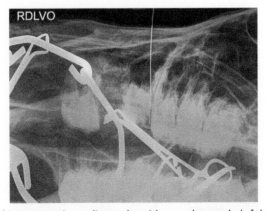

Fig. 24. Additional intraoperative radiographs with a marker are helpful to discern orientation and direction of reserve crown resection.

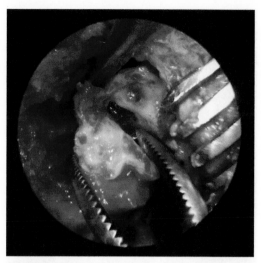

Fig. 25. The remaining reserve/clinical crown is gently elevated and extracted through the osteotomy.

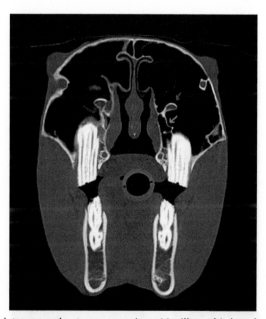

Fig. 26. Computed tomography transverse view. Maxillary third molars (right and left) within the caudal (right and left) maxillary sinus. Normal thin bone (*green arrow*) extending from the left maxillary third molar to the left infraorbital canal (*red arrow*). Infection/reactive bone from the right maxillary third molar extending into the thin bone below the right infraorbital canal (*blue arrow*).

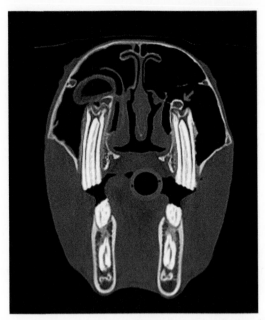

Fig. 27. Computed tomography transverse view. Young developing left third maxillary molar extending into the left infraorbital canal (*red arrow*).

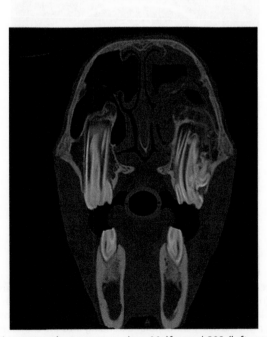

Fig. 28. Computed tomography transverse view. Malformed 209 (left maxillary first molar).

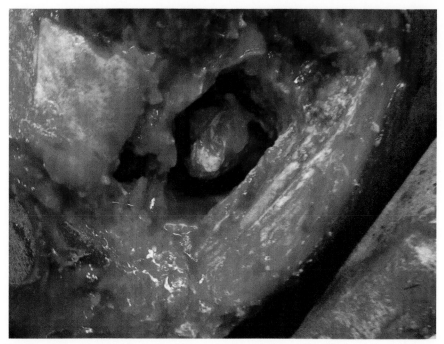

Fig. 29. Intraoperative image of malformed 209. A left maxillary flap has been created, bone is removed from the sinus floor and apical/reserve crown alveolar bone to expose the apical aspect of the malformed left maxillary molar. Noted the thickened/reactive bone along the margins of the maxillary flap.

hard palate are evident (**Fig. 33**). An intraoperative radiograph confirms complete extraction of the diseased first molar (**Fig. 34**). A thin layer of dental packing placed orally into the alveolus is evident from the sinus aspect along with a blood clot starting to form above the packing (**Fig. 35**).

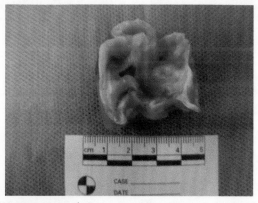

Fig. 30. The remaining portion of the reserve/clinical crown (occlusal view) of the malformed 209 that was luxated and elevated into the oral cavity.

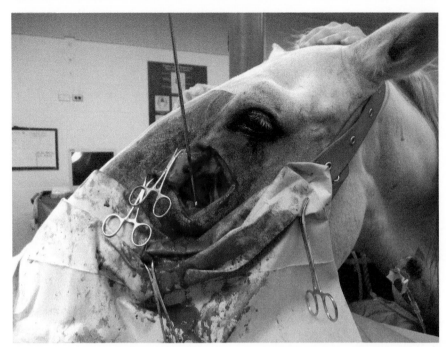

Fig. 31. Left maxillary flap for a surgical approach to 209 (left maxillary first molar) with fractured/fragmented reserve crown. A Steinmann pin is used for intraoperative marking.

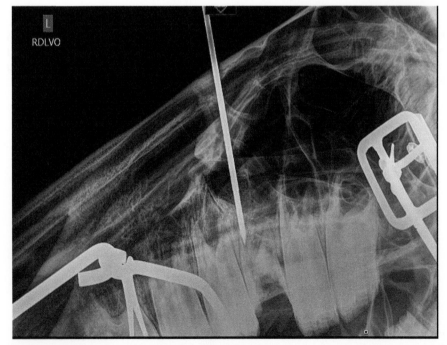

Fig. 32. Intraoperative radiograph shows the Steinmann pin placed directly over the mesial buccal root of 209 (left maxillary first molar).

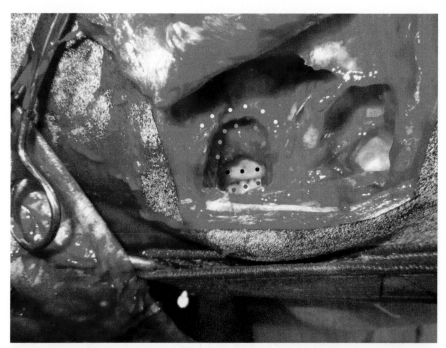

Fig. 33. Intraoperative view through the left maxillary sinus postsurgical extraction of 209. The *white dots* show the remaining floor of the maxillary sinus. The *green dots* show the dorsal aspect of the hard palate. Gentle surgical resection of the palatal root is indicated to avoid damage to the hard palate. The *black dots* mark the tongue and the *purple dots* mark the occlusal surface of 309 (left mandibular first molar) within the oral cavity.

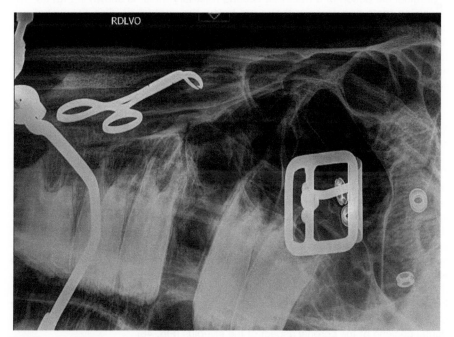

Fig. 34. Intraoperative radiograph confirming complete surgical extraction of 209 (left maxillary first molar).

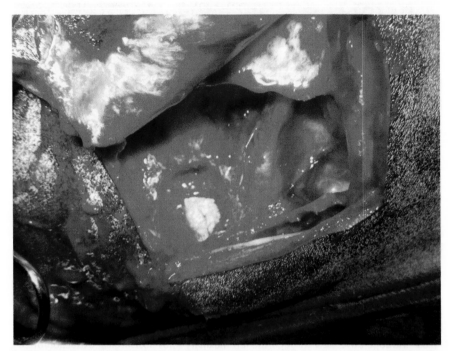

Fig. 35. Placement of a thin layer of dental packing placed from the oral aspect of the alveolus. A blood clot is starting to form above the packing.

Surgical extraction of a fractured second maxillary molar is shown in **Fig. 36**. The remaining roots and reserve crown are below the septum dividing the rostral and caudal components of the maxillary sinus (maxillary septum). Rongeurs[k] are used to remove the septum to expose the roots of the fractured tooth. Needles are placed to radiographically confirm the mesial and distal extent of the tooth roots (**Figs. 37** and **38**). A postextraction radiograph confirms complete extraction of the fractured second maxillary molar (**Fig. 39**).

Surgical extraction of a third maxillary molar is more challenging and may require an additional frontonasal flap. Computed tomography shows an abscessed and malformed developing right third maxillary molar (**Figs. 40** and **41**). The transverse and sagittal view show the long reserve crown extending directly beneath the infraorbital canal. The bone surrounding the tooth and the canal is reactive from the active infection. The sagittal view (see **Fig. 41**) reveals that the apical aspect of developing third molar is bulbous and malformed. A frontonasal and maxillary flap are created to gain adequate surgical exposure to the third molar. The frontonasal flap shows the extensive infection in close association of the apical aspect of the tooth. Extension of the infection into the rostral extent of the caudal maxillary sinus is evident with the maxillary flap (**Fig. 42**). The long reserve crown is sectioned in segments working through the frontonasal and maxillary flaps. The maxillary septum is removed to gain access to the coronal aspect of the alveolus. The remaining clinical crown is sectioned sagittally, luxated into the oral cavity (**Fig. 43**), and removed orally. The alveolus is visually and radiographically (**Fig. 44**) inspected to confirm complete extraction of the right maxillary third molar. A thin layer of dental packing is placed orally (**Fig. 45**). Sinus endoscopy shows the thin layer of dental packing at the coronal aspect of the alveolus (**Fig. 46**).

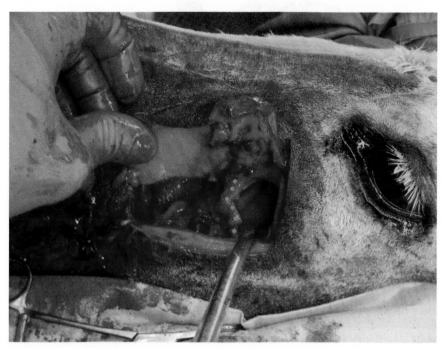

Fig. 36. Left maxillary flap for surgical approach to the retained/fractured roots of 210 (left maxillary second molar). The roots lie directly below the boney septum dividing the rostral and caudal maxillary sinus (*green dots*).

SURGICAL EXTRACTION OF MANDIBULAR PREMOLARS

The surgical approach to the mandibular premolars requires an osteotomy through the lateral mandible dorsal to the mandibular canal and centered over the reserve crown of the diseased tooth. The soft tissue exposure of the mandible should include planning for the final soft tissue closure over approximately 1 cm of bone after completion of the osteotomy. A sharp straight or ventrally curved incision is made through the skin, buccinator muscle, and periosteum in a horizontal (rostrocaudal) direction approximately 2 cm ventral to the vestibule of the cheek and ventral to the depressor labii inferioris muscle. Important regional structures include the ventral branch of the facial nerve, the inferior labial artery, the facial artery and vein, and the parotid duct. Depending on the position of a fourth premolar with respect to the vital structures at the rostral edge of the masseter muscle, a surgical approach with a vertical (dorsoventral) skin incision, as described with the mandibular molars, may provide better access. Following the incision of the peripheral soft tissues and isolation of important structures, the periosteum and overlying soft tissues are elevated dorsally off of the lateral cortex of the mandible. This periosteal elevation is extended under the gingival sulcus. The attached marginal gingiva and gingival sulcus are elevated from the alveolar margin and the clinical crown of the diseased tooth to provide access into the mouth. Hohmann retractors[z] are placed under the elevated soft tissues and onto the occlusal surface of the diseased tooth. Elevation

---

[z] Hohmann retractors, Millennium Surgical.

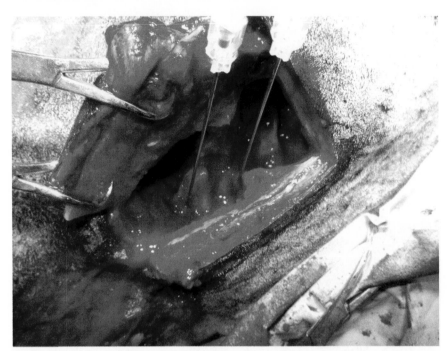

Fig. 37. The boney septum has been removed with rongeurs to expose the alveolar bone overlying the two buccal roots of 210 (left maxillary second M). Two spinal needles are placed to confirm location radiographically.

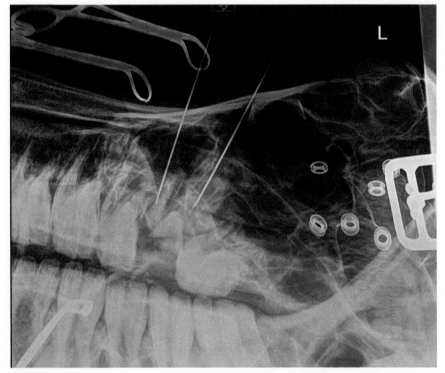

Fig. 38. Intraoperative radiograph shows correct isolation of 210 root fragments.

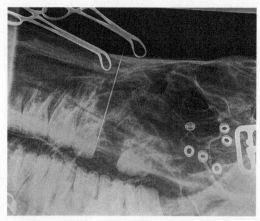

Fig. 39. Intraoperative radiograph confirms complete extraction of the root fragments.

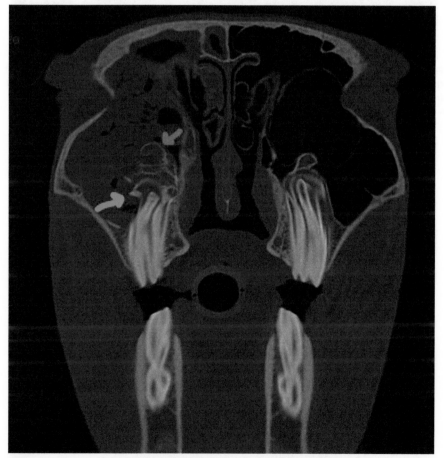

Fig. 40. Computed tomography transverse view. An infected malformed developing 111 (right maxillary third molar; *green arrow*) with reactive bone extending into the infraorbital canal (*red arrow*). Secondary sinusitis is evident in the caudal maxillary and frontal sinus.

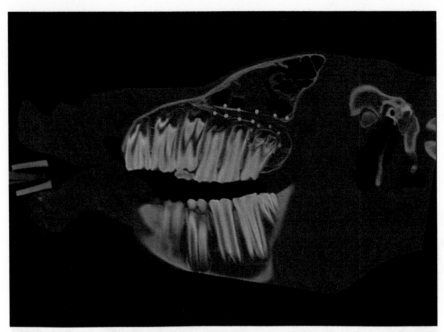

Fig. 41. Computed tomography sagittal view. The infraorbital canal is outlined above all three maxillary molars (*green dots*). *Red dots* outline a bulbous malformed root with 111 (right maxillary third molar).

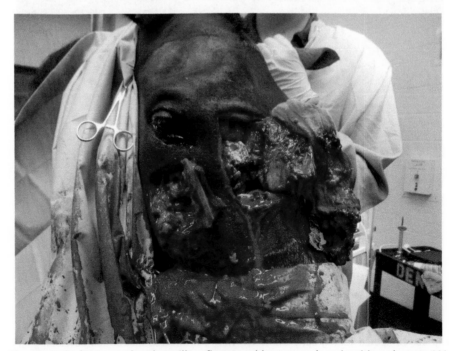

Fig. 42. Right frontonasal and maxillary flaps to address secondary sinusitis and access 111 (right maxillary third molar) for surgical extraction.

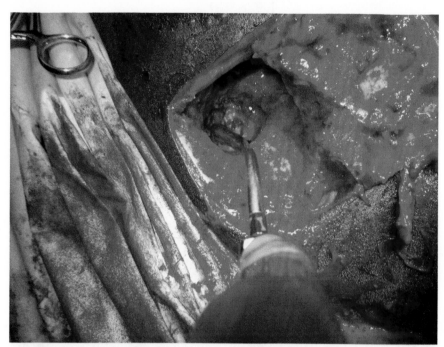

Fig. 43. Following sequential resection of 111 (right maxillary third molar) the remaining reserve/clinical crown is sectioned sagittally and gently luxated into the oral cavity.

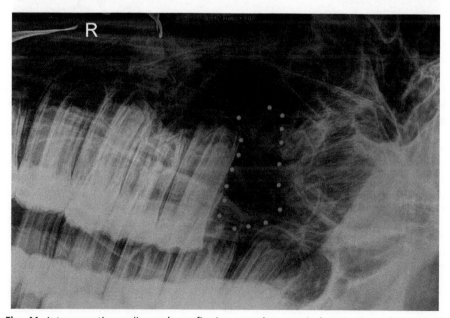

Fig. 44. Intraoperative radiograph confirming complete surgical extraction of 111 (right maxillary third molar; *red dots*).

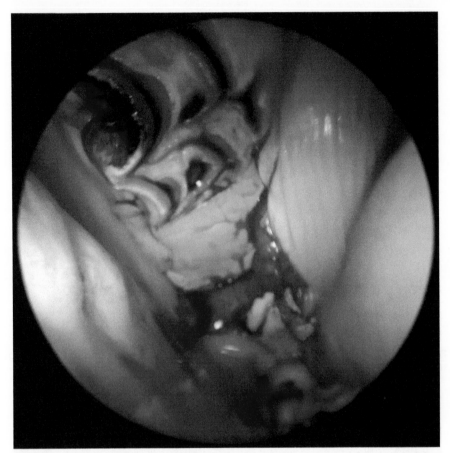

Fig. 45. Oral endoscopy shows a thin layer of dental packing material after it is placed orally into the coronal 2 cm of the 111 alveolus.

with the retractors provides clinical crown visualization of the diseased tooth and alveolar margin for alveolectomy (**Fig. 47**).

Using a surgical drill with an end-cutting carbide bur, saline lavage, and suction[e,f,g] the buccal bone overlying the diseased tooth is removed starting at the alveolar margin and carefully working apically, using the mesial and distal PDL spaces of the reserve crown to identify the limits of alveolectomy (**Fig. 48**). Alveolectomy is usually continued apically until the furcation between the mesial and distal roots is exposed. The tooth is then sectioned transversely from the furcation to the clinical crown taking caution not to damage the lingual alveolar bone (**Fig. 49**). The two sections of the tooth are then luxated and elevated (**Fig. 50**). If resistance to elevation is experienced, the tooth can be further sectioned into additional pieces. Likewise, additional alveolectomy may be required to expose a fractured root; however, aggressive instrumentation and elevation should be avoided to prevent entry into the mandibular canal. Alveolar wound management is similar to that described for maxillary premolars. A coronal alveolar plug is placed as previously described, and the surgical site is closed in two layers.

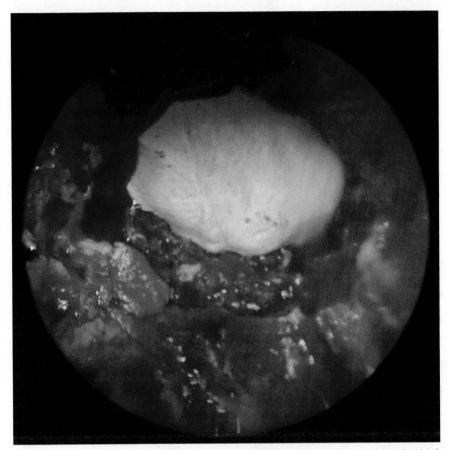

Fig. 46. Sinus endoscopy evaluation of dental packing placed into the 111 alveolus (right maxillary third molar).

SURGICAL EXTRACTION OF MANDIBULAR MOLARS

The soft tissue approach to the mandibular molars (and occasional the fourth premolar) is a vertical incision directly over the affected tooth. Typically, the approach for the first molar (and fourth premolar) is rostral to the masseter muscle (**Fig. 51**). The dorsal extent of the soft tissue incision is ventral to the cheek vestibule, and the ventral extent of the incision is placed at the level of the furcation between the two roots of the affected tooth. The facial artery and vein, parotid salivary duct, and masseter muscle are retracted caudally, and the ventral buccal branch of the facial nerve is isolated and retracted dorsally. The soft tissues are elevated, retracted, and maintained with mechanical retractors (eg, Weitlaner, Gelpi, Balfour)*,**,***, while taking care not to traumatize the facial vein, artery, and parotid duct. As described

---

* Weitlaner retractors, Medco.

** Gelpi retractors, Medco.

*** Balfour retractors, Medco.

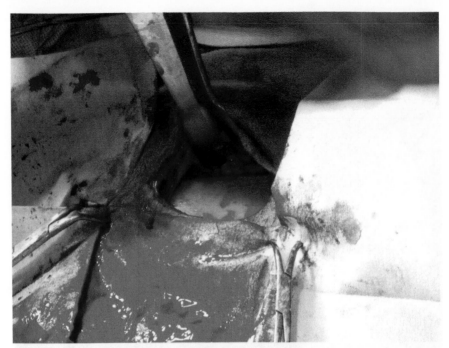

Fig. 47. Horizontal soft tissue approach for surgical extraction of a mandibular premolar. Hohmann retractors are placed into the oral cavity directly over the effected tooth to gain visual access of the clinical crown and alveolar ridge.

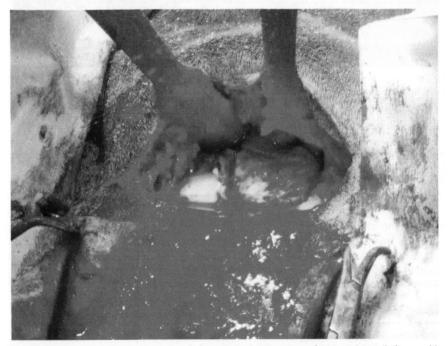

Fig. 48. Horizontal soft tissue approach for surgical extraction of 306 and 307 (left mandibular second and third premolars). Buccal bone is removed from 307 starting at the alveolar ridge and following the mesial and distal margins of the reserve crown.

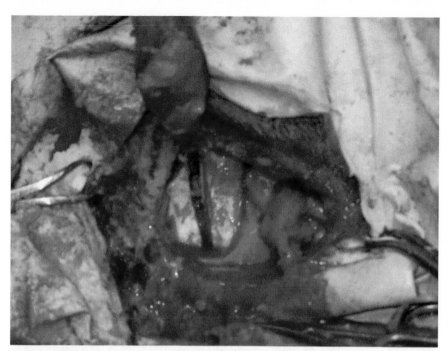

Fig. 49. Horizontal soft tissue approach for surgical extraction of 306 and 307 (left mandibular second and third premolars). The buccal bone is removed over 306 to the furcation between the roots. The tooth is sectioned in a transverse/coronal direction extending from the occlusal surface to the furcation.

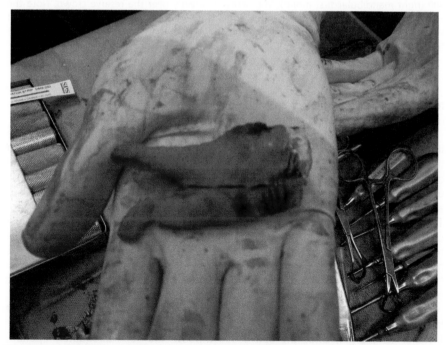

Fig. 50. The 306 (left mandibular second premolar) following tooth sectioning, luxation, and elevation. Note the fractured mesial root tip. If the root tip fractures, root luxation and elevation is indicated. Additional buccal bone resection may be indicated to isolate the root tip. Gentle force is indicated to avoid entering the mandibular canal.

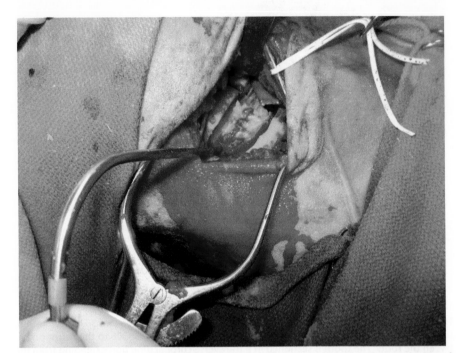

Fig. 51. Vertical soft tissue approach rostral to the masseter muscle for surgical extraction of 409 (right mandibular first molar). The access is directly over the reserve crown. Note the ventral buccal branch of the facial nerve is identified and isolated. Buccal bone is removed starting at the alveolar ridge and following the mesial and distal margins of the reserve crown.

for the mandibular premolars, the oral cavity is fenestrated to provide identification of the diseased tooth and exposure of the alveolar margin for alveolectomy.

The soft tissue approach for the second and third mandibular molars extends through the masseter muscle directly over and in line with the reserve crown of the diseased tooth (**Fig. 52**). The orientation of the mandibular molars is dependent on the curve of Spee; therefore, the ventral margin of the mandible should not be used to align the soft tissue approach. A least one branch of the facial nerve is usually within the surgical field immediately under the skin and can often be palpated. The skin incision should be carefully made and then the facial nerve is bluntly dissected and retracted dorsally out of the field. The masseter muscle and periosteum are sharply transected and retracted to expose the mandible. It may be necessary to remove a segment of masseter muscle for adequate exposure of the buccal bone. As with the other mandibular cheek teeth, the periosteum is elevated and the marginal gingiva is fenestrated providing access into oral cavity; however, this elevation and fenestration must be performed cautiously to prevent lacerating the dilated buccal vein, which lies above the periosteum at the level of the alveolar margin. Once the soft tissue window has been adequately opened, the buccal vein is elevated and protected with Hohmann retractors. The remaining stages of the surgical extraction proceed as previously described for the other mandibular cheek teeth.

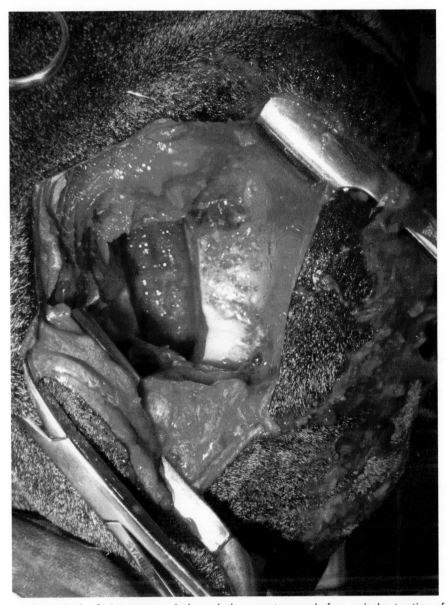

Fig. 52. Vertical soft tissue approach through the masseter muscle for surgical extraction of 410 (right mandibular second molar). The access is directly over the reserve crown. An approximately 1.5-cm wide strip of masseter muscle is removed to improve retraction and visual access. Buccal bone is removed starting at the alveolar ridge and following the mesial and distal margins of the reserve crown.

SUMMARY

Dental repulsion techniques reported in the past decades have an unacceptably high incidence of complications, including iatrogenic damage to surrounding tissues. Although the practice of surgical extractions in horses is limited because of the training, instrumentation, and experience required to perform these techniques, veterinarians should be aware that these procedures are available, that general anesthesia is not required, and when performed by skilled veterinary dentists, have low complication rates. Surgical techniques are often used after the failure of other extraction techniques to remove retained tooth root and fragments or to debride chronically contaminated orofacial lesions. However, surgical extractions should be considered during the initial treatment planning of all complicated cases.

CLINICS CARE POINTS

- Standing surgical extractions can be performed on all equine teeth.
- Surgical extraction techniques are often used after the failure of other extraction techniques but should be considered preoperatively as a definitive treatment in complex cases.
- Training in general and oral surgical principles and techniques, as well as a comprehensive understanding of dental, oral, and regional anatomy, are prerequisite for a successful outcome.
- When performed by a skilled veterinary dentist, surgical extractions produce predictable successful outcomes with rapid healing and low complication rates.
- All veterinarians should be aware that surgical extractions are an available treatment option.

REFERENCES

1. Liuti T, Smith S, Dixon PM. A comparison of computed tomographic, radiographic, gross and histological, dental, and alveolar findings in 30 abnormal cheek teeth from equine cadavers. Front Vet Sci 2018;4:236.
2. Liuti T, Smith S, Dixon PM. Radiographic, computed tomographic, gross pathological and histological findings with suspected apical infection in 32 equine maxillary cheek teeth (2012-2015). Equine Vet J 2018;50(1):41–7.
3. Townsend NB, Hawkes CS, Rex R, et al. Investigation of the sensitivity and specificity of radiological signs for diagnosis of periapical infection of equine cheek teeth. Equine Vet J 2011;43(2):170–8.
4. Weller R, Livesey L, Maierl J, et al. Comparison of radiography and scintigraphy in the diagnosis of dental disorders in the horse. Equine Vet J 2001;33(1):49–58.
5. Caramello V, Zarucco L, Foster D, et al. Equine cheek tooth extraction: comparison of outcomes for five extraction methods. Equine Vet J 2020;52(2):181–6.
6. O'Neil HD, Boussauw B, Bladon BM, et al. Extraction of cheek teeth using a lateral buccotomy approach in 114 horses (1999-2009). Equine Vet J 2011;43(3):348–53.
7. Rawlinson JE. Surgical extraction of mandibular cheek teeth via alveolar bone removal. Proceedings of the American Association of Equine Practitioners Focus Meeting on Dentistry, Albuquerque, NM, September 18-20, 2011. pp. 178–83.
8. Rawlinson JR. Review of surgical extraction of mandibular cheek teeth. Proceedings of the American Association of Equine Practitioners Focus Meeting on Dentistry, Charlotte, NC, August 4-6, 2013. p. 75–9.

9. Rawlinson JR. Review of surgical extraction of maxillary cheek teeth. Proceedings of the American Association of Equine Practitioners Focus Meeting on Dentistry, Charlotte, NC, August 4-6, 2013. p. 80–4.

10. Tremaine WH, McCluskie. Removal of 11 incompletely erupted, impacted cheek teeth in 10 horses using a dental alveolar transcortical osteotomy and buccotomy approach. Vet Surg 2010;39:884–90.

11. Takei H, Carranza FA, Shin K. In: Takei HH, Carranza FA, Shin K, editors. Carranza's clinical periodontology, 12th edition. Chapter 59. The flap technique for pocket therapy. St Louis (MO). Elsevier; 2015. p. 593–603.

12. Takei HH, Azzi RR, Han TJ. Periodontal plastic and esthetic surgery. In: Newman MG, Takei HH, Klokkevold PR, et al, editors. Carranza's clinical periodontology. 10th edition. Philadelphia: Saunders Elsevier; 2006. p. 1025–6.

13. Bula E, Upchurch DA, Wang Y, et al. Comparison of tensile strength and time to closure between an intermittent Aberdeen suture pattern and conventional methods of closure for the body wall of dogs. Am J Vet Res 2018;79(1): 115–23.

14. Coleridge M, Gillen AM, Farag R, et al. Effect of fluid media on the mechanical properties of continuous pattern-ending surgeon's, square, and Aberdeen knots in vitro. Vet Surg 2017;46(2):306–15.

15. Lobprise HB, Dodd JR. Wigg's veterinary dentistry, principles and practice. 2nd edition. Hoboken (NJ): John Wiley & Sons, Inc; 2019. p. 6–9, 200-203.

16. Ashdown RR, Done SH, Evans SA. Color atlas of veterinary anatomy, the horse, vol. 2. Danvers (MA): Elsevier Science Limited; 2002. p. 41–4.

17. Earley ET, Rawlinson JT. A new understanding of oral and dental disorders of the equine incisor and canine teeth. Vet Clin North Am Equine Pract 2013;29(2): 273–300.

18. Rawlinson JT, Earley ET. Advances in the treatment of diseased equine incisor and canine teeth. Vet Clin North Am Equine Pract 2013;29(2):411–40.

19. Budras KD, Sack WO, Rock S, et al. Anatomy of the horse. Sixth edition. Hannover (Germany): Schlutersche Verlagsgesellschaft mbH & Co. KG; 2011. p. 36–9.

20. Tremaine WH, Schumacher J. Chapter 20, Exodontia. In: Easley J, Dixon PM, Schumacher J, editors. Equine dentistry. 3rd edition. Philadelphia: Saunders Elsevier; 2011. p. 331–41.

21. McIlwraith CW, Turner AS. Equine surgery advanced techniques. Philadelphia: Lea & Febiger; 1987. p. 244–9, 260-263.

22. Turner AS, McIlwraith CW. Techniques in large animal surgery. Second edition. Philadelphia: Lea & Febiger; 1989. p. 235–9.

23. Earley ET. How to identify potential complications associated with cheek-teeth extractions in the horse. AAEP Annual Meeting, Baltimore, MD, December 4-8, 2010;56:465–80.

24. Earley ET, Rawlinson JE, Baratt RM. Complications associated with cheek tooth extraction in the horse. J Vet Dent 2013;30(4):220–35.

25. Tiziana L, Reardon R, Dixon PM. Computed tomographic assessment of equine maxillary cheek teeth anatomical relationships, and paranasal sinus volumes. Vet Rec 2017;181(17):452.

26. Barakzai SZ, Dixon PM. Standing equine sinus surgery. Vet Clin North Am Equine Pract 2014;30(1):45–62.

27. Schumacher J, Dutton DM, Murphy DJ, et al. Paranasal sinus surgery through a frontonasal flap in sedated, standing horses. Vet Surg 2000;29(2):173–7.

28. Easley JT, Freeman DE. A single caudally based frontonasal bone flap for treatment of bilateral mucocele in the paranasal sinuses of an American miniature horse. Vet Surg 2013;42(4):427–32.
29. Freeman DE, Orsini PG, Ross MW, et al. A large frontonasal bone flap for sinus surgery in the horse. Vet Surg 1990;19(2):122–30.
30. Robert MP, Stemmet GP, Smit Y. A bilateral sinus cyst treated via a bilateral frontonasal bone flap in a standing horse. J S Afr Vet Assoc 2019;90:e1–6.

Equine Sinus Surgery

John Pigott, DVM, MS

KEYWORDS

- Sinus • Surgery • Trephination • Bone flap • Sinusitis • Horse

KEY POINTS

- An in-depth understanding of equine paranasal sinus anatomy, its communications and drainage is critical for approaching sinus disease.
- Sinocentesis and lavage are simple procedures that can be done in the field with knowledge of anatomic landmarks.
- Sinoscopy via trephination or in combination with a sinus flap is a valuable tool to aid in complete exploration of all sinus compartments.
- Sinus flaps are preferred by some because of the large area of direct visualization, ease of instrument manipulation, and establishment of drainage.
- Complications after sinus surgery are relatively common, but can be reduced with a thorough exploratory, establishing adequate drainage and good surgical technique.

SINUS ANATOMY

The equine paranasal sinuses are traditionally described as having 6 pairs: maxillary, frontal, sphenopalatine, dorsal conchal, middle conchal (ethmoidal), and ventral conchal.[1] However, some publications reference 5 or 7 pairs, with varying interpretations of what constitutes a separate sinus compartment.[2] Functionally, the equine sinuses are separated into a rostral and a caudal system based on communications and drainage into the nasal passage. The maxillary sinus is separated into rostral and caudal compartments via an oblique septum located approximately 5 cm caudal to the rostral end of the facial crest.[1] The septum is typically intact but is thin dorsally and can partially break down with more chronic sinusitis or disease. Alternatively, the septum can thicken with reactive bone subsequent to dental disease (**Fig. 1**).[3]

The nasal conchae are thin, partly ossified scrolls that are covered in mucosa, observed readily during nasal endoscopy. The dorsal and ventral nasal conchae are separated into 2 compartments via a septum, the caudal component of which expands to form the respective dorsal and ventral conchal sinus.[1,4] The ventral conchal sinus extends dorsolaterally in a very thin, friable, boney structure from the maxillary septum.[4] This structure is referred to as the maxillary septal bulla (**Fig. 2**A).[5] The

Cornell Ruffian Equine Specialists, 111 Plainfield Avenue, Elmont, NY 11003, USA
E-mail address: jhp322@gmail.com

Vet Clin Equine 36 (2020) 613–639
https://doi.org/10.1016/j.cveq.2020.08.003
0749-0739/20/© 2020 Elsevier Inc. All rights reserved.

vetequine.theclinics.com

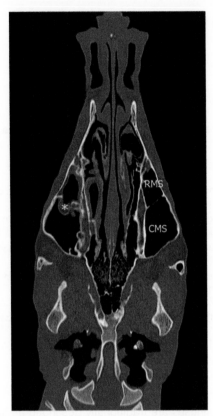

Fig. 1. Dorsal plane computed tomography image showing the rostral maxillary sinus separated by an oblique septum from the caudal maxillary sinus. CMS, caudal maxillary sinus; RMS, rostral maxillary sinus. * A thickened septum on the opposite side owing to rostral maxillary and ventral conchal sinusitis.

ventral conchal sinus, along with the rostral and caudal maxillary sinuses are frequently involved with sinusitis secondary to dental disease (**Fig. 2**B).

The middle conchal sinus is a very small structure, contained within the middle conchus (**Fig. 3**A).[1] The middle conchus is readily observed during routine nasal endoscopy (**Fig. 3**B). The middle conchal sinus should be considered during diagnostic evaluation and treatment but the very small size limits access. In cases of disease (see **Fig. 3**A), sinus access can be gained via laser fenestration of the middle conchus through the nose or direct penetration through a sinus flap or trephine.

The sphenopalatine sinus is composed of a more caudal sphenoidal part and more rostral palatine part, which typically communicate under the ethmoid labyrinth (**Fig. 4**).[1] Although the palatine and sphenoidal parts of the sphenopalatine sinus communicate in many horses, there is considerable anatomic variation with some horses lacking any communication.[2,6]

SINUS COMMUNICATIONS

The equine sinuses form a series of communications that allow drainage into the nasal passage. These communications are important to understand when diagnosing the

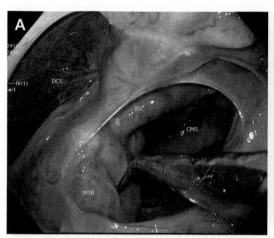
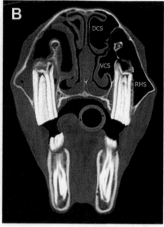

Fig. 2. (*A*) Sinoscopic image from a conchofrontal portal showing the maxillary septal bulla protruding into the frontomaxillary opening, adjacent to the infraorbital canal. (*B*). Transverse CT image showing anatomic relationship of rostral maxillary sinus as it communicates over the infraorbital canal with the ventral conchal sinus. The sinus mucosa of the unlabeled opposite side is thickened from chronic sinusitis. CMS, caudal maxillary sinus; DCS, dorsal conchal sinus; *IOC, infraorbital canal; MSB, maxillary septal bulla; RMS, rostral maxillary sinus.

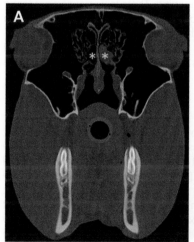
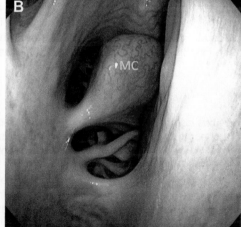

Fig. 3. (*A*) Transverse computed tomography (CT) image showing a normal and abnormal middle conchal sinus. The right middle conchal sinus (*left side* of CT image) is filled with air and seems to be normal. The left middle conchal sinus (*right side* of CT image) is filled with a fluid or soft tissue density material secondary to middle conchal sinusitis. (*B*) Nasal endoscopic image showing the middle conchus where laser fenestration is possible to gain access to the middle conchal sinus. *Middle conchal sinus. MC, middle conchus. ([*A*] *Courtesy of* Dr. Jonathan Cheetham, Ithaca, NY.)

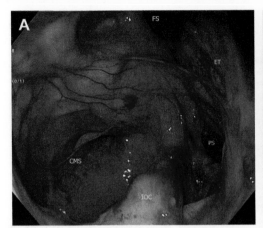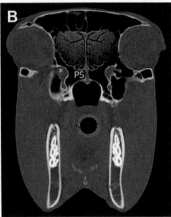

Fig. 4. (A) Sinoscopic image through a sinonasal communication after surgery showing the palatine sinus opening under the ethmoid turbinates. (B) Transverse computed tomography image showing the palatine sinus relative to the infraorbital canal. CMS, caudal maxillary sinus; ET, ethmoid turbinates; FS, frontal sinus; *IOC, infraorbital canal; PS, palatine sinus.

extent of sinusitis, planning surgical approaches and evaluating drainage. The rostral maxillary sinus communicates with the ventral conchal sinus over the dorsal aspect of the infraorbital canal via the conchomaxillary opening (see **Fig. 2**B).[1,7] These 2 sinuses are separated from the more caudal sinuses by the septum between the rostral and caudal maxillary sinuses (see **Fig. 1**). The caudal maxillary sinus communicates with the frontal sinus via the frontomaxillary opening. This opening tends to be large but the exact position is variable (see **Fig. 2**A; **Fig. 5**).[7] The frontal sinus communicates directly with the dorsal conchal sinus via a large opening. There is no defined anatomic separation between the frontal sinus and the dorsal conchal sinus. This extensive communication results in many texts calling it a combined conchofrontal sinus.[1] The caudal maxillary sinus communicates with the sphenopalatine sinus, just axial to the infraorbital canal (see **Fig. 4**), as well as with the middle conchal sinus (see **Fig. 3**A).[1]

SINUS DRAINAGE

The sinus compartments drain through the nasomaxillary aperture into the caudolateral aspect of the middle meatus in the nasal passage.[1] This part of the middle meatus should be inspected thoroughly for any purulent drainage during nasal endoscopy in horses with a history of nasal discharge (**Fig. 6**). The detailed anatomic pathway of the nasomaxillary aperture relative to the equine paranasal sinus system has been described.[8] The rostral maxillary sinus communicates directly with the aperture just medial to the nasolacrimal canal against the maxilla. The caudal maxillary sinus communicates with the nasomaxillary aperture between the roof the maxillary septal bulla of the ventral conchal sinus and the floor of the dorsal conchal sinus. The caudal entrance height was found to be less than 2 mm during this description.[8]

SINUSITIS

Sinusitis is typically described as primary or secondary. Primary sinusitis develops from extension of an upper respiratory infection, most commonly resulting in bacterial

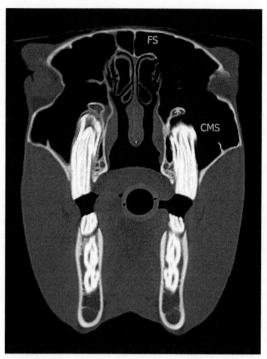

Fig. 5. Transverse computed tomography image showing large communication between the frontal sinus and the caudal maxillary sinus through the frontomaxillary opening. CMS, caudal maxillary sinus; FS, frontal sinus. *Infraorbital canal.

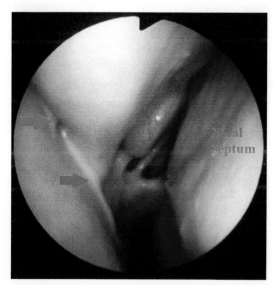

Fig. 6. Bronchoscopic image of purulent material draining from the nasomaxillary aperture. *Green arrow*, nasomaxillary aperture. *Red arrow*, purulent material. (*Courtesy of* Dr. Stephen Galloway, Oakland, TN.)

infection of the sinuses. Secondary sinusitis can be secondary to a number of causes (fracture, neoplasia, ethmoid hematoma, or cyst), although dental disease is a frequent cause.[9] With extension of dental disease to the maxillary sinuses, many horses present with a history of unilateral, malodorous, purulent nasal discharge (**Fig. 7**). However, there is great variation to the amount, character, consistency, and odor of drainage between cases, and this factor should not be used as sole criteria for diagnosing dental sinusitis. Some horses present with bilateral nasal discharge, which could be the result of bilateral dental disease, compromise to the nasal septum and axial sinus walls, or another nonsinus related cause.

LANDMARKS FOR TREPHINATION OR SINOCENTESIS

Making an appropriate surgical approach to the sinus compartments depends on knowing the anatomic landmarks and boundaries of the sinus cavities. Landmarks for sinocentesis using a needle or Steinmann pin, or access via small 15- to 25-mm trephination tend to be similar. For the conchofrontal sinus, the access point is 60% of the distance from midline to the medial canthus, approximately 0.5 cm caudal to this line (**Fig. 8**A).[10] Aiming too far caudally and deep can disrupt the ethmoid labyrinth resulting in prominent hemorrhage. It is important to limit the depth of penetration so that controlled access to the sinus is achieved. The caudal maxillary sinus can be entered at a point approximately 2 cm rostral and ventral to the medial canthus (**Fig. 8**B). The rostral maxillary sinus can be entered by going 40% of the distance along a line drawn from the rostral edge of the facial crest to the medial canthus, and 1 cm ventral to a line between the infraorbital foramen and the medial canthus (**Fig. 8**C).[10] Approaching more caudal to this point runs the risk of penetrating the caudal maxillary sinus instead.[11] In horses younger than 6 years old, approaches to the rostral and caudal maxillary sinus carries risk of iatrogenic damage to the cheek

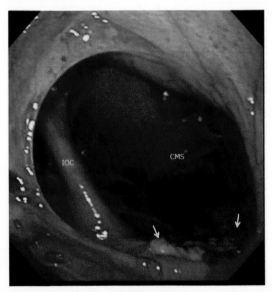

Fig. 7. Sinoscopic image through a conchofrontal portal showing inspissated pus in the caudal maxillary sinus secondary to dental disease. CMS, caudal maxillary sinus; IOC, infraorbital canal. *Yellow arrows,* inspissated pus.

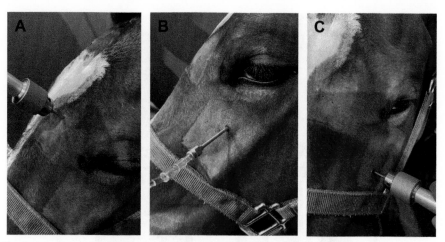

Fig. 8. Landmarks for sinocentesis or lavage of the sinus cavities on a cadaver. (*A*) Concho-frontal sinus. (*B*) Caudal maxillary sinus. (*C*) Rostral maxillary sinus.

teeth reserve crowns that occupy much of the sinus space. Radiographs can aid in assessing tooth position relative to the proposed sinusotomy site to decrease the risk of damage.

SINOCENTESIS PROCEDURE

Access to the sinuses in these locations for simple lavage or aspiration can be done with a 14-gauge needle and a mallet, a Steinmann pin and a Jacobs chuck, or a drill bit. The author prefers the use of a 1/8-inch Steinmann pin and Jacobs chuck to gain access for simple lavage or aspiration. This procedure is simple to do in the field or hospital and is facilitated using light sedation. When using any of these techniques, the area is focally clipped, prepped, and blocked using subcutaneous infiltration of local anesthetic. A 14-gauge needle will bend in some horses with thicker bone, partic-ularly over the rostral maxillary sinus site. With a Steinmann pin, a stab incision is made with a #11 or #15 scalpel blade, just large enough to introduce the pin. For lavage with a teat cannula or smaller bore flush cannula, a hole created with an 1/8-inch Stein-mann pin or slightly larger is usually sufficient (**Fig. 9**). For these locations, only 2.0 to 2.5 cm of the Steinmann pin should be protruding from the Jacobs chuck to mini-mize risk of iatrogenic damage to deeper structures (see **Fig. 8**A). Alternatively, the use of a 3.2-mm or 4.0-mm drill bit is preferred by some, using a hemostat or drill guide to protect the skin while drilling into the sinus. Once sinus access is gained, a sample can be aspirated or the sinus can be lavaged with 1 to 2 L of saline. The skin incision with either technique can either be left open to heal by secondary intention or closed with a single staple or suture.

SINOSCOPY CONSIDERATIONS

Sinoscopy is a valuable tool that provides direct visualization of the sinus cavities. This imaging can be particularly useful when there is question as to the extent of the dis-ease and to further define the cause. It can be performed as a diagnostic or as an adjunctive procedure during surgery to facilitate visualization. Sinoscopy can be per-formed in a minimally invasive fashion using a 14-gauge needle and a 2- to 3-mm rigid

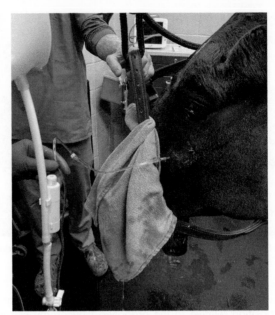

Fig. 9. Lavage of the left rostral maxillary sinus with a teat cannula secondary to oroantral fistula formation after 209 removal.

or flexible endoscope. However, a small field of view and limited visibility in certain sinus compartments are challenges.[12] Some of these limitations can be minimized by making a larger sinusotomy with a 15-mm Galt trephine or larger, for passage of a 12-mm flexible videoendoscope (**Fig. 10**). Although this approach is more invasive

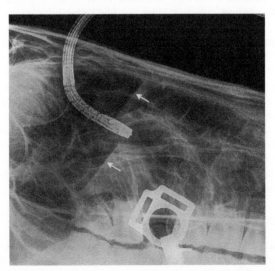

Fig. 10. Lateral sinus radiograph demonstrating fluid in the caudal maxillary and dorsal conchal sinuses (*white arrows*) in a horse with sinusitis. Sinoscopy is being performed through a conchofrontal portal using a flexible endoscope.

than a 14-gauge needle, a larger field of view can be beneficial in certain cases, particularly where instrument manipulation is required.

SINOSCOPY APPROACH

Sinoscopic portals using a Galt trephine are prepared the same as for Steinmann pin trephination. Preoperative antibiotics may be used based on culture and sensitivity results or empirically based on the dental disease present. Preoperative anti-inflammatories typically consist of phenylbutazone or flunixin meglumine. Frequently, the sinus cavities can be fully evaluated through a single portal in the conchofrontal sinus, using the same landmarks as described elsewhere in this article. However, sinoscopy can be performed through any trephine hole if anatomic variation prevents adequate visualization in one location. A small C-shaped skin incision, approximately 10 to 15 mm larger than the trephine, is common (**Fig. 11**A). The skin and periosteum is reflected and the trephination performed (**Fig. 11**B). A larger skin incision relative to the trephine allows for adequate bone support of the skin flap. A linear incision can be used for smaller trephines (15–19 mm). However, linear incisions over larger trephines can result in incisional complications owing to the lack of bone support under the incision.

SINOSCOPY EXPLORATORY

Exploration from the conchofrontal portal requires breaking down the bulla of the maxillary septum to gain access into the ventral conchal sinus and rostral maxillary sinus. The bulla is frequently observed protruding into the frontomaxillary opening and can be broken down through the same portal with a thin rongeur or hemostat (see **Fig. 2**A; **Fig. 12**A). However, in some horses, the bulla does not extend as far caudal and a second portal needs to be created in the caudal maxillary sinus to achieve

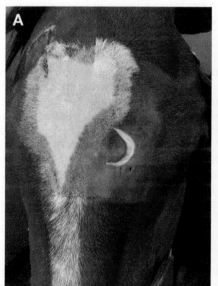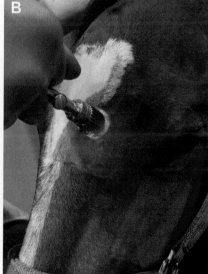

Fig. 11. (*A*) Conchofrontal trephination approach using a C-shaped incision on a cadaver. (*B*) Conchofrontal trephination using a Galt trephine.

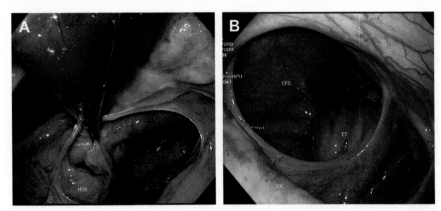

Fig. 12. (*A*) Sinoscopic image through a conchofrontal portal looking down through the frontomaxillary opening. A hemostat is used through the same portal to break down the maxillary septal bulla. (*B*) Sinoscopic image from a caudal maxillary portal looking dorsal through the frontomaxillary opening. CFS, conchofrontal sinus; ET, ethmoid turbinates; IOC, infraorbital canal; MSB, maxillary septal bulla.

adequate visualization to break it down (**Fig. 12**B).[13] Trephination of the caudal maxillary sinus (ventral to the orbit) does not provide consistent sinoscopic access to the rostral maxillary and ventral conchal sinuses. The author uses sinoscopy on every trephination or bone flap procedure to help fully evaluate the sinus compartments. When performing sinoscopy through a smaller trephination, the edges of the sinusotomy should be palpated for any sharp bone edges before endoscope placement. These edges can damage the outside of a flexible endoscope during the procedure. A small bone rasp can smooth any prominent edges before insertion of the scope for sinoscopy. Trephination incisions are typically closed in 2 layers. The author prefers a continuous pattern in the combined subcutaneous tissue and periosteum with either staples or interrupted mattress sutures in the skin.

SMALL VERSUS LARGE SINUS ACCESS

There are several factors to consider when deciding on the degree of sinus access required to complete the anticipated task. Many sinus surgeries can be completed in a less invasive fashion using trephination and sinoscopy. However, hemorrhage and limited visibility for some areas of the sinus can significantly prolong surgical times and increase frustration. The chronicity of the disease process should be considered as unhealthy granulation tissue or mucosa frequently needs to be debrided, which can contribute to hemorrhage and poor visibility (**Fig. 13**). Creation of new drainage into the nasal cavity can result in mild to marked hemorrhage, depending on the location. If encountered, a larger access point facilitates packing or ligating any visible vessels in the sinus wall. Visibility during a surgical dental extraction is paramount, so the author tends to prefer a larger trephination or small bone flap for these procedures.

SINUS FLAP CONSIDERATIONS

Sinus flaps are common standing procedures in dental or surgical practices and are typically created over the conchofrontal sinus (frontonasal flap) or over the maxillary sinus (maxillary flap). The size of the sinus flap is determined by the degree of exposure needed for the procedure. The area is clipped and prepped, and a line block is

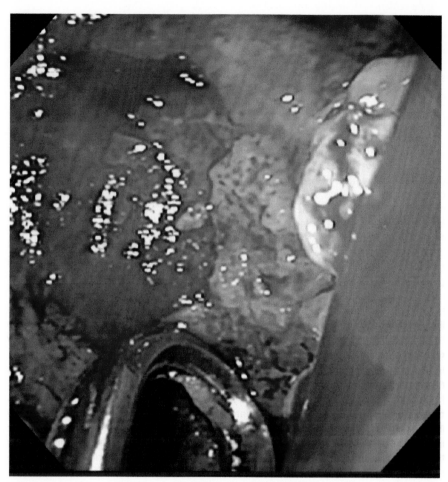

Fig. 13. Sinoscopic image of compromised mucosa secondary to chronic sinusitis in the caudal maxillary sinus that is being debrided using a sponge forceps.

placed around the margin of the anticipated flap site. This procedure can be combined with nerve blocks depending on the flap to be performed. Sinus infiltration with local anesthesia decreases sensitivity during flap creation, sinoscopy, and instrumentation manipulation. The author prefers draping with sterile towels at the margins of the proposed field (**Fig. 14**). Some prefer minimal or no draping considering that purulent material or feed is frequently found in dental sinusitis cases, creating a contaminated field anyway. The use of preoperative antibiotics is case dependent and based on patient-specific considerations. If sampling for bacterial culture and antibiotic sensitivity is anticipated, antibiotics will be delayed until the culture is obtained.

MAXILLARY FLAP VISIBILITY

The maxillary flap will give direct access to both the rostral and caudal maxillary sinuses and is typically used in dental sinusitis cases when additional visualization of this area is required for debridement or surgical extraction of the maxillary molars. The maxillary third molar can be difficult to access through this approach and

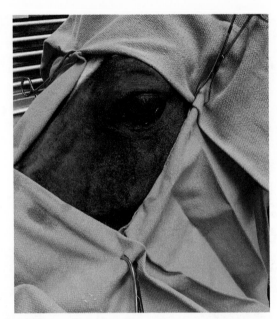

Fig. 14. Draping for a left maxillary sinus flap.

sometimes requires an additional frontonasal approach for instrument manipulation. Improved visualization of the ventral conchal, conchofrontal, and sphenopalatine sinuses can be achieved using sinoscopy through the frontonasal flap. Younger horses have limited space in the rostral maxillary sinus owing to the presence of cheek teeth reserve crown in the sinus. There is anatomic variation in the size of the conchomaxillary opening between the rostral maxillary and ventral conchal sinuses dorsal to the infraorbital canal. This factor can prevent ventral conchal sinus access in some horses through this approach. Trephination of the conchofrontal sinus and removal of the bulla of the maxillary septum may be necessary for adequate visualization of the ventral conchal sinus (see **Fig. 12**A and **Fig. 26**).

MAXILLARY LAP LANDMARKS

Landmarks for the maxillary flap are described to provide maximal visualization. Smaller approaches are frequently made based on the degree of exposure needed for the procedure. The caudal margin is a line from the medial canthus of the eye to the facial crest. The ventrolateral margin is the facial crest and the rostral margin is a line from the end of the facial crest to the infraorbital foramen (**Fig. 15**A).[10] There is no incision on the dorsomedial margin of the flap because this will be the hinge point. The most lateral incision is typically made 5 to 10 mm dorsal to the facial crest and the anticipated fracture line dorsally should remain ventrolateral to the approximate course of the nasolacrimal duct (medial canthus to the nasoincisive notch). The skin incision is carried through the periosteum. The periosteum is then reflected for 5 to 10 mm at the proposed osteotomy site (**Fig. 15**B).

FRONTONASAL FLAP VISIBILITY

The frontonasal flap provides the broadest access to the sinus cavities, but the maxillary flap tends to provide the most direct visualization for surgical extraction of caudal

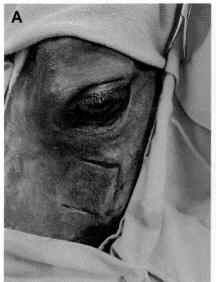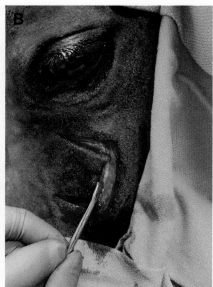

Fig. 15. (*A*) Skin incisions for a left sided maxillary sinus flap. (*B*) The periosteum is being reflected for 5 to 10 mm at the proposed osteotomy site.

cheek teeth. The frontonasal flap gives direct visualization of the conchofrontal sinus with partial visualization of the rostral and caudal maxillary sinuses. The ventral conchal sinus can be visualized after breaking down the maxillary septal bulla, aided by sinoscopy (see **Fig. 12**A) or by removing the rostral floor of the dorsal conchal sinus with subsequent exposure of the middle meatus and the ventral conchal sinus below (**Fig. 16**; see **Fig. 25**).

FRONTONASAL FLAP LANDMARKS

For the frontonasal flap, the caudal landmark is a line running perpendicular to the midline approximately one-half the distance between the supraorbital foramen and the medial canthus of the eye. The lateral landmark is a line coursing rostrally, 2 cm medial to the medial canthus of the eye, extending two-thirds of the distance from the medial canthus of the eye to the infraorbital foramen. The rostral margin connects the lateral margin in a perpendicular line to dorsal midline (**Fig. 17**).[10] The nasolacrimal duct courses approximately along the line from the medial canthus of the eye to the nasoincisive notch of the nasal bone. The skin incision may need to angle medially toward the rostral end to avoid iatrogenic damage to this structure (see **Fig. 17**). The skin incision is carried through the periosteum and the periosteum is reflected for 5 to 10 mm, similar to the maxillary flap.

OSTEOTOMY TECHNIQUE

The osteotomy can be made using an osteotome and mallet, but is more efficient with an oscillating bone saw (**Fig. 18**). The author prefers the use of a microsagittal saw because it creates a very thin cut (see **Fig. 18**B). Longer blades on oscillating saws have more wobble that create a thicker cut and less stability when the flap is closed (see **Fig. 18**A). Regardless of the instrument used, making the osteotomy with an

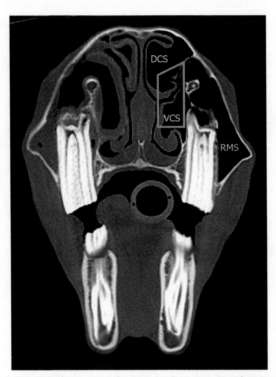

Fig. 16. Transverse computed tomography image showing area (*green box*) that can be removed when establishing access to the ventral conchal sinus and direct communication with the nasal passage. *Infraorbital canal. DCS, dorsal conchal sinus; RMS, rostral maxillary sinus; VCS, ventral conchal sinus.

external bevel at a 30° to 45° angle allows for a more secure closure. Irrigation with saline while using a saw decreases heat generation and improves visualization. Ear plugs in the horse help to mitigate noise sensitivity. After the 3 sides of the osteotomy are complete, a 5 mm wide osteotome is used to create a 90° angle at the corner of the medial fourth side, where you would like the flap to fracture. Osteotomes can be slid under the flap, loosening any septal or soft tissue attachments and are placed as far deep as the anticipated fracture line. Wider osteotomes (10–20 mm) are used to gently lever the flap open, making a controlled fracture along the medial side of the flap (**Fig. 19**).

MAXILLARY SINUS OSTEOTOMY CONSIDERATIONS

In younger horses with a prominent reserve crown, a very controlled osteotomy is required to avoid iatrogenic damage to these structures (**Fig. 20**). The infraorbital canal can be close to the osteotomy site at the rostral and medial edge of the flap. The osteotome is needed to sever the attachment of the maxillary septum to the underside of the flap. Upon entry into the maxillary sinus, the maxillary septum is frequently removed with a rongeur to improve visualization and communication between the rostral and caudal compartments, and to promote improved drainage (**Fig. 21**). The apices of the first and second molars can be present immediately under the septum so care is taken to identify these structures to prevent iatrogenic damage.

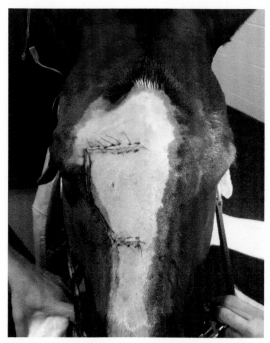

Fig. 17. Right-sided frontonasal sinus flap after closure demonstrating incisional landmarks.

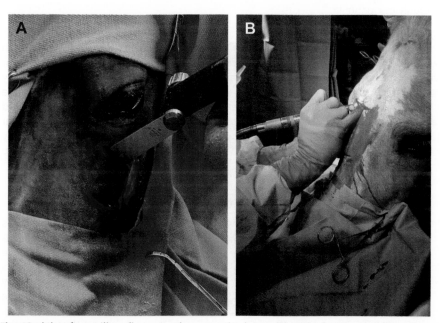

Fig. 18. (*A*) Left maxillary flap using larger sagittal saw. (*B*) Right frontonasal flap using a microsagittal saw.

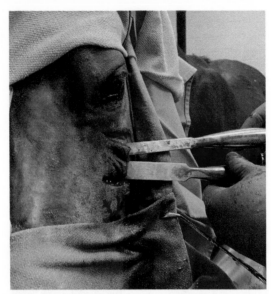

Fig. 19. Left maxillary flap using osteotomes to help elevate the flap and create a controlled fracture along the medial side.

The infraorbital canal should be localized at both margins of the flap to prevent damage to the infraorbital nerve inside. Occasionally the infraorbital canal may be destroyed in cases with chronic maxillary sinusitis, leaving the infraorbital nerve difficult to identify.

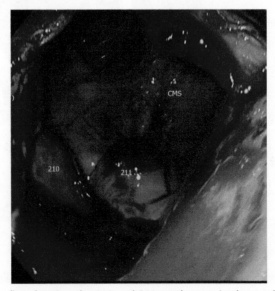

Fig. 20. Maxillary flap showing the 210 and 211 tooth roots in the caudal maxillary sinus (CMS).

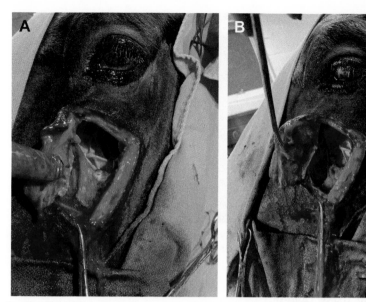

Fig. 21. (*A*) Left maxillary flap with rostral maxillary sinus obliterated by granulation tissue secondary to chronic 209 oroantral fistula. (*B*) The maxillary septum was removed and the unhealthy tissue was debrided from the rostral maxillary sinus.

SINUS EXPLORATION

Once access to the sinus is achieved, it is imperative to perform a full exploratory of all sinus cavities looking for any purulent debris or compromised tissue. Occasionally, a sinus flap over the conchofrontal or maxillary sinus is performed in combination with trephination elsewhere to help optimize visibility and access to certain sinus compartments. Purulent debris is removed via aggressive lavage combined with local debridement if inspissated. Physiologic saline is preferred over tap water for lavage to limit mucosal edema. The ventral conchal sinus should be thoroughly assessed in cases of sinusitis as purulent material in this structure can be missed, leading to persistent purulent nasal discharge postoperatively (**Fig. 22**). Sinusitis involving the ventral conchal sinus has been reported in 75% of dental sinusitis cases. Inspissated pus in the ventral conchal sinus has been demonstrated in 20% of dental sinusitis cases and 46% of all types of sinus disease.[14]

ASSESSMENT OF SINUS DRAINAGE

Sinus drainage is critical to the resolution of sinusitis cases. Drainage through the normal nasomaxillary pathway can be assessed at the time of surgery by instilling saline into the sinus and observing how readily it flows out the ipsilateral nostril. This movement is frequently compromised owing to inflamed mucosa, or bony remodeling secondary to chronic inflammation or the disease process (**Fig. 23**). If compromised, drainage may improve by repeat sinus lavage as mucosal inflammation decreases along the nasomaxillary drainage pathway. Additional drainage may be necessary by creating new sinonasal communications surgically. These 2 techniques are frequently debated as to which is superior. Alternative approaches to reopen the nasomaxillary pathway have been described in cadavers and normal horses in the past using balloon sinuplasty.[15]

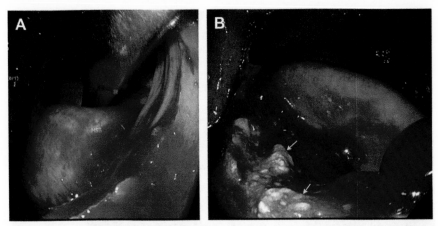

Fig. 22. (*A*) Sinoscopic images of the maxillary septal bulla (MSB) through a conchofrontal portal. (*B*) After breaking down the bulla, inspissated pus was found filling the ventral conchal sinus (*arrows*).

SINUS DRAINAGE USING LAVAGE

More frequent sinus lavage is typically done through an indwelling tube in the sinus cavity (**Fig. 24**). Foley catheters are frequently used, but other types of lavage tubes exist. The tube typically enters the sinus through a trephine, and is tunneled subcutaneously to exit 2 to 3 cm away from the trephination skin incision. These tubes can be left in for days or weeks, allowing for sinus lavage multiple times during the day depending on the horse's behavior. As surgical and sinus inflammation decrease, drainage can improve. However, bone remodeling from chronic disease can result

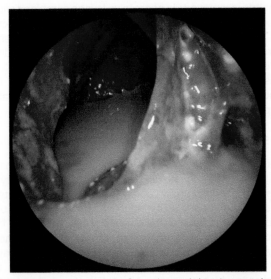

Fig. 23. Sinoscopic image through a conchofrontal portal showing purulent material and inflamed mucosa in the caudal maxillary sinus. (*Courtesy of* Dr. Stephen Galloway, Oakland, TN.)

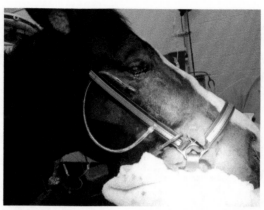

Fig. 24. Indwelling drain present in the right caudal maxillary sinus for daily lavage. (*Courtesy of* Dr. Ed Earley, Ithaca, NY.)

in long-term impairment of drainage. Limited lavage can be performed for 2 to 3 days after surgery, even if new sinonasal communications were created. This process helps to remove residual clot or debris from the sinus compartments. For more chronic sinusitis cases after sinus flap or trephination, the author prefers to make a small sinusotomy with a Steinmann pin at the time of surgery adjacent to the flap or trephination site that can be used for daily postoperative lavage for 2 to 3 days using a teat cannula or needle (see **Fig. 9**). Postoperative lavage might be avoided in some cases to minimize disruption of the alveolar blood clot after a surgical extraction. If adequate drainage is established at the time of surgery, and the purulent material is removed, then postoperative sinus lavage is not essential.

SINUS DRAINAGE THROUGH NEW SINONASAL COMMUNICATION

Surgical creation of new sinonasal drainage sites is frequently performed, particularly with more chronic sinusitis cases. The rostral aspect of the medial wall of the ventral conchal sinus is a common area for establishing nasal drainage (**Fig. 25**). In conjunction, communication can be established between the ventral conchal sinus and the other sinus compartments by removing the bulla of the maxillary septum and the rostral floor of the dorsal conchal sinus (see **Fig. 16**). Larger vessels are present in the caudal aspect of the axial wall of the ventral and dorsal conchal sinuses. These vessels are to be avoided because significant hemorrhage will result when disrupted. Alternate approaches to establishing drainage have been described recently using a combination of transnasal conchotomy of the ventral conchal sinus combined with surgical enlargement of the nasomaxillary aperture.[16] Creating additional sinus drainage using laser and cautery instrumentation via nasal endoscopy is described in the article Elaine F.Claffey and Norm G. Ducharme' article, "Equine Nasal Endoscopy: Treating Bullae Disease and Sinus Disease," in this issue.

SINUS PACKING

Packing the sinus with sterile rolled gauze or a clot promoting bandage will help to control excessive hemorrhage. To pack the sinus, a Chambers catheter or bronchoesophageal forceps is placed nasally and visualized or palpated through the new sinonasal communication with gentle instrument manipulation. Attach the packing to the

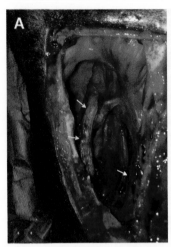 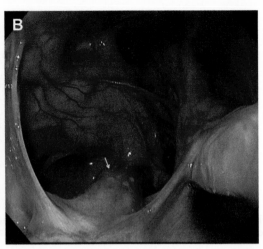

Fig. 25. (A) Right frontonasal sinus flap showing exposure of the infraorbital nerve (*yellow arrows*) secondary to pressure necrosis from an ethmoid hematoma. Poor drainage from chronic sinusitis required removal of the floor of the dorsal conchal sinus, with sinonasal drainage established through the medial wall of the ventral conchal sinus (*white arrow*). (B) Endoscopic image 1 year later showing mucosal covering previously exposed infraorbital nerve (*yellow arrow*) and a persistent sinonasal communication (*red arrows*).

instrument and pull it out the nose. Then, layer the packing in the sinus, starting with the deepest aspect first, close to the sinonasal communication, applying extra packing and pressure over any bleeders. The end of the packing is then sutured to the external nostril (**Fig. 26**). Some surgeons will place the packing inside a stockinette to decrease the risk of dislodging the caudal packing and the horse swallowing it. The packing is typically left in for 24 hours and is then removed through the nostril. Packing the sinus will stop hemorrhage in most cases. If the packing does not stop the hemorrhage after 20 to 25 minutes, then attempts to ligate the vessel or to seal it using an electrocautery device should be attempted before repacking the sinus.

SINUS FLAP CLOSURE

The bone flap is repositioned back into anatomic position. This maneuver sometimes requires mild manipulation along the medial fractured margin, to realign the bone edges. The author prefers to close bone flaps in 3 layers. The deep periosteum is closed using an interrupted pattern with an absorbable monofilament suture. The periosteum frequently tears, so continuous suture patterns are not recommended. The subcutaneous tissue is closed using an absorbable monofilament suture in a continuous pattern along each margin of the flap. The skin is closed with either skin staples or an absorbable monofilament suture in an interrupted horizontal mattress pattern (see **Fig. 17** and **Fig. 26**). The author prefers to maintain a postoperative head bandage for 7 days, changing it every 2 to 3 days. However, bandaging is not considered essential.

SINUS FLAP INTRAOPERATIVE COMPLICATIONS

Extending the frontonasal osteotomy to midline increases risk of the fracture extending to the opposite side of the nasal septum, creating communication with the

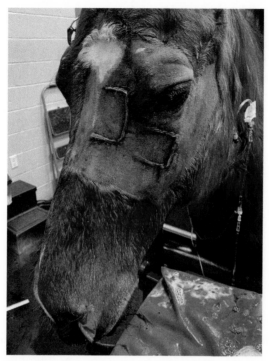

Fig. 26. Left maxillary sinus flap and conchofrontal trephination with packing placed through a new sinonasal communication in the ventral conchal sinus, exiting the left nostril.

opposite sinus. Lavage coming out both nostrils can be a sign of this complication and tends to not have major clinical consequences if the communication is small. However, clients may comment on a bilateral serous nasal discharge after surgery when the horse presented for unilateral nasal discharge before surgery. Occasionally, the flap fractures lateral to the anticipated site (**Fig. 27**). If this happens, visualization can be assessed through the flap obtained and if not adequate, a second fracture can be created further medially using your fingers or an instrument to help elevate. The flap will be less stable with 2 fractures but still tends to heal well if closed securely at the margins. Insecure flap margins are typically stabilized with additional sutures in the periosteal layer. Securing the flap with wire or larger gauge suture through drill holes in the adjacent bones is an option, although this strategy is frequently unnecessary and can result in persistent incisional drainage.

POSTOPERATIVE MANAGEMENT

Postoperatively, the horse is maintained on systemic antibiotics for 3 to 10 days and analgesic and anti-inflammatory medication(s) for 5 to 7 days. Exercise is restricted for bone flap procedures for 30 days consisting of stall rest and hand walking for 7 days, followed by small paddock turnout for 3 weeks. Trephination procedures are stall rested with hand walking for 7 days followed by 7 days of small paddock turnout. Frequently the degree of dental work performed may further limit exercise, beyond that required for healing of the sinus surgery site.

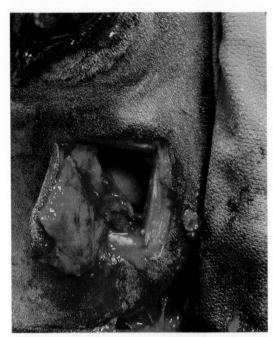

Fig. 27. Left maxillary flap where the medial fourth side fractured obliquely, lateral to the anticipated site.

POSTOPERATIVE COMPLICATIONS: INCISION

Postoperative complications related to the incision may include incisional infection and bone sequestrum formation. Postoperative sinocutaneous fistulas are less common and the incidence can be decreased with good surgical technique. Focal incisional infection is relatively common, particularly when the sinus contains purulent debris (**Fig. 28**). The treatment of incisional infection involves the removal of a staple or suture, local lavage, and continued antibiotic therapy. Bone sequestra can cause more persistent incisional drainage or swelling around the flap margin. Deeper sequestra within the sinus can cause purulent nasal discharge. Additional imaging is suggested for incisions that do not respond to local therapy in 1 to 2 weeks. Postoperative radiographic evaluation of bone flap healing can be difficult owing to the typical reactive appearance of the bone after osteotomy. Ultrasound examination can be very useful for the identification of focal fluid pooling or irregular bone margins (**Fig. 29**). Local debridement with a curette to remove any unhealthy bone, lavage, and sometimes combined with local, absorbable antibiotic bead placement, often fixes the problem if it is superficial. A deeper bone infection may require sinoscopy to evaluate the underside of the flap.

POSTOPERATIVE COMPLICATIONS: POOR DRAINAGE

Sinus drainage may become compromised by mucosal swelling during sinus lavage and debridement. This swelling will usually resolve in 12 to 24 hours. However, persistence of poor drainage often requires the creation of supplemental sinonasal communications. The risk of poor drainage postoperatively has led many surgeons to be more aggressive with establishing drainage at the time of surgery through creation of new

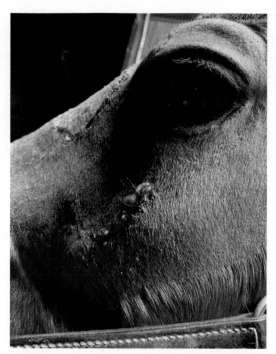

Fig. 28. Postoperative maxillary sinus flap with purulent material draining from the incision.

sinonasal communication. In some sinusitis cases that are particularly reactive, new sinonasal communications can close postoperatively, usually over the course of several months depending on the size of the defect (**Fig. 30**). Additional lavage may help to facilitate drainage postoperatively. With persistent compromise, endoscopic laser procedures can be considered to help create new sinonasal communications into the ventral or dorsal conchal sinus or reopen previously established drainage sites.

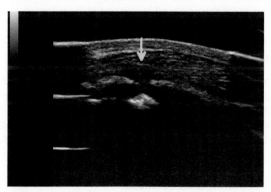

Fig. 29. Ultrasound image of a maxillary sinus flap incision that continues to drain purulent material. A deeper area of bony irregularity surrounded by more hypoechoic fluid (*yellow arrow*) is present at the flap margin, consistent with a bone sequestrum and adjacent purulent debris.

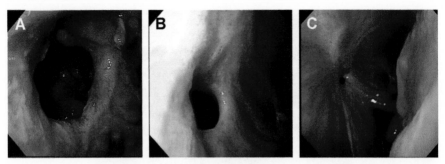

Fig. 30. Nasal endoscopic image showing progressive closure of surgical communication with ventral conchal sinus. (*A*) Three months after surgery. (*B*) Eight months after surgery. (*C*) Thirteen months after surgery.

POSTOPERATIVE COMPLICATIONS: PERSISTENT PURULENT NASAL DISCHARGE

Increased mucus production is a normal healing response after sinus surgery. Nasal discharge should be assessed for odor and presence of pus. Mild mucoserous to serosanguinous nasal discharge is normally expected after sinus surgery and can be observed for 4 to 6 weeks. Persistent purulent nasal discharge after the extraction of a maxillary molar may be related to the loss of the alveolar plug and recontamination of the sinus cavity. Loss of the alveolar plug and/or fluid accumulation within the sinus can be assessed with oral and radiographic examination. If a large sinonasal drainage site has been previously established, nasal endoscopy may be used to determine the source of the sinusitis. If caught quickly, sinus lavage, plug replacement, and antibiotic therapy is often all that is needed to resolve the purulent discharge. Oroantral fistulas can develop after extraction of the caudal maxillary cheek teeth (**Fig. 31**). Oroantral fistula often require epithelial debridement before replacement of the oral plug. Incomplete sinus debridement, lavage, or drainage establishment may leave inspissated pus in portions of the sinus cavity. Additionally, the sinus disease may extend rostral into the nasal bullae causing persistent nasal discharge (see Elaine F.Claffey and Norm G. Ducharme' article, "Equine Nasal Endoscopy: Treating Bullae Disease and Sinus Disease," in this issue). Repeat oral examination, endoscopy, and radiographs should be performed in these cases. If the origin of the drainage remains elusive, additional imaging using a computed tomography scan should be considered.

POSTOPERATIVE COMPLICATIONS: FUNGAL SINUSITIS

Fungal plaques in the sinus or nasal passage are not uncommon after creating new sinonasal communications and can cause purulent nasal discharge. These plaques tend to be focal and respond to topical endoscopic treatment with miconazole after local debridement with an endoscopic biopsy instrument (**Fig. 32**). For small plaques, 1 to 2 topical treatments tends to be effective at resolving the issue. Yearly endoscopy is recommended to monitor for any regrowth.

POSTOPERATIVE COMPLICATIONS: COSMESIS

Suture periostitis causing firm bony swellings around the sinus flap or trephine sites is possible (more common with sinus flaps). They typically are observed around 2 to 4 months postoperatively. Radiographs are performed to evaluate the bone, but

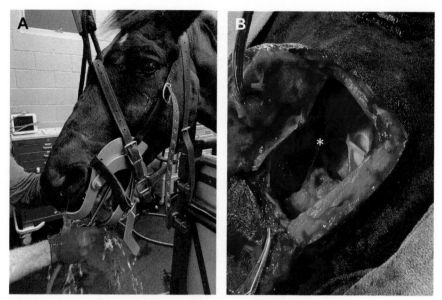

Fig. 31. (*A*) Oroantral fistula after a previous 210 extraction. Water readily comes out the left nostril during lavage of the oral cavity. (*B*) Debridement was elected from a combined oral and sinus approach. Tubing was inserted through oral fistula to determine its entry point into the maxillary sinus. * Tubing through the fistula.

usually no additional treatment is required. Some cases maintain a visible abnormality for several months or longer with a gradual remodeling of the bone over time. Occasionally, the loss of sequestered bone from the sinusotomy site can cause facial disfigurement. White hairs can develop around any healed incision and can be unsightly to some clients (**Fig. 33**). Potential postoperative complications and risks should be discussed with the client (and referring veterinarian) before sinus surgery.

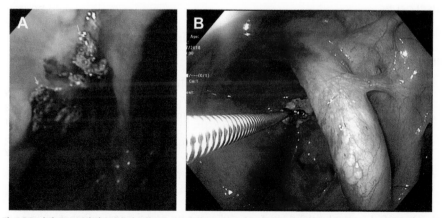

Fig. 32. (*A*) Fungal rhinitis (*yellow arrows*) at the site of surgical fenestration of the ventral conchal sinus into the nasal cavity. (*B*) Focal fungal plaque in caudal maxillary sinus observed via sinoscopy through a previously created sinonasal communication.

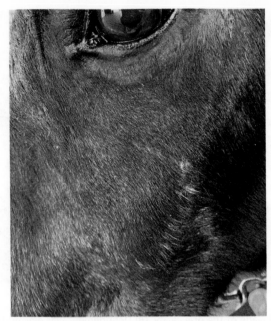

Fig. 33. White hairs visible around the left maxillary sinus flap site, 1 year after surgery.

SUMMARY

The anatomy of the equine paranasal sinus system requires constant review to better understand the origin of clinical disease and the compartments involved. Further, a firm understanding of how sinuses normally drain into the nasal cavity and ways that you can improve drainage will allow you to optimize healing and expedite resolution of sinusitis. Knowledge of the surgical landmarks for sinus access will help to optimize exposure, directly target the cause of sinusitis while facilitating healing and minimizing complications.

DISCLOSURE

No disclosures.

REFERENCES

1. Sisson S, Grossman J, Getty R. 5th edition. The anatomy of domestic animals, Vol. 1. Philadelphia: W.B. Saunders Company; 1975. p. 318–48.
2. McCann J, Dixon P, Mayhew I. Clinical anatomy of the equine sphenopalatine sinus. Equine Vet J 2004;36(6):466–72.
3. Budras K, Sack W, Rock S. Anatomy of the horse. 5th edition. Hannover (Germany): Schluetersche; 2009. p. 32–51.
4. Froydenlund T, Dixon P, Smith S, et al. Anatomical and histological study of the dorsal and ventral nasal conchal bullae in normal horses. Vet Rec 2015; 177(21):1–5.
5. Dixon P, Froydenlund T, Liuti T, et al. Empyema of the nasal conchal bulla as a cause of chronic unilateral nasal discharge in the horse: 10 cases (2013-2014). Equine Vet J 2015;47(4):445–9.

6. Tucker R, Windley Z, Abernethy A, et al. Radiographic, computed tomographic and surgical anatomy of the equine sphenopalatine sinus in normal and diseased horses. Equine Vet J 2016;48(5):578–84.
7. Probst A, Henninger W, Willmann M. Communications of normal nasal and paranasal cavities in computed tomography in horses. Vet Radiol Ultrasound 2005; 46(1):44–8.
8. Tatarniuk D, Bell C, Carmalt J. A description of the relationship between the nasomaxillary aperture and the paranasal sinus system of horses. Vet J 2010; 186(2):216–20.
9. Tremaine W, Dixon P. A long-term study of 277 cases of equine sinonasal disease. Part 1: details of horses, historical, clinical and ancillary diagnostic findings. Equine Vet J 2001;33(3):274–82.
10. Auer J, Stick J. Equine surgery. 4th edition. St. Louis (MO): Elsevier; 2012. p. 557–68.
11. Barakzai S, Kane-Smyth J, Lowles J, et al. Trephination of the equine rostral maxillary sinus: efficacy and safety of two trephine sites. Vet Surg 2008;37(3):278–82.
12. Pouyet M, Bonilla A. Validation of a 2-mm videoendoscope for the evaluation of the paranasal sinuses with a minimally invasive technique. Vet Surg 2020;49 Suppl 1:O60–70.
13. Perkins J, Bennett C, Windley Z, et al. Comparison of sinoscopic techniques for examining the rostral maxillary and ventral conchal sinuses of horses. Vet Surg 2009;38(5):607–12.
14. Dixon P, Parkin T, Collins N, et al. Equine paranasal sinus disease: a long-term study of 200 cases (1997-2009): ancillary diagnostic findings and involvement of the various sinus compartments. Equine Vet J 2012;44(3):267–71.
15. Bell C, Tatarniuk D, Carmalt J. Endoscope-guided balloon sinuplasty of the equine nasomaxillary opening. Vet Surg 2009;38(7):791–7.
16. Bach F, Bohler A, Schieder K, et al. Surgical enlargement of the nasomaxillary aperture and transnasal conchotomy of the ventral conchal sinus: two surgical techniques to improve sinus drainage in horses. Vet Surg 2019;48(6):1019–31.

Minimizing Equine Tooth Extraction Complications

Stephen S. Galloway, DVM[a],*, Edward T. Earley, DVM[b]

KEYWORDS

- Equine • Tooth extraction • Outcome • Complications • Instrumentation
- Treatment planning

KEY POINTS

- Iatrogenic complications are minimized by an experienced veterinarian and a trained staff using appropriate instrumentation and practicing within their level of clinical competency.
- Preoperative evaluation and treatment planning allow the dentist to predict intraoperative complications and prepare for the best extraction procedure.
- An understanding of extraction principles allows the dentist to recognize procedural difficulties.
- An understanding of alveolar wound healing allows the dentist to establish appropriate postoperative follow-up evaluations and recognize postoperative complications.

INTRODUCTION
Extractions Are Awfully Simple or Simply Awful!

Merillat predicted in1906 that "when dentistry in animals is more generally recognized as an important if not essential feature of animal therapeutics, and when dental operations by reasons of greater skill are made easier, veterinarians will then treat the art of dentistry with the same dignity as other branches of surgery."[1] This prediction was followed by a century of equine tooth extractions with unacceptably high major complications as a direct result of poor procedural technique, poor instrumentation, and poor operator training and experience. Although extractions should always be considered a major oral surgery procedure, they would rarely be considered an emergency; yet, postoperative complication rates as high as 70% have been reported,[2] and patients have been euthanized because of untreatable iatrogenic complications.

Historically, some surgeons have reluctantly performed extractions out of necessity and compassion rather than having an interest in dentistry. The resurgence in professional equine dentistry was started by Dr Paddy Dixon during the 1990s and was followed by significant improvements in dentistry training and equipment. Equine

[a] Animal Dental Care Specialist, 8565 Highway 64, Somerville, TN 38068, USA; [b] Large Animal Dentistry, Equine Farm Animal Hospital, Cornell University, Ithaca, NY, USA
* Corresponding author.
E-mail address: achvet@yahoo.com

Vet Clin Equine 36 (2020) 641–658
https://doi.org/10.1016/j.cveq.2020.08.004
0749-0739/20/© 2020 Elsevier Inc. All rights reserved.
vetequine.theclinics.com

veterinary dentistry was recognized as a unique veterinary specialty in North America and Europe in 2014, and the incidence of major postoperative complication has been markedly decreased to less than 10% in procedures performed by veterinary dentists.[3-6]

A variety of extraction complications ranging in severity from mild and transient to major and permanent have been documented or suspected; however, based on the inherent biases of case reporting and the lack of standardization for follow-up evaluation methods, these complications and rates may under-represent actual complications. Soft tissue complications result from iatrogenic laceration of the oral (palate, tongue, cheeks) and regional (parotid salivary duct) structures. Hemorrhage or hematoma result from laceration of the infraorabital, lingual, and palatine vasculature. Dental complications include retained roots and dental fragments and iatrogenic damage to nondiseased teeth. Bone complications include alveolar osteitis; sequestration; fracture of the mandible, hard palate, and facial bones; and oronasal, oroantral, and orocutaneous fistulae. Neuropathies have resulted secondary to trauma to the facial (paralysis), infraorbital (headshaking), and lingual nerves (tongue maceration). Secondary regional infections (sinusitis, mandibular osteitis, fascial space infection, cellulitis) and systemic infections (endocarditis) have also been reported as complications of exodontia. This list does not include the often-significant complication secondary to general anesthesia.

HOSPITAL, DOCTOR, AND STAFF FACTORS

In human medicine, hospital and surgeon factors are investigated with respect to specific surgical procedures. Although the authors could not find similar investigations in veterinary medicine or human dentistry and oral surgery, the conclusions of these reports are relevant (**Box 1**). Investigations of both hospital and surgeon caseload volume suggest that complications decrease as the caseload of a procedure increases, and the conclusion of these investigations is that increased doctor and staff experience and preparation for a specific procedure decreases complications. Hospitals that routinely perform extractions schedule appropriate time for a comprehensive preoperative assessment, treatment planning, and the procedure. Inappropriate scheduling precipitates rushed procedures, staff frustration, and intraoperative complications.

It is generally accepted that the golden period to minimize anesthesia and procedural complications is 2 hours. Extended procedures precipitate fatigue, frustration, and impatience. Procedural efficiency is optimized through the training and experience of a dedicated team. Ergonomic studies show that a full-time dental assistant reduces procedural time by 20%; therefore, the authors recommend that the minimum dedicated staff for an extraction case be a veterinary dentist and 2 technicians or

---

Box 1
Factors effecting procedural outcomes

Hospital factors: caseload and scheduling

Dentist and staff factors: training, experience, and caseload

Procedural factors: dental principles, instrumentation, and treatment planning

Patient factors: concomitant regional and systemic disease, and compliance

Owner factors: compliance and procedural expectations

assistants. The veterinarian is responsible for case management and performing the extraction. The senior technician is responsible for patient care and administering sedation, and the assistant manages the instrumentation and assists with the extraction procedure. The American Veterinary Dental College and American Association of Equine Practitioners have published guidelines on the ethical practices of different veterinary healthcare providers.

The training and experience of the veterinarian and staff for a specific procedure is prerequisite to successful procedural outcomes. Although dentistry training and instrumentation has some overlap with general hard tissue surgery, both the academic and practical trainings differ significantly. One such example in dentistry training is the emphasis on dental and surgical drill skills, which are required during oral surgery. Training teaches a dentist how to perform a procedure, whereas experience teaches the dentist how to perform the procedure efficiently as well as when the procedure is inappropriate. Overall complication rates should decrease as a dentist's experience increases and his or her skills and case selection criteria improve. Ironically, investigations reporting the association between surgeon experience and outcome in human procedures often finds the opposite association, probably because of the recognized bias that experienced surgeons perform the most difficult procedures, which inherently have the most complications. A recent report comparing the outcomes of different equine extraction techniques performed over a 16-year period in an academic referral center investigated the association between outcome and surgeon experience, but found no significant association, other than transient postoperative pyrexia, owing to the large number of rotating residents and the variability of their roles as the either the primary or assisting surgeon.[7]

PROCEDURAL FACTORS

Whether simple or surgical extraction is elected, an understanding of the fundamental principles of oral surgery and exodontia promotes successful outcomes and minimizes complications. Principles specific to surgical extractions and mucoperiosteal flap design are presented in the Edward T. Earley and Stephen S. Galloway's article, "Equine Standing Surgical Extraction Techniques," elsewhere in this issue. General tooth extraction principles include:

1. Preoperative treatment planning is based on both clinical and radiologic evaluation.
2. The operator must have adequate visualization of the operative field (tooth to be extracted).
3. Vital structures and adjacent tissues/teeth should not be damaged.
4. The tooth being extracted must have an unimpeded extraction pathway.
5. Controlled force is applied to fatigue and tear the periodontal ligament (PDL) before the tooth is extracted from the alveolus.
6. The tooth must be mobilized before removal from the alveolus.
7. The extracted tooth is visually examined, and the alveolus is radiographed to confirm complete extraction of the tooth.
8. The alveolus is debrided to produce a clean wound.

Adherence to principles 4, 5, and 6 will prevent the majority of intraoperative complications. For example, bone sequestration is the most common postoperative complication of the intraoral extraction techniques. Tissue ischemia typically results secondary to aggressive instrumentation or to a tooth being forcibly extracted through an anatomically restrictive extraction pathway. Although minor alveolar sequestration is often acceptable and easily removed between 2 and 3 weeks postoperatively, prolonged intraoral extraction procedures can produce sequestra that require additional procedures to remove (**Fig. 1**).

Instrumentation

Selection of instrumentation is largely a matter of personal preference, but many improvements in the design and quality of equine extraction instruments have occurred over the past decade. Unfortunately, although many veterinarians focus their attention on extraction instrumentation, some do not possess the minimum instrumentation required to perform a professional oral examination, which includes a full-mouth speculum, a bright, targeted light, a mirror, a dental explorer, and a periodontal probe. The examination is the foundation of ethical, professional veterinary practice. A veterinarian must examine the patient and make a diagnosis before prescribing a treatment.

Oral Endoscopy (see Claudia K. True and Allison R Dotzel's article, "Equine Oral Endoscopy," in this issue) provides superior diagnostic viewing of the oral tissues and is now affordable. The authors consider oral endoscopic examination and intraoperative monitoring a prerequisite to cheek tooth extractions other than significantly mobile teeth as described by Duncanson.[3] Visualization of the operating field is a surgical and extraction principle. Ramzan and colleagues[8] demonstrated that oral endoscopy optimizes instrument placement during oral extraction procedures, and Langeneckert and colleagues[5] attributed the low incidence of morbidity in their case series to the direct endoscopic guidance of the drill. The authors consider the blind cutting of oral hard tissues with motorized instruments to be below the current standard of care.

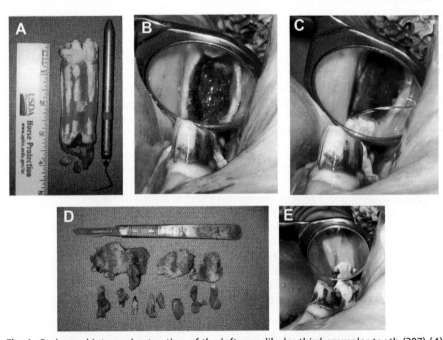

Fig. 1. Prolonged intraoral extraction of the left mandibular third premolar tooth (307) (*A*) in a 5-year-old TN Walking Horse caused significant alveolar sequestration. At day 7 after extraction, sequestration of the alveolus was evident (*B*). Four subsequent follow-up procedures (days 15, 22, 27, and 44 postoperatively) were required to debride the alveolus (*C, D*). Complete epithelialization was confirmed 3 months postoperatively (*E*).

Mechanical principles and tooth extraction instruments

Dental extraction instruments use simple machine technology (lever, wheel and axle, inclined plane, and wedge) to gain mechanical advantage when applying manual force to a tooth (**Box 2**).

The application of mechanical advantage with dental instruments should follow the 3 Ps: Purchase, Persistence, and Patience. To maximize mechanical advantage, dental instrument selection should be based on the best contact between the instrument head and the tooth surface. Because tooth shape and diameter vary greatly, a selection of luxators, elevators, molar spreaders, and extraction forceps should be available to maximize instrument purchase. (See also the Jon M. Gieche's article "Equine Oral Extraction Techniques," elsewhere in this issue.) The mechanical advantage provided by dental instruments requires the application of incrementally increasing, persistent force. The PDL is designed to withstand heavy, short duration masticatory forces; therefore, PDL fatigue and rupture is achieved through the application of lighter, long duration force. Force is gradually increased as the PDL fails. The operator must use finesse and patience to prevent iatrogenic damage such as alveolar bone and root fractures. Properly performed tooth extractions take time, and frustration precipitates poor operator technique.

Luxation is the process by which the PDL is cut to loosen a tooth from the surrounding alveolar bone. A luxator is wedged into the PDL spaces between the root and alveolar bone, and then apically directed pressure is held for 10 to 15 seconds. Proper luxation should elicit PDL hemorrhage. The luxator is moved to another aspect of the root, and the process is continued circumferential around the tooth.

Elevation is the process by which the PDL is stretched, fatigued, and torn, while the alveolar bone is expanded to facilitate removal of the tooth from the alveolus. After luxation, an elevator is placed into the PDL space, advanced apically until it stops, and then rotated (torqued) and held for 15 seconds to apply leverage. The process is then repeated in the opposite PDL space. Elevation is alternated between different aspects of the tooth until finger-loose mobilization is achieved.

Extraction forceps (small animal, wolf tooth) are used to remove the "finger loose" tooth from the alveolus. The beaks should grip the root as far apically as possible. The tooth is then extruded with gentle traction as the tooth is rotated axially in a clockwise or counterclockwise direction. Significant mechanical advantage is achieved with extraction forceps, and attempting to extract an immobile tooth often results in root fracture.

A molar spreader is a ramp designed to be placed between the crowns of a base cheek tooth and the diseased cheek tooth. Application of force would ideally tilt the diseased tooth mesiodistally away from the base tooth, stretching the PDL of the diseased tooth. In reality, molar spreaders work like a wedge to separate both

---

Box 2
Extraction instruments and simple machines

Lever (class 1): dental forceps and scissors. A dental elevator when bone is used as fulcrum.

Lever (class 3): Tissue forceps.

Wheel and axle: molar extractor. Dental elevators when axially torqued between the tooth and bone.

Ramp (inclined plane): screw, molar spreaders, and chisel.

Wedge (2 back-to-back ramps): dental luxators and osteotome.

the base and target teeth. Caution must be exercised to ensure that nontarget teeth are not mobilized during the spreading process.

Molar extractors use wheel and axle technology to apply significant torsion (rotational force) or lingual/vestibular transverse force (coronal tipping) to the crown of a diseased cheek tooth. This force stretches the PDL, but also severely deforms the alveolar bone, which creates an unobstructed eruption pathway for the eventual removal of the tooth. This bone deformation is often responsible for ischemic necrosis, which results in alveolar sequestration, the most common postoperative complication of oral extraction.

When treatment planning for the oral extraction of a cheek tooth, dentists should consider the physiologic resistance of the PDL to directional movements. The PDL is designed to withstand significant compressive (intrusive) and shearing (coronal tipping) forces during mastication while providing eruptive (extruding) forces to maintain occlusion secondary to physiologic attrition. Using a molar extractor and a fulcrum to apply a vertical extruding force to the diseased cheek tooth over an extended period of time will help to fatigue the PDL in the direction of the extraction pathway while minimizing alveolar bone damage.

Almost all dental instruments are sharp tools that rapidly dull owing to intentional hard tissue contact. Dull instruments are inefficient and precipitate impatience, frustration, and poor technique. Instrument sharpening instructions and videos are available (free) online. Synthetic and natural stones in flat and conical shapes are used to manually sharpen instruments. Practices that have a significant dentistry or oral surgical caseload should consider purchasing an instrument sharpening machine (**Fig. 2**).

Gas-driven, high-speed (100,000–400,000 rpm) dental and surgical drills are autoclavable, low-torque handpieces that are specifically designed for cutting teeth and bone in a confined wet space (see also the Edward T. Earley and Stephen S. Galloway's article, "Equine Standing Surgical Extraction Techniques," in this issue). Low-torque handpieces stall when the bur binds, preventing bur kick back or jumping, which minimizes iatrogenic damage. Because the surgical field in dental surgery is often measured in millimeters, not centimeters, these precision drills are the hard tissue cutting instruments of choice. Some operators are currently using general surgical instruments (eg, chisels, osteotomes, gouges) or electric, low-speed (<60,000 rpm), motors for hard tissue instrumentation. These hand instruments are not designed for the precise cutting required to prevent collateral iatrogenic damage, and low-

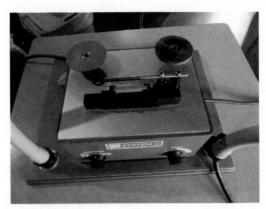

Fig. 2. Motorized instrument sharpener capable of sharpening dental luxators, dental elevators, and periosteal elevators.

speed motors are inefficient and overheat. Increased complication rates should be expected with inappropriate instrumentation (**Fig. 3**).

Treatment Planning Considerations

A comprehensive preoperative assessment and treatment planning facilitate accurate procedural estimates and scheduling, reduce procedural time, and prevent unexpected intraoperative complications. Prerequisite to any tooth extraction procedure is an understanding of dental, oral, and regional anatomy. Detailed anatomic considerations are discussed in the Edward T. Earley and Stephen S. Galloway's article, "Equine Standing Surgical Extraction Techniques," in this issue.

Sedation, Anesthesia, and Patient Care

Each patient's anesthesia and analgesia plan should be individualized based on a preanesthetic evaluation consisting of a clinical and diagnostic evaluation (see also Luis Campoy and Samantha R. Sedgwick's article, "Standing Sedation and Analgesia in Equine Dental Surgery," in this issue). The veterinary profession has adopted the American Society of Anesthesiology's Physical Status Classification System to guide anesthetic treatment planning. All staff members should be trained to recognize critical monitoring parameters that dictate evaluation by a veterinarian. Wet conditions can predispose dentistry patients to hypothermia, which affects multiple organ systems and makes the patient less responsive to emergency treatments.

General anesthesia is associated with significant complications and significant expense. Head surgeries have been safely performed in standing, sedated horses for more than 25 years,[9] and oral extraction techniques have routinely been performed standing for more than 20 years.[4] Contrary to reports in the current literature, opining the necessity of general anesthesia for surgical extraction techniques, the authors have been safely performing a modified transcutaneous lateral alveolar ostectomy technique in standing horses for more than 10 years (see Edward T. Earley and Stephen S. Galloway's article, "Equine Standing

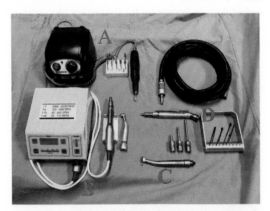

Fig. 3. Dentistry Motors and Handpieces. Electric, low-speed engines, handpieces, and burs designed for dental laboratory use (A) and endodontic procedures (B) are inappropriate for oral surgery. A gas-driven, high-speed handpiece (C), designed for human operative dentistry, works well for small animal oral surgery, but the heavier workload of equine oral surgery predisposes these handpieces to turbine failure. A gas-driven, high-speed surgical drill system (D), designed for cranio-maxillofacial surgery, allows for precision hard tissue cutting at depths up to 7cm. Pictured are the gas supply hose, the drill handpiece, bur guards (3 lengths), and assorted carbide burs.

Surgical Extraction Techniques," in this issue). A recent study documented the complications associated with regional nerve blocks performed by experienced veterinarians in equine dental patients were minimal (2.96%) and transient. Hematoma was the most common complications (62.5%), which resolved within 48 hours in all cases. Lingual self-trauma occurred in 2 cases of 51 mandibular nerve blocks and resolved completely by 3 months postoperatively.[10] Based on overwhelming evidence, general anesthesia should be reserved for patients in which behavior or pain is unmanageable.

Dental Radiology and Computed Tomography Scans

The primary factors used to determine the best extraction technique(s) to minimize intraoperative and postoperative complications are (1) the morphology of the diseased tooth's reserve crown and root and the degree of root resorption or ankylosis (**Fig. 4**), (2) the clinical periodontal attachment level, and (3) potential obstruction of the extraction pathway (**Fig. 5**) (see also the Robert M. Baratt's article "Dental Radiography and Radiographic Signs of Equine Dental Disease"; and Erin Epperly and Justin A. Whitty's article, "Equine Imaging: Computed Tomography Interpretation," elsewhere in this issue). Because the tooth must have an unobstructed extraction pathway, reserve crown and root morphology are critical for extraction treatment planning. Anatomic variations such as an abnormal curvature of the reserve crown or root dilaceration could indicate surgical extraction regardless of periodontal status. Similarly, pathologic conditions such as hypercementosis or ankylosis (**Fig. 6**) commonly cause intraoperative difficultly regardless of the extraction technique used.

The portable digital radiograph systems and light-weight, high frequency x-ray generators available today produce high-quality diagnostic radiographs acceptable for treatment planning in the majority of extraction cases. For more difficult cases, especially those with regional extension into the sinuses, computed tomography scanning is the imaging modality of choice.

In addition to preoperative radiographs for treatment planning, radiographs should be taken intraoperatively any time an extraction is not progressing as expected and postoperatively to confirm complete extraction of all tooth fragments (**Fig. 7**).

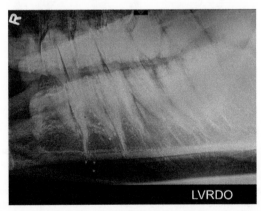

Fig. 4. Radiograph of a right mandibular third premolar (407) with a long thin curved mesial root (*red dots*) and an ankylosed resorbing distal root (*green dots*). Both root morphologic features predispose this tooth to intraoperative complications during intraoral extraction.

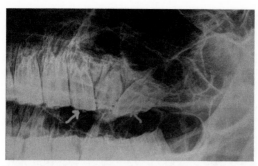

Fig. 5. A radiograph demonstrating an intraoral extraction eruption pathway that is block by adjacent teeth. The left maxillary second molar (210) is block (*red dots*) by the distally tipped of 209 (*green arrow*) and the mesial tipped of 211 (*red arrow*). Alternative or surgical extraction techniques will be required to extract 210.

ORAL EXTRACTION

A standard oral extraction using gingival elevators, molar spreaders, and forceps has been practiced for more than a century and is the preferred technique for extraction owing to its lack of invasiveness, high success rate, and low incidence of complications (see also Jon M. Gieche's article, "Equine Oral Extraction Techniques," in this issue). Additionally, standard oral extraction techniques are almost always used for the initial mobilization of a cheek tooth, even when a crown fracture is expected and an additional procedure will be required to ultimately remove the tooth. Reported complication rates range from 2.4% to 8.0%, with the most common, and expected, complication being alveolar sequestration. The case series with the lowest reported complication rate emphasized appropriate case selection and was performed by a general practitioner whose cases were primarily limited to senior horses with advanced periodontal disease. Three of 125 cases experienced intraoperative root fractures, and none required additional corrective procedures.[3] Other authors emphasize that adequate time and patience are required to prevent complications and also recognize that space limitation in the back of the mouth as well as crown morphology (abnormal shape, low height, fracture) can make the standard procedure technically difficult.[8,11,12] Inappropriate instrument placement and overly aggressive

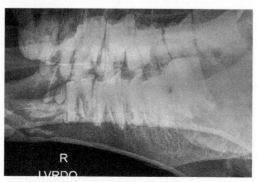

Fig. 6. A radiograph of the right mandible demonstrating resorption and hypercementosis involving all the roots of the left mandibular cheek teeth. Difficulty during intraoral extraction should be anticipated.

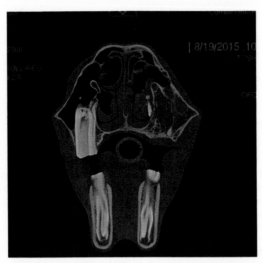

Fig. 7. This computed tomography (axial plane) demonstrates postoperative sinusitis caused by the retention of a dental fragment (*red dot*) from the left maxillary first molar (209) embedded in the conchal scroll (adjacent to the junction of the left ventral conchal sinus and left ventral conchal bullae) after dental repulsion.

instrumentation are almost exclusively the cause of major complications, such as palatine artery laceration, soft palate tear, damage to other teeth, and iatrogenic oronasal or antral fistula.

MINIMALLY INVASIVE BUCCOTOMY TECHNIQUES

Stoll[13] introduced the minimally invasive buccal approach to the cheek teeth and the screw extraction technique in 2007. This approach provides access for straight line instrumentation of cheek teeth. The dentist must avoid several significant neurovascular and salivary structures during the surgical approach. Instrumentation of the molars is challenging owing to the restrictions of the masseter muscle making the placement of the buccotomy site critical for success. Also, instrumentation of the mandibular cheek teeth can be difficult to impossible, the farther caudal the tooth position, owing the anisognathic conformation of the jaw. When performed by an experienced dentist with proper case selection and instrumentation, significant complications are uncommon, but secondary sinusitis owing to perforation with the drill or threaded pin may occur; therefore, endoscopic guidance and frequent intraoperative radiography are recommended to confirm screw and drill placement (**Fig. 8**). The most common minor complications are skin edema at the buccotomy site and transient facial nerve paralysis, which typically resolve within a few days.[5,14]

PARTIAL CORONECTOMY AND TOOTH SECTIONING

Coronectomy, tooth sectioning, and alveolectomy are advanced procedures that are commonly used in small animal dentistry and have been adapted to equine cheek teeth.[15] (See Travis Henry and Ian Bishop' article, "Adjunct Extraction Techniques in Equine Dentistry," in this issue.) Coronectomy provides space within the alveolus for luxation of the tooth, sectioning divides a multirooted tooth into single-rooted fragments, and alveolectomy opens an obstructed extraction pathway. A recent case

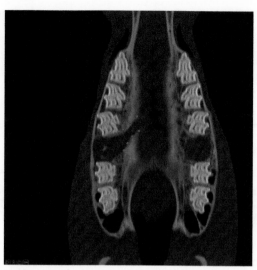

Fig. 8. A computed tomography (coronal plane) demonstrating hard palate damage owing to inappropriate drill placement during a minimally invasive buccotomy technique. Red dots outline the hard palate damage.

series on coronectomy reported an excellent success rate (99.4%) with minimal postoperative complications (3.6%)[6]; however, it should be recognized that the authors presenting these procedures are board-certified veterinary dentists and that these procedures require competency in advanced drill skills to perform without causing iatrogenic damage to the surrounding oral tissues. These procedures in small animals are performed with extreme caution under direct visualization, and the same standard of care should be applied to equine patients. Performing intraoral hard tissue cutting procedures on equine molars without endoscopic guidance is below the current veterinary standard of care. Inappropriate use of this technique has caused severe iatrogenic damage to equine patients (**Fig. 9**).

COMMISSUROTOMY

A board-certified veterinary dentist reported performing a bilateral commissurotomy in a 39 kg, 19-month-old dwarf miniature pony to gain access to the maxillary first molars for oral extraction. The mouth was too restrictive for per os instrumentation and the tooth's position under the orbit prevented a dorsal surgical approach. Regional vital structures were identified, and no complications were reported.[16]

SURGICAL BUCCOTOMY APPROACHES TO THE CHEEK TEETH

Three case series in the last decade have reported the outcomes of buccotomy techniques, as an alternative to repulsion, for the removal of cheek teeth when oral extraction was inappropriate (eg, imbedded or fractured teeth) or failed or when indicated by preoperative planning.[7,17,18] Like other oral surgical techniques, these procedures require advanced skills and instrumentation to perform competently without significant iatrogenic damage (**Fig. 10**). The procedures reported were all performed under general anesthesia and associated complications were reported. The overall procedural complication rates ranged from 30% to 53%, and the most common

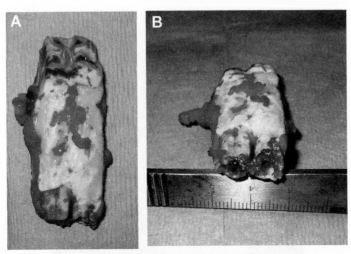

Fig. 9. The right mandibular second molar (410) extracted from a 4-year-old Miniature Horse that presented with an orocutaneous fistula and a history of having the third molar (411) extracted approximately 3 months prior. A coronectomy cut through the 2 caudal pulp horns (*A*) and caused iatrogenic irreversible pulpitis (*B*). Surgical extraction of 410 and debridement of the 411 alveolus was required to correct the iatrogenic damage from the first extraction procedure.

complication associated with these techniques was, expectedly, transient facial nerve neuropathy, which was the only statistically significant complication in one study. However, permanent facial nerve paralysis was also reported. Other complications included intraoperative hemorrhage, nonhealing alveoli, oroantral fistulae, persistent sinusitis, wound dehiscence, and long-term nonpainful mandibular swelling. General surgical instrumentation (osteotome and mallet) was used, and 1 group of authors acknowledged its imprecision. Rawlinson[19] reported a transcutaneous surgical

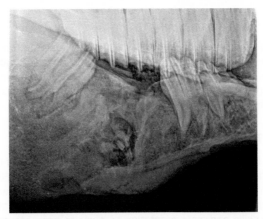

Fig. 10. Radiograph demonstrating iatrogenic damage secondary to an inappropriate buccotomy technique. A large bone sequestration is present with dental fragments from the right mandibular first molar (409) (*red dots*). Retained roots and reserve crown of the right mandibular second molar (410) are present from an incomplete extraction (*green arrows*).

approach in 2011, which the authors have used in standing horses with only minor complications (see the Edward T. Earley and Stephen S. Galloway's article, "Equine Standing Surgical Extraction Techniques," elsewhere in this issue.)

REPULSION

Cheek tooth repulsion is an extraction technique that has been practiced for over a century and that has been associated with an unacceptably high rate of major iatrogenic complications which frequently require other major procedures to correct. Most veterinary dentist currently consider repulsion techniques contraindicated unless the tooth has first been fully mobilized using other extraction techniques. A recent case series of cheek teeth repulsed in standing horses after intraoral extraction failure reported no iatrogenic complications. However, persistent sinusitis and mandibular draining tracts were reported in 54% of the treated horses and 41% of the cases required follow-up medical or surgical treatments[20] (**Fig. 11**).

ALVEOLAR WOUND HEALING

An understanding of the physiology of wound healing helps to explain the impact of extraction techniques, alveolar treatments, and postoperative management upon the quality and rate of alveolar wound healing. This knowledge can be used by the dentist to predict appropriate times for follow-up evaluations to minimize complications. All mammalian tissues follow a similar, predictable sequence of events regardless of the specific tissue affected, and studies investigating extraction wound healing have establish that the rate of healing is similar regardless of the species.[21] Alveolar wound healing can be divided into three overlapping phases.

The first phase of healing, the inflammatory phase, begins immediately after injury and is characterized by the formation of a fibrocellular blood clot. Cytokines released primarily by platelets attract inflammatory cells to the wound. Neutrophils are the predominant cell during the first few days after injury but are soon replaced by macrophages, which remove damaged tissue, debris, and bacteria. Within a day of injury,

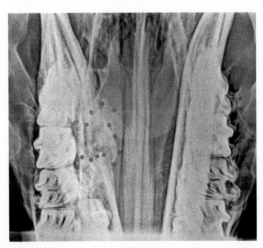

Fig. 11. Radiograph demonstrating extensive iatrogenic damage secondary to cheek tooth repulsion of the right mandibular third molar (411). The medial cortex of the right mandible is fractured after a repulsion extraction (*red dots*).

the proliferation phase of healing begins as macrophages release cytokines, which stimulate fibroblasts to produce collagen, initiating the formation of disorganized granulation tissue. Fibroblasts also differentiate into osteoblast, which produce osteoid. Simultaneous neoangiogenisis provides oxygen and nutrients to the newly formed collagen matrix. During this phase, epithelial cells along the margin of the wound proliferate and migrate across the granulation tissue to close and protect the wound from further oral contamination. During the maturation phase of healing, the disorganized collagen fibers are broken down, realigned, and cross-linked to improve the tensile strength of the wounded tissue. Epithelialization of the mucosa is completed, and osteoblasts mineralize and reorganize the osteoid into bone.

In a healthy patient with a clean alveolus, the blot clot usually fills the extraction site for the first 3 days of healing and is replaced by granulation tissue in the coronal one-third of the alveolus by the end of second week (**Table 1**). Epithelialization of all effected wound margins begins after stabilization of the blood clot, progresses over the surface of the blood clot or granulation tissue,[22] and continues to migrate until coming into contact with another epithelial edge. Oral epithelium migrates at a rate of 0.3 to 0.5 mm per day,[23] and mucosal epithelialization from the gingival margin should be significant within 2 weeks and complete within 1 month. In the apical two-thirds of the alveolus the blot clot is replaced by osteoid. The osteoid fully mineralizes into woven bone by the beginning of the second month, and remodeling into cortical and trabecular bone is complete by 6 months.[24]

Thorough alveolar wound debridement to produce a clean environment is the foundation of wound healing; however, evidence suggests that the PDL should not be indiscriminately stripped from the alveolus[25] because it provides fibroblasts for the wound healing. Also, chlorhexidine solutions and other disinfectants should be used judiciously to rinse alveolar wounds because they are cytotoxic to fibroblasts and other stem cells.[26,27] Because primary closure of extraction sites is rarely achieved in the horse, obturating the occlusal aspect of the alveolus while allowing space for apical blood clot formation is critical during the first 2 phases of healing to prevent wound contamination while allowing space for granulation tissue and osteoid production. Once a healthy granulation bed is established on the occlusal aspect of the wound (week 2), further retention of the obturator may interfere with tissue remodeling and delay healing (**Fig. 12**). Alveolar sequestration[28] and the inability to remove alveolar plug[29] have been report secondary to the use of exothermic, hard-setting methyl methacrylate materials; therefore, most dentists prefer to use a cold-setting medium-body polyvinylsiloxane impression material to fabricate the obturator.

Local factors that prolong the inflammatory phase of healing include contamination, retained tooth fragments and roots, and damage to alveolar bone. Completely filling

Table 1	
Table of alveolar wound healing	
Time After Procedure	**Stage**
Day 1–3	Blot clot
Week 1	Granulation tissue
Week 2	Bone replacement begins
Week 3–4	Epithelialization complete
Month 2	Bone replacement complete
Month 6	Bone remodeling complete

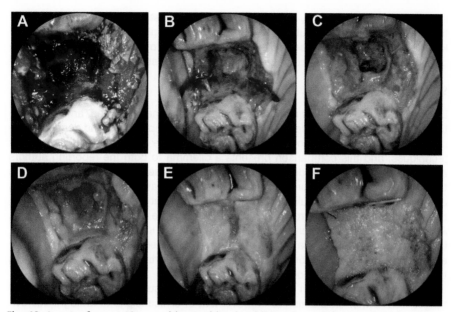

Fig. 12. Images from a 10-year-old warmblood gelding whose right maxillary first molar (109) was extracted using intraoral and minimally invasive buccotomy techniques. The patient had a preexisting and persistent sinusitis originating from a pulp expose through the palatal root into the ventral conchal sinus. Alveolar debridement of the oroantral fistula was perform on the day of extraction, but the entire alveolus was not curetted. (A) A blood clot is established in the apex. On postoperative days 7 (B), 13 (C), and 27 (D), images were taken immediately after removing the polyvinylsiloxane obturator to document the level of oral contamination and healing. The alveolus was rinsed with a pulsating irrigator, and spot curetted to remove debris and granulomatous tissue, and the apex of the obturator was progressively trimmed to allow room for continued development of granulation tissue. Note that the walls of the alveolus are lined with granulation tissue by day 7 (B) and that epithelialization is functionally complete by day 27 (D), at which time the obturator was removed. Images on days 38 (E) and 128 (F) demonstrate continued remodeling of the alveolus.

the alveolus with obturation material interferes with the formation of the blood clot. Aggressive or prolonged oral or sinus lavage can destabilize the blood clot. Overfilling an alveolus, that has a fistulous tract, with obturation material predisposes the tract to re-epithelialize with the oral mucosal.

Systemic disease, systemic inflammation, endocrine conditions, age, and nutritional deficiencies suppress tissue perfusion, the inflammatory response, and immune system. These systemic conditions delay or inhibit wound healing and ideally should be addressed before extractions. Local infection and the systemic use of antibiotics is an issue of constant debate; therefore, antibiotic therapy should be used judiciously. Antibiotics are not indicated in healthy patients when the extraction procedure adheres to extraction principles.

POSTOPERATIVE CARE

The owner should be provided with written discharge instructions discussing the procedures performed, postoperative wound care (eg, oral rinses), expected recovery and postoperative evaluations, medications dispensed (antibiotics, analgesics, anti-inflammatories), restrictions, and dietary guidelines. Postoperative care and evaluation following extraction is subjectively prescribed and highly variable. To the authors' knowledge, no significant research has been conducted to investigate the contribution of postoperative care to the outcome of extraction procedures.

STANDARDIZATION OF CASE REPORTING

During the last decade, new instrumentation has been manufactured, and extraction techniques have been modified in an effort to reduce complications and decrease procedural times. Authors are now beginning to compare the outcomes of these different techniques, and this comparison presents a dilemma to both the reporting authors and the readers. Veterinary dentists often plan for and use multiple techniques during the same extraction procedure. For example, most alternative and surgical techniques are preceded by oral manipulation to provide initial mobility to the tooth. The contribution of each technique toward the ultimate removal of the disease tooth is subjective. Although most veterinary dentist have the experience to interpret these case reports, the inherent subjectivity can confuse less experienced readers trying to make educated health care decisions. Standardization of reporting would make interpreting the conclusions of case reports easier for all.

Additionally, the definition of procedural success is currently very subjective and ranges from owner satisfaction to improvement of clinical signs to radiographic evidence of hard tissue healing. It is generally accepted that, as pray animals, horse will mask signs of pain, disease, and injury and that people without medical training are not qualified to accurately assess medical outcomes; therefore, the authors recommend that case reporting exclude owner reported outcomes. The authors recommend that the minimum standard for reporting of dentistry and oral surgery procedural outcomes be based on the American Veterinary Dental College standard for case reporting. An oral examination should be performed by an experienced veterinary dentist after the epithelialization of oral mucosa is complete at least 1 month postoperatively. For small animals, the American Veterinary Dental College requires radiograph evidence of bone healing 6 months postoperatively. Evidence of both soft and hard tissue healing should be the goal for all dentistry case reporting.

The authors recommend dividing complications into categories as preexisting, minor, or major. Although a preexisting condition that persists after tooth extraction should be reported, it should not be considered a complication of the extraction procedure. The classic example of this is chronic dental sinusitis. If the dental alveolus completely heals, the persistence of sinusitis may not be related to the extraction procedure. A minor complication would include a self-resolving complication (mild alveolar osteitis, transient facial neuropathy) or a complication that is easily corrected during the first follow-up visit using a single sedative bolus and no additional anesthesia (eg, loose alveolar sequestration debridement, sinus flush without debridement). A major complication is iatrogenic or permanent or requires an extended or additional procedure to correct (eg, retained root extraction, treatment of oroantral fistula or sinusitis, when this was not a preexisting condition).

SUMMARY

Oral extraction and tooth repulsion techniques have been practiced for over a century. Although oral extraction has become the most popular extraction technique owing to its high rate of success with a low rate of major complication, repulsion continues to produce an unacceptably high rate of major complications. In an effort to avoid tooth repulsion, veterinary dentists have introduced procedures to facilitate difficult intraoral extractions and surgical extraction techniques. Improvements in dentistry and oral surgery instrumentation and training over the last 20 years are now mitigating complications that previous resulted from deficiencies in these areas.

Minimizing tooth extraction complications is best achieved preoperatively. A trained staff and experienced veterinary dentist with proper instrumentation work efficiently minimizing fatigue and mistakes. A comprehensive preoperative evaluation and treatment plan allow the dentist to predict intraoperative complication and prepare for procedures that will produce the best outcome. With proper case selection and adherence to extraction principles, both the primary veterinarian and the veterinary dentist can perform equine tooth extractions with minimal complications.

DISCLOSURE

No funding sources, financial interests, or conflicts of interest to disclose.

REFERENCES

1. Merillat LA. Veterinary surgery, vol I, animal dentistry and diseases of the mouth. Chicago: Haussmann and Dunn Co; 1905. p. 13.
2. Earley ET, Rawlinson JE, Baratt RM. Complications associated with cheek tooth extraction in the horse. J Vet Dent 2013;30(4):220–35.
3. Duncanson GR. A case study of 125 horses presented to a general practitioner in the UK for cheek teeth removal. Equine Vet Educ 2004;6(3):212–6.
4. Dixon PM, Dacre I, Dacre K, et al. Standing oral extraction of cheek teeth in 100 horses (1998–2003). Equine Vet J 2005;37(2):105–12.
5. Langeneckert F, Witte T, Schellenberger F, et al. Cheek tooth extraction via a minimally invasive transbuccal approach and intradental screw placement in 54 equids. Vet Surg 2015;44:1012–20.
6. Rice MK, Henry TJ. Standing intraoral extractions of cheek teeth aided by partial crown removal in 165 horses (2010-2016). Equine Vet J 2018;50(1):48–53.
7. Caramello V, Zarucco L, Foster D, et al. Equine cheek tooth extraction: comparison of outcomes for five extraction methods. Equine Vet J 2020;52(2):181–6.
8. Ramzan PHL, Dallas RS, Palmer L. Extraction of fractured cheek teeth under oral endoscopic guidance in standing horses. Vet Surg 2011;40:586–9.
9. Scrutchfield WL, Schumacher J, Walker M, et al. Removal of an osteoma from the paranasal sinuses of a standing horse. Equine Pract 1994;16:24–8.
10. Tanner RB, Hubbell JAE. A retrospective study of the incidence and management of complications associated with regional nerve blocks in equine dental patients. J Vet Dent 2019;36(1):40–5.
11. Dixon PM, Tremaine WH, Pickles K, et al. Equine dental disease Part 4: a long term study of 400 cases: apical infections of cheek teeth. Equine Vet J 2000; 32:182–94.
12. Tremaine WH. Oral extraction of equine cheek teeth. Equine Vet Educ 2004;6(3): 191–8.
13. Stoll M. How to Perform a Buccal Approach for Different Dental Procedures. In: Proceedings. Am Assoc Eq Pract 2007;53:507–11.
14. Stoll M. Minimally invasive transbuccal surgery and screw extraction. In: Proceedings. Am Assoc Eq Pract-Focus Dent 2011;170–6.
15. Rice MK. Removal of difficult teeth: intraoral tooth sectioning, alveolectomy and partial crown removal techniques. In: Proceedings. Am Assoc Eq Pract-Focus Dent 2017;75–7.

16. Wilson G. Commissurotomy for oral access and tooth extraction in a dwarf miniature pony. J Vet Dent 2012;29(4):250–2.

17. Tremaine WH, McCluskie LK. Removal of 11 incompletely erupted, impacted cheek teeth in 10 horses using a dental alveolar transcortical osteotomy and buccotomy approach. Vet Surg 2010;39(7):884–90.

18. O'Neill HD, Boussauw B, Bladon BM, et al. Extraction of cheek teeth using a lateral buccotomy approach in 114 horses (1999-2009). Equine Vet J 2011; 43(3):348–53.

19. Rawlinson JE. Surgical extraction of mandibular cheek teeth via alveolar bone removal. In: Proceedings. Am Assoc Eq Pract-Focus Dent 2011;178–83.

20. Coomer RP, Fowke GS, McKane S. Repulsion of maxillary and mandibular cheek teeth in standing horses. Vet Surg 2011;40(5):590–5.

21. Amler MH. The time sequence of tissue regeneration in human extraction wounds. Oral Surg Oral Med Oral Pathol 1969;27:309–18.

22. Hupp JR, Ellis E III, Tucker MR. Contemporary oral and maxillofacial surgery. Sixth Edition. St. Louis (MO): Elsevier Mosby; 2014. p. 43–50.

23. Nanci A. Ten Cate's Oral histology, development, structure and function. sixth edition. St. Louis (MO): Mosby; 2003. p. 400–5.

24. Cardaropoli G, Araujo M, Lindhe J. Dynamics of bone tissue formation in tooth extraction sites. An experimental study in dogs. J Clin Periodontol 2003;30: 809–18.

25. Lin WL, McCulloch CA, Cho MI. Differentiation of periodontal ligament fibroblasts into osteoblasts during socket healing after tooth extraction in the rat. Anat Rec 1994;1240:492–506.

26. Liu JX, Werner J, Kirsch T, et al. Cytotoxicity evaluation of chlorhexidine gluconate on human fibroblasts, myoblasts, and osteoblasts. J Bone Jt Infect 2018;3(4): 165–72.

27. Coelho AS, Laranjo M, Gonçalves AC, et al. Cytotoxic effects of a chlorhexidine mouthwash and of an enzymatic mouthwash on human gingival fibroblasts. Odontology 2020;108(2):260–70.

28. Carmalt JL. Complications of Intra-oral Extraction. In: Proceedings. Am Assoc Eq Pract-Focus Dent 2017;81–2.

29. Gordon DL, Radtke CL. Treatment of chronic sinusitis in a horse with systemic and intra-sinus antimicrobials. Can Vet J 2017;58(3):289–92.

Equine Nasal Endoscopy
Treating Bullae Disease and Sinus Disease

Elaine F. Claffey, DVM[a],*, Norm G. Ducharme, DVM, MS[a,b]

KEYWORDS

- Sinusitis • Conchal bulla/bullae • Endoscopy • Nasal concha/conchae
- Ventral conchal sinus

KEY POINTS

- The nasal conchal bullae (dorsal and ventral) are distinct, air-filled structures contained within the dorsal and ventral nasal conchae.
- They are adjacent to, but do not communicate with, the corresponding conchal sinuses (dorsal and ventral).
- With the use of computed tomography, empyema of the conchal bullae is increasingly recognized with dental and sinus disease.
- The ventral conchal bullae are accessed endoscopically through the ventral conchal recess at the rostral aspect of the middle nasal meatus.
- Fenestrations of the bullae can be created with a diode laser, equine laryngeal forceps, or bipolar vessel sealing devices; access to the ventral conchal sinus is created with fenestration of the mucosal septum separating the bulla and sinus.

Video content accompanies this article at http://www.vetequine.theclinics. com.

A greater understanding of sinus anatomy and dental disease provided by the increased use of computed tomographic (CT) examinations and recent publications has highlighted the importance of the nasal conchal bullae as contributory to sinus and dental disease.[1–3] Dixon and colleagues[3] (2015) showed that 20% of horses with paranasal sinus disease also had involvement of the dorsal and/or ventral conchal bullae (VCB) on CT examinations. This article reviews the anatomic locations of the dorsal and ventral nasal conchal bullae, their nasal communications, disease of these bullae and the relationship with dental disease, and visualization through nasal endoscopy, as well as surgical options for treatment of empyema of the nasal conchal bullae.

[a] Cornell Ruffian Equine Specialists, 111 Plainfield Avenue, Elmont, NY 11003, USA; [b] Department of Clinical Sciences, Cornell University, College of Veterinary Medicine, 930 Campus Road, Box 25, Ithaca, NY 14853, USA
* Corresponding author.
E-mail address: elf66@cornell.edu

Vet Clin Equine 36 (2020) 659–669
https://doi.org/10.1016/j.cveq.2020.08.005
0749-0739/20/© 2020 Elsevier Inc. All rights reserved.

vetequine.theclinics.com

ANATOMY AND LOCATION OF THE NASAL CONCHAL BULLAE

The nasal conchae in the horse consist of large paired (left and right) dorsal and ventral conchae that are attached laterally within the nasal cavity. These ventral and dorsal nasal conchae create the dorsal, middle, and ventral meatuses (openings) commonly referenced during nasal endoscopy. The conchae consist of scrolls of thin bone covered with mucosa. The dorsal concha scrolls ventrally and the ventral concha scrolls dorsally in direction, each coiling toward the middle meatus. The caudal aspect of each dorsal and ventral concha extends to the well-described dorsal conchal sinus and ventral conchal sinus, respectively. These sinuses are separated from the conchae by distinct, vertical to obliquely oriented septa; the caudal wall of the dorsal conchal bulla (DCB) is immediately rostral to the distinct rostral wall of the dorsal conchal sinus.[1,2] In contrast, the VCB is usually only separated from the ventral conchal sinus by a thin mucosal septum.[1,2]

Rostral to these septa, both the dorsal and ventral conchae contain a distinct, separate air-filled structures, known as the DCB and VCB. Recent updates in nomenclature recommend that these bullae be referred to as the bulla conchalis dorsalis and bulla conchalis ventralis. These structures should not be confused with the dorsal aspect of the maxillary septum, which has in the past been called the ventral conchal bulla, because this entity is more appropriately called the maxillary septal bulla (bulla of the septum sinuum maxillarium). In fact, the nasal conchal bullae do not have any obvious communication with the paranasal sinuses, although communication is often present in the setting of dental disease or empyema of the paranasal sinuses.[3]

The conchal bullae are overlapped medially by the scrolling nasal conchae, but laterally they are not fully covered. The ventromedial aspect of the DCB and the dorsomedial aspect of the VCB are not covered by nasal conchae; these areas are both within the middle nasal meatus. Surgical drainage of affected bullae generally requires an approach through the middle nasal meatus, so the vascular nasal conchae can be avoided.[1]

Both nasal conchae are continued rostrally by mucosal folds; the ventral concha mucosal fold contains a thick venous plexus. There is a small recess between the external surface of each bulla and the overlying nasal concha, and this area is open to the middle meatus.[2]

The DCB and VCB are each divided by small transverse septa into 2 to 7 cells. These cells or cellulae communicate through small openings with the nasal cavity, opening into the recess of the middle meatus as noted elsewhere in this article. The DCB has slightly more cellulae than the VCB. The septa dividing them vary from a thin layer of mucosa to some containing thin bone that provides a more robust separation. The DCB also has more apertures or drainage passages into the middle meatus than the VCB. These apertures are ventrally located in the DCB, whereas in the VCB they exit from the dorsal or dorsorostral aspects. It should be noted that the VCB occasionally does have a wide drainage aperture at the rostral aspect. When examining drainage from separate cellulae within the bullae in a cadaver study, a total of 7.1% of the VCB and 3.6% of the DCB lacked a visual drainage aperture on anatomic studies of cadavers; however, it was noted that, owing to the secretory nature of the epithelium of the bullae, drainage apertures were likely present but not detected in this study.[2]

The DCB is generally longer in rostrocaudal length and located dorsally along the maxillary triadan 07-09s/10s.[4] The VCB is smaller, with less septae and cellulae, and most commonly located dorsal to the maxillary 07s-08s/09s.[4] The VCB is often significantly compressed laterally in younger horses by the large reserve alveoli of the developing maxillary cheek teeth. In fact, both the DCB and VCB have smaller volumes on CT examination in horses 0 to 5 years old versus those that are greater than 16 years old, with the average volume of the DCB in the younger group being 15.6 cm^3 and 24.7 cm^3 in the older group. For the VCB, the younger horses had an average volume of 8.5 cm^3 versus 17.2 cm^3 in the older horses.[1]

Summary

- The dorsal and VCB are small, distinct air-filled structures contained within the dorsal and ventral conchae of the nasal passages, located rostrally to the conchal sinuses (dorsal conchal sinus, ventral conchal sinus) within their respective nasal conchae
- The DCB and VCB do not normally communicate with the paranasal sinuses, but communication is often present with paranasal sinus disease
- Each bulla is divided into multiple compartments by thin septae composed of mucosa or mucosa with a thin layer of bone; each compartment, or cellula, likely has an aperture for drainage into the nasal passages via the middle meatus
- Both bullae (DCB and VCB) are most accessible to surgical intervention through the middle meatus, where they are not covered by the vascular nasal conchae

IMAGING OF THE NASAL CONCHAL BULLAE

Identification of the conchal bullae with plain radiography of the skull is challenging owing to the anatomic complexity of the area and superimposition of structures in conventional radiographs. If clearly visible, they are roughly oval radiolucent structures with a thin bony wall; the septae dividing the interior of the bullae into cellulae may also be visible on a lateral radiograph projection as small, thin, radiopaque divisions.[4]

The VCB are positioned medial to the maxillary sinuses but cannot be reliably visualized on plain dorsoventral projections. On a lateral view, the position of the VCB is more variable, because it can be located either rostral to the most rostral aspect of the maxillary sinus or superimposed on the rostral aspect of the rostral maxillary sinus. The rostral aspect of the VCB is easier to identify than its caudal limit; the rostral mucosal fold that extends from the VCB is typically visible as a well-defined soft tissue opacity and is a useful landmark for identification of the VCB. This structure can be obscured in younger horses owing to the larger alveoli of the maxillary cheek teeth.

The DCB is more easily identified and evaluated with radiography. In a lateral projection, the DCB dorsal border was visible as a thin line parallel to the dorsal nasal meatus and nasal bone (**Fig. 1**A). Rostrally, the DCB has a similar rostral mucosal fold as the VCB, visible as a soft tissue opacity extending from the rostral DCB to the caudal nasoincisive notch (**Fig. 1**B).

In the dorsal 30° ventral lateral oblique projection, it is more difficult to identify the bullae owing to superimposition of the nasal meatuses and contralateral bulla. The dorsoventral view is also not as useful, because only the caudomedial part of the DCB can be seen owing to the superimposition of the mandible and cheek teeth. There is also frequent superimposition of the DCB and the ventral conchal sinus in the dorsoventral view.[4]

CT examinations have greatly increased our understanding of the nasal conchal bullae (**Fig. 2**). In the only reported case series of empyema of the nasal conchal bullae, all cases were identified using CT imaging.[3] Disease of the conchal bullae is indicated by fluid and/or soft tissue density within the bullae (**Fig. 3**). CT scans are also useful for defining associated paranasal sinus disease, dental disease, and other abnormalities that are often present with nasal conchal bulla disease.[5]

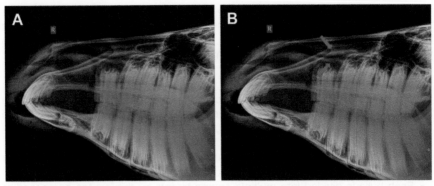

Fig. 1. Lateral radiograph of a 4-year-old horse. (*A*) The visible portion of the DCB is out-lined. The VCB is obscured from the reserve alveolus of the maxillary cheek teeth. (*B*) The rostral mucosal folds extending from the dorsal and VCB are indicated with *arrows*.

Summary

- Evaluation of the nasal conchal bullae is challenging on plain radiography; lateral projections are the most useful and the DCB are most easily visible.
- CT scans provide 3-dimensional imaging and the most accurate diagnosis of bulla disease, as well as defining associated paranasal sinus or dental disease.

NASAL ENDOSCOPY

To visualize the rostral aspect of the VCB, the endoscope is placed into the ventral conchal recess (the space between the external surface of the bullae and the internal surface of the nasal conchae). To enter the recess, the endoscope is retracted rostrally to the very rostral aspect of the middle meatus. The scope must be directed laterally and ventrally to follow the direction of the coiling ventral nasal concha. The scope is advanced as it is directed ventrally until the scope is within the concha. Sedation

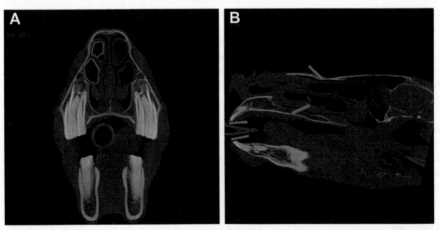

Fig. 2. (*A*) A frontal section of a normal horse skull CT scan shows the dorsal and VCB at the level of the maxillary 108/208 cheek teeth. Both bullae on the right side of the horse are highlighted in *red*. (*B*) A sagittal section of the same horse shows the normal dorsal and VCB, which are indicated by *arrows*.

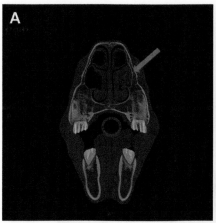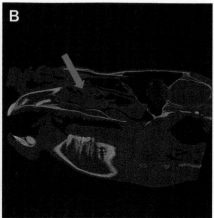

Fig. 3. CT images of a 16-year-old horse with empyema of the left VCB. Tooth 209 had been extracted 2 years prior, but left-sided nasal discharge recurred. (*A*) A frontal section of the skull, the VCB has increased soft tissue opacity indicated by the *arrow*. The right VCB and both DCB are normal. (*B*) A sagittal section of the skull of the same horse, the VCB indicated by the *arrow* is irregular and has increased soft tissue opacity.

and topical application of lidocaine are helpful to decrease sensation and patient resistance. As the scope is advanced caudally within the recess of the ventral concha, the rostral end of the VCB will become visible (**Fig. 4**). Care must be taken to distinguish the rostral end of the bulla itself from the thick folded mucosa that continues rostrally from the bulla; this process can be more difficult with disease and swelling of the VCB. This maneuver can be difficult (or impossible) in younger horses because the VCB and recess are both compressed by the maxillary cheek teeth. See Video 1 for an example of passage of the endoscope to view the right VCB.

With empyema of the conchal bullae, purulent debris or gross distortion or swelling of the bullae may be noted from visualization in the middle meatus. A fistula with purulent drainage may be present from the bullae into the nasal passages or can be obvious when examined from the ventral conchal recess.

Once the endoscope has been passed to the level of the rostral VCB, it can often be passed underneath the VCB (passing ventral and medial to the bulla, between the bulla and the overlying nasal concha). At the caudal aspect of the VCB, a small septum is visible ventral and medial to the bulla. This septum is variable in thickness, from a thin mucosal layer to mucosa overlying thin bone, and divides the ventral conchal recess from the rostral aspect of the ventral conchal sinus. This septum can be penetrated using either the endoscope itself, a biopsy forceps, or a diode laser and the endoscope passed into the ventral conchal sinus (**Fig. 5**).

The DCB can be visualized in a similar fashion, but often requires a smaller diameter endoscope than the standard 10-mm diameter flexible videoendoscope. The rostral scroll of the dorsal concha is supported by bone (unlike the more flexible mucosal component of the ventral nasal concha), which adds to the difficulty of endoscopic passage through this area.[6]

Summary

- A standard 10-mm endoscope can be used to evaluate the rostral aspect of the VCB, by starting in the middle meatus and introducing the endoscope into the ventral conchal recess.

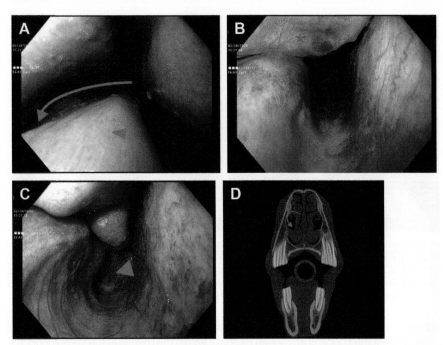

Fig. 4. Passage of the endoscope around the ventral conchae of the right nostril to visualize the right VCB. (*A*) The endoscope is passed 10 to 15 cm caudal to the nares where the middle meatus is clearly visible. The nasal septum is on the right (*starred*) and the ventral concha is visible on the bottom (*arrowhead*). The *arrow* indicates the path of the endoscope to pass around the ventral conchal scroll. (*B*) The scope has been passed around the ventral concha and is now in the ventral conchal recess. The rostral mucosa fold extending from the VCB is visible (*starred*). (*C*) The endoscope has been advanced caudally within the ventral conchal recess until the VCB is visible (*starred*). The thin septum separating the ventral conchal recess from the ventral conchal sinus is visible (*arrowhead*). (*D*) A sagittal CT image taken rostral to the VCB. The *arrow* indicates the path taken by the endoscope around the ventral concha into the ventral conchal recess. This is at the level of the maxillary 06 teeth.

- In younger horses, it can be difficult to impossible to pass the scope to the VCB owing to external compression from the maxillary cheek teeth.
- Once the endoscope has reached the VCB, in some horses it can be passed underneath the VCB to reach the rostral septum of the ventral conchal sinus.
- Entry into the ventral conchal sinus can often be obtained by penetration through the thin septum between the ventral conchal recess and the ventral conchal sinus.

DISEASE OF THE NASAL CONCHAL BULLAE

Disease of the nasal conchal bullae was first described by Dixon and colleagues in 2014.[3] In this publication, of the 103 head CT scans that were reviewed, 44 horses had paranasal sinus disease. Of the horses with paranasal sinus disease, 20% also had disease of the conchal bullae. Only 1 horse in this series had VCB disease without accompanying paranasal sinus disease. Of the 8 horses that were treated by the authors, 7 of them were diagnosed with infected teeth (triadan 109 in 2 cases, 110 in 1 case, 209 in 2 cases or 210 in 1 case and 207 in 1 case). The horse with the infected

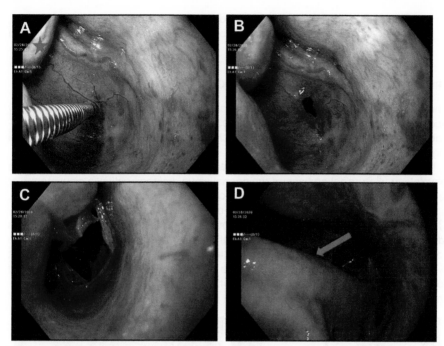

Fig. 5. (*A*) The endoscope has been passed under the VCB of the right nasal passage to the thin membrane separating the ventral conchal recess from the ventral conchal sinus (some of the bullae is still visible, *starred*). An endoscopic biopsy forceps has been used to penetrate the membrane. (*B*) The initial fenestration from the biopsy forceps is visible. In some horses, this membrane has a thicker mucosa and may be more vascular. In these cases, a diode laser may be needed to assist with the fenestration. (*C*) The fenestration from the ventral conchal recess into the ventral conchal sinus is open. In this horse, the membrane was composed of thin mucosa and bone and bled minimally. (*D*) The endoscope has been passed into the ventral conchal sinus. The infraorbital canal is visible (*arrow*).

207 was the only case where the VCB was affected without associated paranasal sinus disease.

Because conchal bulla disease is almost always diagnosed in conjunction with dental pathology or sinusitis, signs are those typically associated with dental sinusitis (mucopurulent or purulent, malodorous, unilateral nasal discharge). On nasal endoscopy, exudate may be noted from the sinonasal drainage aperture owing to concurrent paranasal sinus disease. Purulent drainage can be noted directly from the conchal bulla itself and often sequestered bone may be present as well. Distortion of the outline of the bullae can also be noted on nasal endoscopy, from the middle meatus view of the conchal bulla. If severe, the swelling may distort the nasal conchae sufficiently that the nasal passages themselves are distorted or narrowed.

Temporary improvement of clinical signs is often reported with antimicrobial therapy, although signs recur when treatment is stopped or soon after.

Summary

- Empyema of the nasal conchal bullae is commonly associated with primary dental disease.
- Clinical signs are those associated with sinusitis or dental disease, such as foul smelling unilateral mucopurulent discharge.

- Although the treatment of the primary disease and paranasal sinuses is required, failure to address the nasal conchal bullae may result in treatment failure and recurrence of clinical signs.

TREATMENT OF EMPYEMA OF THE NASAL CONCHAL BULLAE

The treatment of empyema of the nasal conchal bullae must start with treatment of any accompanying dental disease and sinusitis. However, failure to also address inspissated purulent debris within the nasal conchal bullae may result in persistent clinical signs (nasal discharge, etc).

In human medicine, drainage is considered critical for maintenance of normal sinus physiology.[7,8] Surgical opening of the normal sinus drainage ostia via sinusotomy, or less invasive measures, such as endoscopic surgery or balloon dilation of those ostia, are used restore normal drainage in cases of chronic sinusitis.[9,10]

To treat ventral conchal bulla disease though an endoscopic approach, the bulla is identified as described elsewhere in this article by passing the endoscope into the rostral aspect of the middle meatus, then lateral and ventral until the endoscope is within the ventral conchal recess. Once the bulla is identified, it should be evaluated for swelling, purulent debris, or drainage, which may indicate a fistula or other abnormalities (**Fig. 6**).

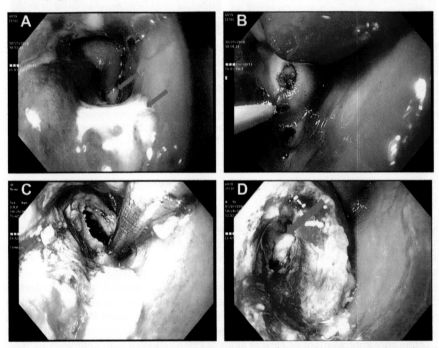

Fig. 6. Images from a 16-year-old horse with empyema of the right VCB, ventral conchal sinus, and maxillary sinus owing to a periapical infection associated with tooth 109. (*A*) The endoscope has been passed into the right ventral conchal recess. The VCB is visible (*starred*). Mucopurulent discharge is visible ventral and rostral to the bullae, likely draining from the rostral aspect of the ventral conchal sinus (*arrows*). (*B*) A diode laser is used to create a fenestration into the VCB. (*C*) An equine laryngeal forceps has been passed into the right ventral conchal recess to continue the fenestration into the VCB. (*D*) Fenestration with purulent material within the lumen of the right VCB (*arrow*).

If a fistula from the affected bulla into the nasal passages or into the nasal conchal recess is already present on endoscopy, transendoscopic lavage may be sufficient for treatment. Repeated lavage is generally recommended until endoscopic resolution of purulent material and debris. Sequestered bone may also be present and can be removed using endoscopic biopsy or basket forceps, high-pressure transendoscopic lavage, equine laryngeal forceps, or a combination of the three.

If a fistula is not present, or if the existing fistula is not large enough to provide sufficient drainage, transendoscopic fenestration with a diode laser is recommended. The VCB is approached through the middle nasal meatus and the bulla fenestrated in the visible free portion where there is not overlying nasal concha. Note that hemorrhage sometimes impedes endoscopic visualization and the procedure may need to be performed in multiple steps to create a large enough fenestration for drainage. Equine laryngeal forceps can be passed into the ventral conchal recess (guided by the endoscope) and used to assist with fenestration of the bulla or removal of sequestered bone fragments. See **Fig. 6** for an example in a clinical case. Using the diode laser initially at lower settings to help promote coagulation of the mucosal vasculature to decrease hemorrhage is recommended.[3]

If larger fenestration of the bulla is required, or the laser fenestration is unsuccessful, an electrothermal bipolar vessel sealing device (eg, LigaSure Covidien, Covidien, Boulder, CO) can also be used to open the rostral aspect of the VCB (author's experience). The LigaSure is passed caudally, similarly to the standard endoscopic

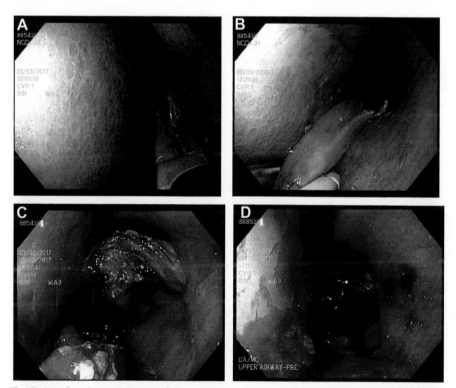

Fig. 7. Nasal endoscopy images from a 12-year-old horse diagnosed with empyema of the right VCB on a CT examination. (*A, B*) The bipolar vessel sealing device is being used within the ventral conchal recess to open the rostral aspect of the VCB. (*C, D*) Right VCB after fenestration with the device.

approach to visualize the VCB and used to grasp, cauterize, and excise the rostral portion of the VCB. See **Fig. 7** for an example in a clinical case.

Occasionally, owing to swelling or difficulty visualizing the bulla, surgical fenestration of the ventral aspect of the bulla may be required. This procedure has been described using a long-handled curved blade for the VCB.[3] Fenestration of the ventral and dorsal conchal sinuses using an electrosurgical conchotomes (450 mm long, 6-mm circular steel shafts with variously shaped tips that provide electrocautery) has been described and could potentially be used as well for the nasal conchal bullae, although there is a risk of hemorrhage at the rostal aspect of the ventral conchal sinus.[11] Laser fenestration of the DCB via a contralateral nostril approach has also been described.[12]

Summary

- Preexisting fistulas between the bullae and the nasal passages provide access for transendoscopic lavage; in some cases, this may be sufficient for debridement and lavage treatment.
- If increased drainage is required, transendoscopic fenestration using a diode laser or LigaSure is recommended; if access or visualization is not possible, direct surgical techniques may also be used transnasally

SUMMARY

Empyema of the conchal bullae is an increasingly recognized clinical condition of the horse. Disease of the conchal bullae should be suspected with persistent or recurrent nasal discharge especially when associated with chronic dental or sinus disease. It is most easily identified on CT examination though careful scrutiny of skull radiographs may provide suspicion of disease. Fenestration of the affected bulla through nasal endoscopic visualization is recommended to establish sufficient drainage of the bulla. Access to the paranasal sinuses (specifically the ventral conchal sinus) via the ventral conchal recess with nasal endoscopy provides an additional entry point to create nasal drainage for the paranasal sinus system.

DISCLOSURE

The authors have no conflicts of interest to disclose.

SUPPLEMENTARY DATA

Supplementary data related to this article can be found online at https://doi.org/10.1016/j.cveq.2020.08.005.

REFERENCES

1. Liuti T, Reardon R, Smith S, et al. An anatomical study of the dorsal and ventral nasal conchal bullae in normal horses: computed tomographic anatomical and morphometric findings. Equine Vet J 2016;48(6):749–55.
2. Froydenlund TJ, Dixon PM, Smith SH, et al. Anatomical and histological study of the dorsal and ventral nasal conchal bullae in normal horses. Vet Rec 2015;177(21):542.
3. Dixon PM, Froydenlund T, Luiti T, et al. Empyema of the nasal conchal bulla as a cause of chronic unilateral nasal discharge in the horse : 10 cases (2013 – 2014). Equine Vet J 2014;445–9. https://doi.org/10.1111/evj.12322.

4. Giavitto AE, Barakzai SZ. Radiographic identification of the equine dorsal and ventral nasal conchal bullae. Equine Vet Educ 2019;31(5):264–70.
5. Henninger W, Frame EM, Willmann M, et al. CT features of alveolitis and sinusitis in horses. Vet Radiol Ultrasound 2003;44(3):269–76.
6. Hubert S. Trans Nasal Sinoscopy. ACVS Proc 2019;46–50.
7. Bajaj V, Singh B, Purohit JP. Prevalence of anatomical variations of lateral wall of nose in chronic sinusitis patients. J Evol Med Dent Sci 2015;4(32):5492–505.
8. Butaric LN, Wadle M, Gascon J. Anatomical variation in maxillary sinus ostium positioning: implications for nasal-sinus disease. Anat Rec 2019;302(6):917–30.
9. Hathorn IF, Pace-Asciak P, Habib ARR, et al. Randomized controlled trial: hybrid technique using balloon dilation of the frontal sinus drainage pathway. Int Forum Allergy Rhinol 2015;5(2):167–73.
10. Thottam PJ, Haupert M, Saraiya S, et al. Functional endoscopic sinus surgery (FESS) alone versus balloon catheter sinuplasty (BCS) and ethmoidectomy: a comparative outcome analysis in pediatric chronic rhinosinusitis. Int J Pediatr Otorhinolaryngol 2012;76(9):1355–60.
11. Bach FS, Böhler A, Schieder K, et al. Surgical enlargement of the nasomaxillary aperture and transnasal conchotomy of the ventral conchal sinus: two surgical techniques to improve sinus drainage in horses. Vet Surg 2019;48(6):1019–31.
12. Kološ F, Bodeček Š, Žert Z. Trans-endoscopic diode laser fenestration of equine conchae via contralateral nostril approach. Vet Surg 2017;46(7):915–24.

Update on Equine Odontoclastic Tooth Resorption and Hypercementosis

Leah E. Limone, DVM

KEYWORDS

- Equine • Tooth resorption • Hypercementosis • EOTRH

KEY POINTS

- Tooth resorption and hypercementosis is a relatively common clinical finding in middle age to geriatric horses.
- Radiography is necessary for diagnosis and treatment planning for EOTRH-affected teeth.
- Staging tooth resorption objectively can aid the decision-making process for when to pursue extractions in mild to moderate cases.
- Extraction of all diseased teeth is a reasonable and effective treatment approach and requires client communication to achieve compliance and improved quality of life for the horse.
- Dental sequelae should be considered as a potential long-term complication of bisphosphonate use in the horse.

 Video content accompanies this article at http://www.vetequine.theclinics.com.

INTRODUCTION

Equine odontoclastic tooth resorption and hypercementosis (EOTRH) is a relatively recently described disorder of unknown etiology affecting the teeth of older horses.[1] The condition was first described as an uncommon disorder of canine and incisor teeth,[2] and then subsequently described histologically and given a descriptive name.[1] Recognized most often in horses more than 15 years old, EOTRH is characterized by internal and external tooth resorption and destruction in combination with excessive cemental deposition.[1,3–7] Hypercementosis is considered a reparative rather than the primary pathologic process.[4] Older age is a risk factor for EOTRH, but moderate-to-severe radiographic changes have been identified in middle-aged horses (11–13 years).[8,9] Concurrent periodontal disease is typically associated with

Northeast Equine Veterinary Dental Services, LLC, PO Box 264, Topsfield, MA 01983, USA
E-mail address: leahlimonedvm@gmail.com

Vet Clin Equine 36 (2020) 671–689
https://doi.org/10.1016/j.cveq.2020.08.006
0749-0739/20/© 2020 Elsevier Inc. All rights reserved.

vetequine.theclinics.com

clinical presentation,[1,5,10–12] and seems to affect incisors and canine teeth more commonly than premolars and molars.[5,13] EOTRH is painful, although often asymptomatic, until associated periodontitis becomes severe.[5] Diagnosis of EOTRH is based on clinical findings and dental radiographs, and histopathology can help to differentiate the disease from other proliferative dental diseases.[6,14]

ETIOLOGY

While no single etiology for EOTRH has been established, there have been several theories suggested.[3,5,14,15] EOTRH is likely to be multifactorial. Current EOTRH research lacks control-based studies along with the identification of a normal resorptive process in aging dentition. With very limited evidence of disease origin, hypotheses include immune-mediated disease, bacterial infection, periodontal disease, masticatory forces iatrogenic odontoplasty, ischemic necrosis, genetics, and systemic/endocrine disease.[1,7,14]

- Immune-mediated syndrome, similar to feline and human immune-mediated syndromes.[16–20] In human and feline syndromes, resorptive lesions are the main feature. In the horse, the condition is mixed with both resorptive and proliferative (hypercementosis) changes.[1,15]
- Increased occlusal force in aging teeth putting excessive mechanical stress on the periodontal ligament.[1,21,22] Aged equine teeth have proportionally less periodontal ligament to occlusal area than younger teeth, but are exposed to the same masticatory forces.[23] This stress causes focal micronecrosis and cytokine release, recruiting and activating clastic cells. Odontoclasts subsequently cause tooth resorption that ultimately affects tooth integrity.[6] This then leads to a reparative reaction by cementoblasts depositing reparative irregular cementum. Irregular cementum deposition is unregulated and causes bulbous enlargements of affected teeth.[1,21] There are still unknown components to this disease since this hypothesis does not account for absence of occlusal force with canines nor how occlusal force has changed since 2004 when the disease was first reported.
- Bacterial members of the red complex and other *Treponema* sp. have been associated with affected equines.[7] Oral infections by *Treponema* and *Tannerella* sp. were reported in 23 of 23 EOTRH-affected horses, suggesting a role in the pathogenesis of the periodontal component of EOTRH.[7] However, control horses were also found to have *Treponema* sp.[7]
- Canine teeth affected by EOTRH present a challenge to the proposed strain-related etiology, as they have no masticatory forces exerted on them.[3] A transfer of strain energies along the jaw bone into the periodontal area of the canines has been demonstrated, but the force is very mild compared with the incisors.[23]

Premolars and molars affected by EOTRH have been reported to have a disproportionate quantity of cementum relative to dentine and enamel.[13,15] Deposition of irregular cementum was noted on the palatal side of maxillary cheek teeth and the buccal side of mandibular cheek teeth.[13,15] These locations were found to be affected by high biomechanical stresses and strains during the power stroke of the masticatory cycle, especially in older horses.[24]

CLINICAL DIAGNOSIS

EOTRH has been shown to affect the aged equine; studies have identified horses older than 15 years are primarily affected.[1,6,15] In a study looking at horses presenting for primary care and no previously diagnosed dental disease, it was shown that tooth resorption started before age 15 years and that tooth resorption of all types and hypercementosis significantly increased after age 15 years.[4] No statistical difference was found for individual breeds or sex of horses having any type of resorption.[4] There is an overrepresentation in the literature of neutered males, warmbloods, and thoroughbreds, and this may represent a biased population of horses receiving dental examinations.[15] There are no known breed, genetic, nutritional, or management predispositions.[6,15]

Affected horses may be asymptomatic or have variable clinical signs when diagnosed. These include pain, masticatory difficulty, quidding, hypersalivation, halitosis, bitting problems, head shaking, behavioral changes, periodic inappetence, and weight loss.[5,6] Older horses may present with fractured or avulsed teeth as a consequence of the resorptive disease.[25,26]

Oral examination findings typically include gingival inflammation and edema, gingival hyperplasia, or recession and loss of interdental papillae[5] (**Fig. 1A–D**). Prominent juga secondary to tooth expansion/extrusion may be present with or without associated draining tracts (**Figs. 1E and 1F**). It seems that the disorder first affects the third incisors (triadan 03s) and then progresses to the second and first incisors (triadan 02s and then 01s).[5] Coronal areas of tooth resorption may have tooth discoloration or granulation tissue (**Fig. 2**). These findings may be concealed beneath calculus deposition and feed accumulation and are easily missed on examination if the calculus and feed are not removed. As the disease progresses additional clinical findings may include pulp exposure, advanced periodontal disease, bone disease, tooth mobility, tooth or bone fracture, or tooth absence[5] (**Fig. 3**). A fine periodontal probe is used to evaluate the gingival sulcus for periodontal pockets and draining tracts (**Fig. 4**), and this may elicit a pain response. A response, such as tooth chattering or sensitivity to light touch with the probe, indicates pain. A comprehensive visual oral examination should be completed on all dental patients, and similar clinical findings may be noted with cheek teeth.[13] EOTRH affecting cheek teeth has been described with only

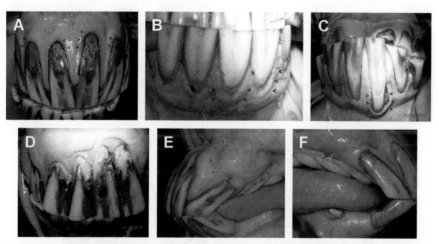

Fig. 1. (*A–F*). Oral examination findings typically include gingival inflammation and edema (*arrows, A*), gingival hyperplasia (*arrows, B*) or recession (*arrows, C*), and loss of interdental papillae (*arrows, D*). Prominent juga secondary to tooth expansion/extrusion present at tooth 203 (*arrows, E*) without draining tract. Draining tract present and identified by an arrow (*F*).

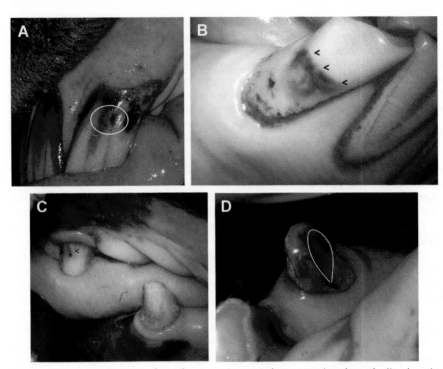

Fig. 2. (*A–D*). Coronal areas of tooth resorption may have associated tooth discoloration (*circled area, A; arrows, B; arrows, C*) or granulation tissue present (*asterisk, C; circled area, D*).

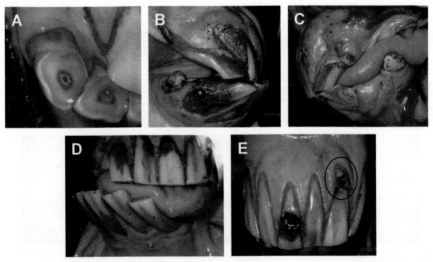

Fig. 3. (*A–E*) With advanced disease, pulp horn defects (*arrow, A*), bulbous enlargement of dental structures (*arrows, B; arrows, C*), tooth displacement (*asterisks, all mandibular incisors displaced to the horses, right, D*), associated periodontal disease, and finally pathologic tooth fracture (*circle, E*) may be present.

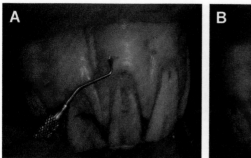
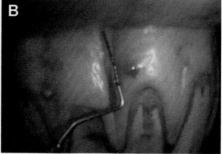

Fig. 4. (A, B) A fine periodontal probe is used to evaluate the gingival margin for periodontal pockets and draining tracts.

moderate periodontal changes and distinguishing changes in clinical crown cementum (**Fig. 5**).[13] It is currently unclear whether EOTRH affecting cheek teeth has a lower prevalence than incisors or whether it is currently underdiagnosed.[13] Examination of each tooth using an intraoral mirror or oral endoscopy can identify areas of gingivitis, hypercementosis, draining tracts, pulp horn defects, tooth fracture, or mobility that would guide the veterinarian to pursue radiographic imaging for disease confirmation and assessment.

HISTOPATHOLOGIC DIAGNOSIS

Histopathologic changes have been reported and help to elucidate the radiographic findings in advanced disease. Two separate cellular processes characterize EOTRH, odontoclastic tooth resorption and unregulated deposition of cementum (hypercementosis).[1,6,7,13] Grossly the periodontium component (alveolus, cementum, periodontal ligament, gingiva) of a tooth is affected initially; with enlargement of peripheral cementum and external tooth resorption.[3,15] Macroscopically, odontoclasts are responsible for resorptive lesions that extend into peripheral cementum, then progress into enamel, dentine, and eventually even the pulp, causing destruction of dental architecture.[5]

There have been 3 different manifestations of EOTRH previously reported: predominant tooth resorption, predominant hypercementosis, and combined resorption and hypercementosis.[4-6,12] (**Fig. 6**) Histologic findings suggest a chronologic sequence of tooth resorption, which is followed by reparative irregular cementum, but that this sequence of events is not synchronized along the entire tooth,[1] and this has led to the above-mentioned 3 types of disease.[14] The resorptive type is considered to be dominated by odontoclast cells resulting in inflammation of the periodontal ligament, and subsequent prolonged odontoclastic resorption.[14] The hypercementotic type predominantly shows a reparative process in deposition of unregulated cementum.[14] In all 3 types of EOTRH reported, histologic studies have always shown some degree of resorption and hypercementosis in every affected tooth.[1,6] These 3 manifestations of EOTRH may be related to altered phases within the periodontium, of inflammatory (resorption) and reparative (cementosis) processes.[14]

RADIOGRAPHIC DIAGNOSIS

Studies have shown that clinical signs may be subtle even in the presence of marked radiographic changes[6,26] (**Fig. 7**). While the clinical crown of the tooth may appear

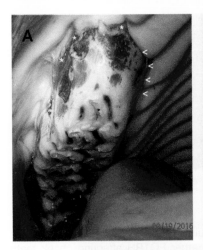
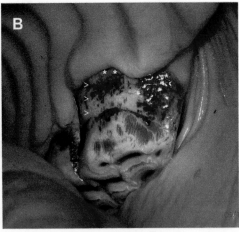
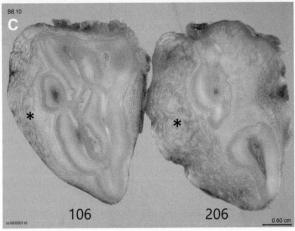

Fig. 5. (*A–C*) Changes in clinical crown cementum (*arrows*) and gingival recession (*asterisks*) may be present in cheek teeth affected by EOTRH (*A, B*). Gross histopathological sections on the affected teeth in this case demonstrate excessive peripheral cementum deposition (*asterisk, C*).

healthy, there may be advanced lesions along the reserve crown and root(s).[26] By the time clinical signs are present, EOTRH is often radiographically at an advanced stage. Screening radiographs will identify subclinical, yet clinically relevant, dental pathological processes.[4] Radiography is required to assess subgingival disease.[27]

Intraoral radiographs of incisors and canines and extraoral radiographs of premolars and molars are readily obtainable in the well-sedated patient using portable radiographic equipment.[28,29] To minimize superimposition of teeth, multiple radiographs are indicated for accurate assessment. Radiographic findings include resorptive lesions of the reserve crown, root(s), and/or surrounding bone, hypercementosis of the reserve crown/root(s), widening of the periodontal ligament space, expansion of alveolar bone, periapical alveolar bone lysis and areas of condensing osteitis (periapical alveolar bone sclerosis), and tooth fracture[6] (**Fig. 8**). Depending on the case, the extent and degree of radiographic changes are variable. Similar radiographic findings may be seen with

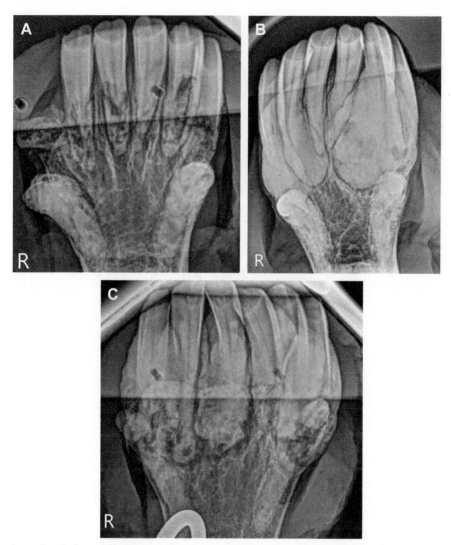

Fig. 6. (*A–C*) Three different manifestations of EOTRH previously reported are predominant tooth resorption (*A*), predominant hypercementosis (*B*), and combined resorption and hypercementosis (*C*).

affected cheek teeth (**Fig. 9**). These findings need to be distinguished from other age-related normal or pathologic radiographic changes that may not be specifically caused by EOTRH, such as apical blunting, widening of periodontal ligament space, alveolar sclerosis, and alveolar bone loss secondary to periodontal disease.[14]

A recent study proposed that external replacement resorption and external inflammatory resorption are frequent in equine incisor teeth.[4] Research aligning histopathology with radiographic interpretation is needed for confirmation. Classifying tooth resorption in horses may be clinically important as external inflammatory resorption typically requires treatment, whereas external replacement resorption usually does not require treatment.[4] Hypercementosis is most likely a reparative or secondary process associated with external inflammatory resorption.[1,4]

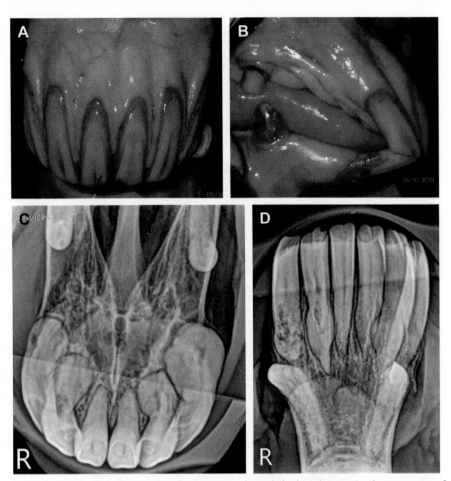

Fig. 7. (*A–D*) Clinical examination findings may be subtle (*A, B*) even in the presence of marked radiographic changes, note advanced tooth resorption and hypercementosis radiographically (*C, D*).

- External replacement resorption is evident radiographically as a gradual disappearance of the periodontal ligament space with progressive replacement of root tissues by the surrounding alveolar bone. It is associated with injuries that lead to necrosis of the periodontal ligament fibers. In humans, clinical signs are minimal to absent and it is considered untreatable with a poor long-term prognosis[4,5,30] (**Fig. 10**).
- External inflammatory resorption: radiographic characteristic is loss of dental tissues adjacent to areas of loss of alveolar bone secondary to inflammatory conditions. Endodontically compromised teeth are considered to have some degree of external inflammatory resorption[4,5,30] (see **Fig. 10**).

Stages of tooth resorption have been classified by the American College of Veterinary Dentistry and are based on the assumption that tooth resorption is a progressive condition.[31]

Stages of tooth resorption are classified as (**Fig. 11**):

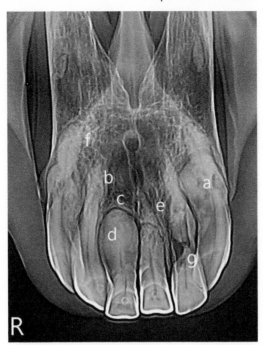

Fig. 8. Radiographic findings seen with EOTRH include resorptive lesions of the reserve crown (a), apex (b), widening of the periodontal ligament space (c), bulbous enlargement of the intra-alveolar crown–root (d), periapical alveolar bone lysis (e), areas of condensing osteitis (periapical alveolar bone sclerosis, f), and tooth fracture (g).

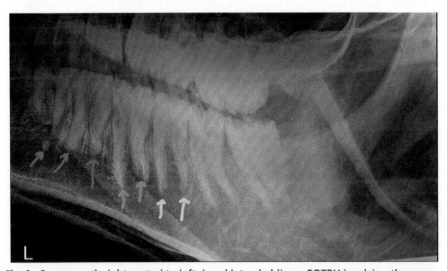

Fig. 9. Open-mouth right ventral to left dorsal lateral oblique. EOTRH involving the premolars and molars. Resorption and root blunting of the left mandibular second premolar (306, *blue arrows*). Primarily hypercementosis evident with the left mandibular third premolar (307, *red arrows*). A combination of resorption and hypercementosis is noted with the left mandibular fourth premolar (308, *green arrows*). The presentation in the left mandibular first molar seems to be primarily resorptive disease (309, *yellow arrows*). A small root fragment/cementum is evident apical to the distal root of the left mandibular second premolar (*orange arrow*).

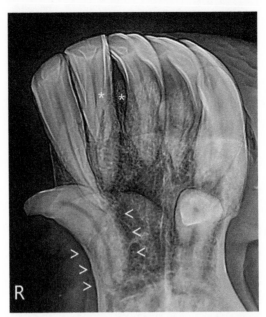

Fig. 10. Intraoral radiograph demonstrating both external inflammatory resorption with loss of both tooth structure and alveolar bone causing a widened periodontal ligament space (*asterisks*), and external replacement resorption with loss of the periodontal ligament space with surrounding alveolar bone replacing the tooth structure (*arrows*).

- Stage 1: mild dental hard tissue loss (cementum or cementum and enamel);
- Stage 2: moderate dental hard tissue loss (cementum or cementum and enamel with loss of dentin that does not extend to the pulp cavity);
- Stage 3: deep dental hard tissue loss (cementum or cementum and enamel with loss of dentin that extends to the pulp cavity); most of the tooth retains its integrity;
- Stage 4: extensive dental hard tissue loss (cementum or cementum and enamel with loss of dentin that extends to the pulp cavity); most of the tooth has lost its integrity;
  - Stage 4a: crown and root equally affected;
  - Stage 4b: crown is more affected than root;
  - Stage 4c: root is more affected than crown
- Stage 5: remnants of dental hard tissue are visible only as irregular radiopacities, and gingival covering is complete. This is rare in equine tooth resorption.

Staging tooth resorption based on radiographic changes provides an objective scale for case evaluation, treatment planning, and disease progression. Dentin is considered a physically sensitive living tissue,[32] and so horses may feel pain in teeth affected by stage 2 lesions. Stage 3, 4a, 4b, and 4c lesions have resorption involving the pulp cavity. Severe endodontically compromised teeth should be considered for extraction.[4] Using this objective scale can help the decision-making process for when to pursue extractions in mild to moderate cases.

CASE MANAGEMENT

The management goals of EOTRH is early recognition, radiographic diagnosis, monitoring disease progression, and client communication.[14] Careful monitoring with

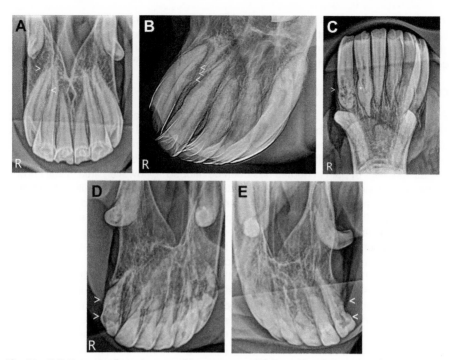

Fig. 11. AVDC stages of tooth resorption: stage 1, mild dental hard tissue loss (cementum or cementum and enamel) in tooth 103 (*arrows, A*); stage 2, moderate dental hard tissue loss (cementum or cementum and enamel with loss of dentin that does not extend to the pulp cavity) in tooth 103 (*arrows, B*); stage 3, deep dental hard tissue loss (cementum or cementum and enamel with loss of dentin that extends to the pulp cavity; tooth retains most of its integrity) in tooth 402 (*asterisk, C*); stage 4, extensive dental hard tissue loss (cementum or cementum and enamel with loss of dentin that extends to the pulp cavity with most of the tooth having lost its integrity, *arrows, C, D, E*). Stage 4a, crown and root equally affected in tooth 103 (*arrows, D*); stage 4b, crown is more affected than root in tooth 203 (*arrows, E*); stage 4c, root is more affected than crown in tooth 403 (*arrows, C*).

regular oral and radiographic examinations is essential as the progression of the disease varies significantly between both teeth and individuals.[5] Pain relief and improved quality of life are the primary treatment goals. Currently, since there is no cure, extraction of the affected teeth is the only viable treatment option.[6,26,33,34] Because this disease is progressive, the importance of documenting early lesions with radiography gives the veterinarian the ability to plan future treatment and to prevent the patient from having a painful lesion for a prolonged period of time.[35] Previously reported options for management of mild cases involves a combination of home care, including removal of interdental food accumulation, tooth brushing, and topical administration of 0.12% chlorhexidine gluconate solution.[12] Other proposed therapies include analgesia, antibiotics, dietary modification, incisor reductions, corticosteroids, gingivoplasty, surgical curettage and debridement, and intraoral splinting.[3,5,12,22,36] However, these reported treatment options have minimal to no effect on the disease progression.[3,5,12,36] Extraction is recommended when pain, and dental and bone lesions, become severe. Pain is subjective and difficult to measure. Dental and bone pathology are monitored radiographically. Severe lesions indicating extraction include alveolitis, osteomyelitis, periodontal disease, endodontic disease, tooth and bone fractures, and tooth and bone resorption.[4,5] Further research is needed to identify options for early treatment and prevention of EOTRH. While the prognosis for the affected teeth is poor in most cases,[37] complete removal of affected teeth carries a good prognosis for an improved quality of life for the horse.[6]

CLIENT COMMUNICATION

Educating owners about EOTRH and how it affects the whole horse is an important consideration when establishing a treatment plan. Advanced disease may be present although the clinical crown and surrounding soft tissues may not necessarily look severely diseased. It is difficult to correlate radiographic lesions with pain.[26] Systematic assessment of pain in horses has been developed[38]; however, little is still known about dental pain. Chronic pain is undetected, especially with a gradually progressing condition such as EOTRH.[26] Pain is underestimated by people involved in the horse's daily care, and the owner's perception of pain is often not considered severe enough to warrant extractions when recommended.[26] Owners may also have financial constraints in pursuing extractions as typically these horses are older and no longer working, and may have other unrelated health concerns.

Extraction of the affected teeth (frequently all incisors and canine teeth in moderate to severe cases) may be considered radical by the owner. Unfortunately, this is currently the only effective treatment option, and client education is crucial to achieving treatment compliance and thus improvement of quality of life for the horse. Significant time may be spent counseling owners about the disease and anticipated progression, surgery, postoperative care (see **Fig. 15**B), and procedural complications.[33] Extracting a few diseased incisors when all are severely affected will not significantly improve the horse's level of pain. Staged extractions entail multiple major procedures and recoveries. Communicate to the client that the prognosis for complete extractions is very good.[35] Directing owners to previous case photos, radiographs, and educational information helps them to better understand the disease and need for treatment. The author has found it helpful to refer owners to previous clients who have already been through the diagnosis and extractions to help alleviate concern and answer additional questions.

EXTRACTION TECHNIQUES

Severe cases involving all incisors should be referred to an experienced veterinary dentist because complete extraction of severely affected teeth often requires surgical extraction techniques.[33] A thorough physical examination and baseline laboratory testing (complete blood count, serum biochemistry, corcticotropin baseline, and/or thyrotropin-stimulating hormone stimulation test) is recommended to systemically evaluate the patient and to allow for additional diagnostics if necessary. Because most of these patients are geriatric, it is not uncommon to identify undiagnosed pituitary pars intermedia dysfunction (PPID), heart murmurs, renal or hepatic insufficiency, and underlying musculoskeletal disease that should be addressed before a major procedure. Potential procedural complications include flap dehiscence, tongue protrusion, bleeding, and postoperative inappetence.[33]

Depending on the severity of the case, either simple or surgical extraction may be performed. Regardless of the extraction technique, all diseased tissue should be debrided on extraction of EOTRH-affected teeth. Single incisor extraction can often be accomplished by simple extraction. Complete incisor and canine extractions can be performed in the standing sedated horse with appropriate regional nerve blocks and local subgingival anesthesia by a skilled veterinary dentist, as previously described.[33] In cases of moderate to severe disease affecting multiple teeth, a surgical approach is preferred and may be efficiently performed in the standing patient. Surgical extraction facilitates complete removal of all dental tissue of affected teeth by allowing improved visualization, debridement, fragment removal (**Fig. 12**), and closure.[33] The alveolus and gingiva should be debrided and intraoperative radiographs (**Fig. 13**) taken to confirm removal of all tooth fragments.[6,33] Retained fragments can cause persistent pain due to inflammation, infection, and draining tracts (**Fig. 14**). Primary closure of mucogingival flaps are ideal; however, they notoriously dehisce.[33] The author prefers to close via partial apposition with 1 suture layer to stabilize the alveolar blood clot (**Fig. 15**). While less cosmetic, this approach decreases surgical time spent closing a wound that has a high likelihood of dehiscence. The owner should be advised that dehiscence can occur and that the wound will heal by second intention in 3 to 6 weeks. Sutures should then be removed and the owner instructed to rinse the extraction sites daily with saline solution.

POSTPROCEDURE CARE

In the author's experience, following partial or complete incisor extractions horses typically exhibit minimal discomfort. Analgesia with nonsteroidal anti-inflammatory drugs effectively manage surgical pain (Video 1). Antimicrobials are recommended for 7 to 10 days to prevent infection and should be utilized in PPID-affected horses.[33] The author also recommends daily oral rinse until the extraction sites are healed with normal gingiva (**Fig. 16**). In the absence of cheek teeth comorbidity, most horses are able to eat their normal diet of hay and processed feed within 24 to 48 hours of multiple incisor extractions and are able to go on to live normal lives free of chronic dental pain and infection.[6,33] Anecdotal reports from owners following multiple or complete incisor extractions frequently include a noted improved condition and appearance, disposition, increased energy, improvement in eating and weight gain, and a generalized improvement in quality of life.

BISPHOSPHONATE (BP) USE IN THE HORSE AND POTENTIAL ORAL/DENTAL CONSEQUENCES

The use of BPs in the horse has become common in recent years to treat degenerative pathologies, such as arthritis, because of their anti-inflammatory and analgesic properties for musculoskeletal pain and lameness. There are 3 BPs that have been reported for use in the horse: tiludronate, clodronate, and zoledronate.[39–44] BPs

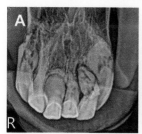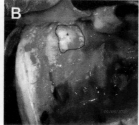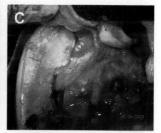

Fig. 12. (*A–C*) Preextraction radiograph indicates a separate cemental fragment apically at tooth 101 (*asterisk, A*). Surgical extraction facilitates complete removal of all dental tissue of affected teeth by allowing improved visualization and removal of 101 apical fragment (outlined and *asterisk, B*). Apical fragment removed, allowing improved visualization of 102 (*C*).

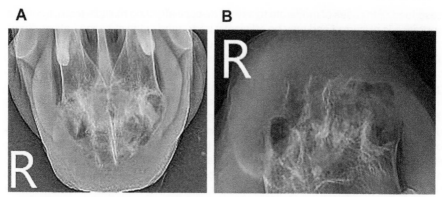

Fig. 13. (*A*, *B*) Maxillary (*A*) and mandibular (*B*) postextraction radiographs confirming extraction of all dental material.

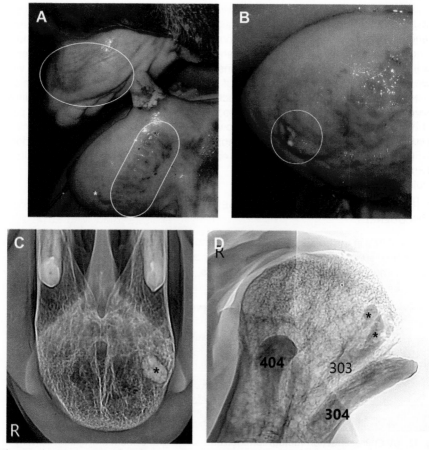

Fig. 14. (*A–D*) Retained fragments following EOTRH extractions can cause persistent pain due to inflammation, infection, and draining tracts (circled areas, *asterisk* draining tract *A*, circled fragment *B*). Intraoral radiographs identify retained fragments in the areas of 203 (*asterisk, C*) and 302/303 (*asterisks, D*) and 303 retained root.

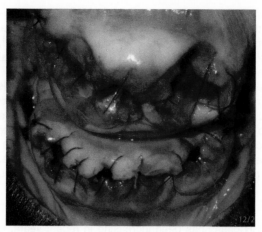

Fig. 15. Surgical closure via partial apposition with 1 suture layer to stabilize the alveolar blood clot.

inhibit bone resorption through their intracellular effects on osteoclasts. After uptake by endocytosis, BPs disrupt the normal function of these cells, decreasing resorption of bone and eventually causing osteoclast apoptosis.[45] The disruption of osteoclast activity has spurred speculation of BP use as a treatment of dental resorption. Zoledronate has a longer duration of action and increased potency in humans when compared with tiludronate and other nonnitrogen-containing BPs.[40,44,45] Tiludronate disodium (Tildren, Ceva Animal Health, Lenexa, KS, USA) and clodronate disodium (Osphos, Dechra, Staffordshire, UK) are BP drugs that are licensed for use in horses to reduce lameness associated with navicular disease[46–50] Zoledronate is currently not Food and Drug Administration approved for use in the horse. To date, we do not know the long-term consequences that BP therapy may have on the current horse population as they age. A serious side effect known as osteonecrosis of the jaw (ONJ) has been observed and associated to IV administration of nonnitrogen-containing BPs, including zoledronate in humans with concomitant dental disease.[51,52] ONJ after

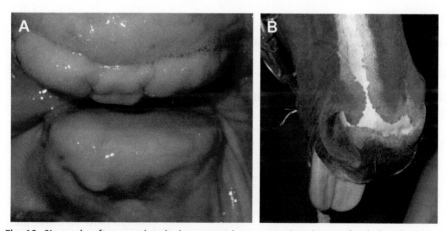

Fig. 16. Six weeks after complete incisor extractions, extraction sites are healed with normal gingiva (*A*). Owners should be advised before extraction that tongue protrusion often occurs following incisor extractions (*B*).

zoledronic acid administration is observed after high doses and long-term administration in patients with cancer or after dental procedures.[53–59] ONJ has a multifactorial pathology, so cannot be directly attributed to zoledrondate use[60–63]; however, veterinarians should be aware of this potential adverse effect when a history of BP use is present in patients with dental disease.

A recent study evaluating zoledronate in horses did not identify dental problems in horses in the study for a year after treatment; however, it was not specified if complete visual oral or dental radiographic examinations were performed.[44] The study authors recommended that no dental procedures be performed immediately before zoledronic acid administration or for 6 months afterward based on extrapolation from the human literature.[44] Zoledronic acid is reported to be the strongest BP currently available, and equine studies evaluating potential benefits of zoledronic acid in clinical cases are warranted.[44]

SUMMARY

Diagnosis of EOTRH cases has been increasing in recent years, partly because of increased awareness of the disease and partly unknown because of lack of an identified etiologic origin. Owner awareness has also increased, and it is important that veterinarians are aware of the clinical signs, examination findings, and radiographic diagnosis so that they can effectively guide clients with case management and treatment planning. Since first noted in 2004, this resorptive disease has rapidly progressed to a painful debilitating disease affecting a wide range of the horse population around the world. Currently the only known treatment is dental extraction of affected teeth. It is hoped that, with additional research, we will be able to ascertain the multiple contributing factors causing this severe and debilitating disease. As the cause of the disease becomes more evident, protocols for early treatment and intervention will develop.

CLINICS CARE POINTS

- EOTRH affects incisors, canines, premolars and molars of horses.
- EOTRH is a progressive and painful disease.
- Horses with complete or multiple extractions have a favorable prognosis.

DISCLOSURE

No funding sources, financial interests, or conflicts of interest to disclose.

SUPPLEMENTARY DATA

Supplementary data related to this article can be found online at https://doi.org/10.1016/j.cveq.2020.08.006.

REFERENCES

1. Staszyk C, Bienert A, Kreutzer R, et al. Equine odontoclastic tooth resorption and hypercementosis. Vet J 2008;178:372–9.
2. Klugh, D. Incisor and canine periodontal disease. Proceedings of the 18th Annual Veterinary Dental Forum, Fort Worth, TX. 2004;166-169.
3. Hole, S.L. Equine odontoclastic tooth resorption and hypercementosis (EOTRH): a review. Handbook of Proceedings, 21st ECVD, Lisbon, Portugal. May 24-27, 2012;148.

4. Henry TJ, Puchalski SM, Arzi B, et al. Radiographic evaluation in clinical practice of the types and stage of incisor tooth resorption and hypercementosis in horses. Equine Vet J 2017;49:486–92.
5. Earley E, Rawlinson JT. A new understanding of oral and dental disorders of the equine incisor and canine teeth. Vet Clin North Am Equine Pract 2013;29:273–300.
6. Lorello O, Foster DL, Levine DG, et al. Clinical treatment and prognosis of equine odontoclastic tooth resorption and hypercementosis. Equine Vet J 2016;48:188–94.
7. Sykora S, Pieber K, Simhofer H, et al. Isolation of *Treponema* and *Tannerella* spp. from equine odontoclastic tooth resorption and hypercementosis related periodontal disease. Equine Vet J 2014;46:358–63.
8. Pearson AM, Mansfield G, Conaway M. Associated risk factors of equine odontoclastic tooth resorption and hypercementosis. In: Proceedings of the 59th annual convention of the American association of equine practitioners. Nashville, TN, December 7-13, 2013;59:65–70.
9. Rehrl S, Schröder W, Müller C, et al. Radiological prevalence of equine odontoclastic tooth resorption and hypercementosis. Equine Vet J 2018;50:481–7.
10. Gregory, R., Fehr, J. and Bryant, J. Chronic incisor periodontal disease with cemental hyperplasia and hypoplasia in horses. Proceedings of AAEP Focus on Dentistry, Indianapolis, IN. August 1, 2006;312-316.
11. Baratt, R. Equine incisor resorptive lesions. Proceedings of the 21st Annual Veterinary Dental Forum, Minneapolis, MN. 2007;23-30.
12. du Toit N, Rucker BA. The gold standard of dental care: the geriatric horse. Vet Clin North Am Equine Pract 2013;29:521–7.
13. Moore NT, Schroeder W, Staszyk C. Equine odontoclastic tooth resorption and hypercementosis affecting all cheek teeth in two horses: clinical and histopathological findings. Equine Vet Educ 2016;28:123–30.
14. Hole SL, Staszyk C. Equine odontoclastic tooth resorption and hypercementosis. Equine Vet Educ 2018;30(7):386–91.
15. Smedley RC, Earley ET, Galloway SS, et al. Equine odontoclastic tooth resorption and hypercementosis: histopathologic features. Vet Pathol 2015;52:903–9.
16. Dixon P, du Toit N. Equine dental pathology. In: Easley J, Dixon PM, Schumacher J, editors. Equine dentistry. 3rd ediiton. Edinburgh (Scotland): Saunders Elsevier; 2011. p. 144.
17. Moody G, Muir K. Multiple idiopathic root resorption. J Clin Periodontol 1991;18: 577–80.
18. Okuda A, Harvey C. Etiopathogenesis of feline dental resorptive lesions. Vet Clin North Am Small Anim Pract 1992;22:1385–404.
19. Reiter A, Mendoza K. Feline odontoclastic resorptive lesions an unsolved enigma in veterinary dentistry. Vet Clin North Am Small Anim Pract 2002;32:791–837.
20. Reiter A, Lewis J, Okuda A. Update on the etiology of tooth resorption in domestic cats. Vet Clin North Am Small Anim Pract 2005;35:913–42.
21. Staszyk, C., Bienert, A., H€uls, et al. EOTRH: macroscopical and pathohistological investigations. In: Proceedings of AAEP Focus on Dentistry, Albuquerque, NM. September 20, 2011;105.
22. Klugh D. Principles of equine dentistry. London: Manson Publishing; 2010. p. 195–8.
23. Schrock P, L€upke M, Seifert H, et al. Finite element analysis of equine incisor teeth. Part 2: investigation of stresses and strain energy densities in the periodontal ligament and surrounding bone during tooth movement. Vet J 2013; 198:590–8.

24. Cordes V, Luepke M, Gardemin M, et al. Periodontal biomechanics: finite element simulations of closing stroke and power stroke in equine cheek teeth. BMC Vet Res 2012;8:60.
25. Caldwell, L. Clinical features of chronic disease of the anterior dentition in horses. In: Proceedings of the 21st Annual Veterinary Dental Forum, Minneapolis, MN. 2007;18-21.
26. Rahmani V, Häyrinen L, Kareinen I, et al. History, clinical findings and outcome of horses with radiographical signs of equine odontoclastic tooth resorption and hypercementosis veterinary. Record 2019;185:730.
27. Tremaine H. A modern approach to equine dentistry 3: imaging. In Pract 2012;34:114–27.
28. Baratt RM. Advances in equine dental radiology. Vet Clin Equine 2013;29:367–95.
29. Limone LE, Baratt RM. Dental radiography of the horse. J Vet Dentistry 2018;35:37–41.
30. DuPont GA. Radiographic evaluation and treatment of feline dental resorptive lesions. Vet Clin North Am Small Anim Pract 2005;35:943–62, vii–viii.
31. Veterinary Dental Nomenclature—Home American Veterinary Dental College. p. 11. Available at: https://avdc.org/avdc-nomenclature/.
32. Dacre IT. Equine dental pathology. In: Baker GJ, Easley J, editors. Equine dentistry. 2nd ediiton. Oxford (UK): W.B: Saunders; 2005. p. 91–109.
33. Rawlinson JT, Earley E. Advances in the treatment of diseased equine incisor and canine teeth. Vet Clin North Am Equine Pract 2013;29:411–40, vi–vii.
34. Foster DL. The gold standard of dental care for the adult performance horse. Vet Clin North Am Equine Pract 2013;29:505–19.
35. Henry, TJ. Equine tooth resorption: what is all the fuss? Proc AAEP RESORT symposium. january 25-27, 2016;23-27.
36. Baratt, R. Clinical management of equine odontoclastic tooth resorption and hypercementosis. Proceedings of AAEP Focus on Dentistry, Albuquerque, NM. September 20, 2011;112.
37. Tremaine H, Casey M. A modern approach to equine dentistry 2: identifying lesions. In Pract 2012;34:78–89.
38. de Grauw JC, van Loon JPAM. Systematic pain assessment in horses. Vet J 2016;209:14–22.
39. McLellan J. Science-in-brief: bisphosphonate use in the racehorse: safe or unsafe? Equine Vet J 2017;49:404–7.
40. Soto SA, Chiappe Barbará A. Bisphosphonates: pharmacology and clinical approach to their use in equine osteoarticular diseases. J Equine Vet Sci 2014;34:727–37.
41. Katzman SA, Nieto JE, Arens AM, et al. Use of zoledronate for treatment of a bone fragility disorder in horses. J Am Vet Med Assoc 2012;240:1323–8.
42. Mitchell A, Wright G, Sampson SN, et al. Clodronate improves lameness in horses without changing bone turnover markers. Equine Vet J 2019;51:356–63.
43. Richbourg HA, Mitchell CF, Gillett AN, et al. Tiludronate and clodronate do not affect bone structure or remodeling kinetics over a 60 day randomized trial. BMC Vet Res 2018;14:105–11.
44. Nieto JE, Maher O, Stanley SD, et al. Pharmacokinetics, pharmacodynamics, and safety of zoledronic acid in horses. Am J Vet Res 2013;74:550–6.
45. Russell RG, Xia Z, Dunford JE, et al. Bisphosphonates: an update on mechanisms of action and how these relate to clinical efficacy. Ann N Y Acad Sci 2007;1117:209–57.
46. Freedom of Information Summary: for the control of clinical signs associated with navicular syndrome in horses. Available at: https://animaldrugsatfda.fda.gov/adafda/app/search/public/document/downloadFoi/923.

47. Freedom of Information Summary: For the control of clinical signs associated with navicular syndrome in horses. Available at: https://animaldrugsatfda.fda.gov/adafda/app/search/public/document/downloadFoi/918.

48. Gough MR, Thibaud D, Smith RK. Tiludronate infusion in the treatment of bone spavin: a double blind placebo-controlled trial. Equine Vet J 2010;42:381–7.

49. Coudry V, Thibaud D, Riccio B, et al. Efficacy of tiludronate in the treatment of horses with signs of pain associated with osteoarthritic lesions of the thoracolumbar vertebral column. Am J Vet Res 2007;68:329–37.

50. Carpenter R. How to treat dorsal metacarpal disease with regional tiludronate and extracorporeal shock wave therapies in thoroughbred racehorses. In: Proceeding AAEP Annual Convention 2012. Lexington (KY): American Association of Equine Practitioners; 2012. p. 546–9.

51. Lesclous P, Abi Najm S, Carrel J, et al. Bisphosphonate-associated osteonecrosis of the jaw: a key role of inflammation? Bone 2009;45:843–52.

52. Robichaux C, Ong M, Veillon D, et al. Bisphosphonate-related osteonecrosis of the jaw. J La State Med Soc 2014;166:200–2.

53. Kohno N, Aogi K, Minami H, et al. Zoledronic acid significantly reduces skeletal complications compared with placebo in Japanese women with bone metastases from breast cancer: a randomized, placebo-controlled trial. J Clin Oncol 2005;23:3314–21.

54. Woo SB, Hellstein JW, Kalmar JR. Narrative [corrected] review: bisphosphonates and osteonecrosis of the jaws. Ann Intern Med 2006;144:753–61 [Erratum appears in Ann Intern Med 2006;145:235].

55. Black DM, Delmas PD, Eastell R, et al. Once-yearly zoledronic acid for treatment of postmenopausal osteoporosis. N Engl J Med 2007;356:1809–22.

56. Rosen LS, Gordon D, Kaminski M, et al. Long-term efficacy and safety of zoledronic acid compared with pamidronate disodium in the treatment of skeletal complications in patients with advanced multiple myeloma or breast carcinoma: a randomized, double-blind, multicenter, comparative trial. Cancer 2003;98:1735–44.

57. Rosen LS, Gordon D, Tchekmedyian S, et al. Zoledronic acid versus placebo in the treatment of skeletal metastases in patients with lung cancer and other solid tumors: a phase III, doubleblind, randomized trial—the Zoledronic Acid Lung Cancer and Other Solid Tumors Study Group. J Clin Oncol 2003;21:3150–7.

58. Lyles KW, Colon-Emeric CS, Magaziner JS, et al. Zoledronic acid and clinical fractures and mortality after hip fracture. N Engl J Med 2007;357:1799–809.

59. Hoff AO, Toth BB, Altundag K, et al. Frequency and risk factors associated with osteonecrosis of the jaw in cancer patients treated with intravenous bisphosphonates. J Bone Miner Res 2008;23:826–36.

60. Pazianas M, Abrahamsen B. Safety of bisphosphonates. Bone 2011;49:103–10.

61. Pazianas M, Cooper C, Ebetino FH, et al. Long-term treatment with bisphosphonates and their safety in postmenopausal osteoporosis. Ther Clin Risk Manag 2010;6:325–43.

62. Otto S, Pautke C, Opelz C, et al. Osteonecrosis of the jaw: effect of bisphosphonate type, local concentration, and acidic milieu on the pathomechanism. J Oral Maxillofac Surg 2010;68:2837–45.

63. Walter C, Klein MO, Pabst A, et al. Influence of bisphosphonates on endothelial cells, fibroblasts, and osteogenic cells. Clin Oral Investig 2010;14:35–41.

Printed and bound by CPI Group (UK) Ltd, Croydon, CR0 4YY

03/10/2024

01040407-0008